MEASUREMENT IN CLINICAL RESPIRATORY PHYSIOLOGY

MEDICAL PHYSICS SERIES

P. N. T. WELLS. Physical Principles of Ultrasonic Diagnosis. 1969

D. W. HILL and A. M. DOLAN. Intensive Care Instrumentation. (2nd edition) 1982

P. N. T. WELLS. Biomedical Ultrasonics. 1977

P. ROLFE. Non-invasive Physiological Measurements, Volume 1. 1979

P. ATKINSON and J. P. WOODCOCK. Doppler Ultrasound and its Use in Clinical Measurement. 1981

P. ROLFE. Non-invasive Physiological Measurements, Volume 2. 1983

A. R. WILLIAMS. Ultrasound: Biological Effects and Potential Hazards. 1983

MEASUREMENT IN CLINICAL RESPIRATORY PHYSIOLOGY

Edited by

Gabriel Laszlo

*Respiratory Department, Bristol Royal Infirmary,
Bristol*

Michael F. Sudlow

*Department of Respiratory Medicine, City Hospital
Edinburgh*

1983

ACADEMIC PRESS

A Subsidiary of Harcourt Brace Jovanovich, Publishers
London   New York
Paris   San Diego   San Francisco   São Paulo
Sydney   Tokyo   Toronto

ACADEMIC PRESS INC. (LONDON) LTD.
24/28 Oval Road,
London NW1

United States Edition published by
ACADEMIC PRESS INC.
111 Fifth Avenue
New York, New York 10003

British Library Cataloguing in Publication Data

Measurement in clinical respiratory physiology.—
(Medical physics, ISSN 0076-5953)
1. Respiratory system—Examination
I. Laszlo, G.   II. Sudlow, M.   III. Series
616.2'065   RC734.R3

ISBN 0-12-437080-2
LCCCN 83-70715

Printed by W. & G. Baird Ltd., Greystone Press, Antrim, Northern Ireland.

CONTRIBUTORS

DAVID T. DELPY *Medical Physicist, University College Hospital, London, U.K.*

STANLEY FREEDMAN *Physician, Chase Farm Hospital, Enfield, London, U.K.*

G. JOHN GIBSON *Physician, Freeman Hospital, Newcastle upon Tyne, U.K.*

ANDREW GUYATT *Physiologist, Midhurst Medical Research Institute, Midhurst, Sussex, U.K.*

JAMES W. KANE *Technologist, Ambrose Cardio-respiratory Unit, McMaster University Medical Centre, Hamilton, Ontario, Canada*

GABRIEL LASZLO *Physician, Bristol Royal Infirmary, Bristol, U.K.*

A. GORDON LEITCH *Physician, City Hospital, Edinburgh, U.K.*

G. J. ROSS MCHARDY *Senior Lecturer in Respiratory Medicine and Physician, City Hospital, Edinburgh, U.K.*

PHILIP MORGAN *Managing Director, P. K. Morgan Ltd, Rainham, Kent, U.K.*

DAWOOD PARKER *Medical Physicist, University College Hospital, London, U.K.*

KEITH PROWSE *Physician, City General Hospital, Stoke-on-Trent, U.K.*

PETER SCHEID *Professor of Physiology, University of Bochum, Bochum, Federal Republic of Germany*

MICHAEL SILVERMAN *Senior Lecturer in Child Health and Paediatrician, Royal Postgraduate Medical School, Hammersmith Hospital, London, U.K.*

MICHAEL F. SUDLOW *Senior Lecturer in Respiratory Medicine and Physician, City Hospital, Edinburgh, U.K.*

PATRICIA M. TWEEDDALE *Physiologist, City Hospital, Edinburgh, U.K.*

PATRICIA WARREN *Physiologist, City Hospital, Edinburgh, U.K.*

PREFACE

This book is intended to be a practical handbook for those working in a respiratory function laboratory. We hope it will be of use in the laboratory and find a place there as well as in the reference library. The authors are all active research workers and we have invited them to contribute because of their practical experience in the topics they discuss.

The book falls into two parts. In the first, we discuss instrumentations; in the second, the assembly of equipment for specific purposes.

In writing, we had in mind the hospital physicist, technician or physiologist who has to equip, organise and run and service a respiratory function laboratory for routine clinical or research purposes. Except for the briefest account in Chapter 1, we have not included any systematic discussion of pulmonary physiology and have avoided details of the interpretation of respiratory function tests or their role in clinical management. Several recent texts listed at the end of Chapter 1 deal with these problems.

We have not attempted a comprehensive review of all the possible measurements of lung function but have dealt with the more important aspects in current practice and emphasized those of growing importance.

We would like to thank all who contributed for their time and effort. Many medical illustrators and secretaries have contributed to the volume, but we particularly thank Claire Douglas, Russell Harvey, Gary James, Anne McAuley, Judy Seward and Morag Wells. We are grateful to Jeanette Dennison for preparing the index.

May 1983

Michael F. Sudlow
Gabriel Laszlo

CONTENTS

Contributors v
Preface vii

1. The Work of the Respiratory Laboratory
   G. Laszlo and M. F. Sudlow 1

2. Design of Respiratory Circuits and Spirometry
   S. Freedman 9

3. Measurement of Pressure and Flow
   A. R. Guyatt 25

4. Respiratory Gas Analysis and Blood pH
   P. M. Tweeddale 57

5. Blood Gas Analysis by Invasive and Non-invasive
   Techniques
   D. Parker and D. T. Delpy 75

6. Physical Gas Analysers
   P. K. Morgan 113

7. Respiratory Mass Spectrometry
   P. Scheid 131

8. Treadmills and Cycle Ergometers
   J. W. Kane 167

9. Measurement of the Mechanical Properties of the
   Thorax, Lungs and Airways
   G. J. Gibson 185

10. Intrapulmonary Distribution of Insoluble Gases
    K. Prowse 217

11. Measurement of Carbon Monoxide Transfer
    P. WARREN   227

12. Assessment of the Control of Breathing and Monitoring
    during Sleep
    A. G. LEITCH   251

13. Exercise Testing
    G. LASZLO and G. J. R. McHARDY   .   .   .   271

14. Respiratory Function Testing in Infancy and Childhood
    M. SILVERMAN   293

Subject Index   329

1. THE WORK OF THE RESPIRATORY LABORATORY

G. Laszlo and M. F. Sudlow

Bristol Royal Infirmary, Bristol, U.K.
City Hospital, Edinburgh, U.K.

INTRODUCTION

Clinical respiratory physiology is concerned with the investigation of pulmonary function when it is disturbed. The investigator may need to:

(1) identify normality or abnormality;
(2) identify the disordered component or components of the respiratory system;
(3) measure the severity of the abnormality identified.

The functions and architectural features of the lungs which may be tested are:

(1) pulmonary ventilation and the work of breathing: the mechanical properties of the lungs;
(2) pulmonary gas exchange and the integrity of the gas exchanging surface;
(3) Neural control of the rate and depth of breathing.

Most respiratory disorders can be diagnosed by clinical means, from the patient's history and medical examination. Occasionally, the condition is complex and a careful study of the components of the respiratory system is required to elucidate the diagnosis fully. Such sessions are not readily repeatable. Many of the procedures described in this book, therefore, are selected for simplicity and repeatability, so that patients can be asked to perform them at intervals to judge the progress of the disorder or the response to treatment. Thus, some tests are chosen for their ability to measure the overall impairment of the system while others, more complex, are designed to reveal more specifically the nature of the abnormality.

Ventilation

Normal individuals can breathe in and out and thus ventilate the lungs at a much greater rate than is necessary to supply oxygen for most purposes. Severe exercise is normally limited by the ability of the heart and circulation to deliver oxygen to exercising tissues, rather than by the ventilatory capacity. However, a disease may reduce the ventilatory capacity by several mechanisms:

(1) weakness of the respiratory muscles;
(2) narrowing of the air passages, thus reducing maximum rate of air flow than can be achieved;
(3) reduction in lung volume or lung elasticity;
(4) deformity of the thorax.

These may be identified by measuring air movement in relation to maximum effort, or by examining the relationship between pressure generated by the respiratory muscles and movement of air in and out of the thorax achieved as a result of these pressure changes. A large section of this book, therefore, is concerned with the techniques which have been developed to examine the relationship between air flow and the effort of the respiratory muscles.

The simplest tests of ventilation are those derived from the *timed forced vital capacity*. The vital capacity is the maximum volume of air which can be delivered during expiration after a full inspiration. This test identifies the reduction in the size of the accessible portion of the lung and the patency of the airways (Chapter 9).

Normally, 80% of the vital capacity can be exhaled forcibly in one second. If the vital capacity is normal but the ratio that can be exhaled in one second is reduced, we deduce that obstruction to air flow is present.

If the vital capacity is small, it is necessary to distinguish between several causes of this abnormality:

(1) Premature closure of airways because of obstruction. In this situation, the total lung volume is normal and the air left in the lungs at the end of a full expiration (residual volume) is increased.
(2) So-called *restrictive* diseases in which the total lung volume is reduced after maximal inspiratory effort. There are three main types of abnormality which produce this result:
(a) reduced numbers of alveoli;
(b) increase in the density of the lung tissue in relation to the volume of air within the lungs;

    (c) deformity of the thoracic cage;

    (d) weakness of the inspiratory muscles.

The last two may often be recognized by examination of the patient. These conditions are not easy to investigate physiologically but may be distinguished by the measurement of pressure within the thorax (oesophageal pressure, Chapter 9) in relation to lung volume. In the case of (b), relaxation pressure is increased in relation to lung size, whereas in (a), (c) and (d) it is normal. The distending pressure of the thorax as distinct from the lungs is best measured under an anaesthetic by relating lung volume to pressure, but under certain circumstances it may be measured if the patient can learn to relax all the respiratory muscles while expiration is obstructed at the mouth. Weakness of the respiratory muscles may be shown by the inability of the patient to generate the normal negative inspiratory and positive expiratory pressures while the breathing is obstructed.

The inspiratory muscles work by enlarging the thoracic volume and distending the lungs. The *diaphragm* forms the floor of the thorax. When it contracts, it generates a positive pressure within the abdomen and a negative pressure in the chest. The difference between these pressures, measured in the stomach and oesophagus respectively, reflect the force of diaphragmatic contraction.

Knowledge of the *lung volumes* is an important component of physiological interpretation of ventilatory tests. These may be measured by introducing a known volume of an insoluble foreign gas into a closed breathing circuit and measuring its dilution. Alternatively, there is a technique using Boyle's law to study the changes of pressure as the subject pants against an obstruction at the mouth in a body plethysmograph (Chapters 9 and 14).

Gas Exchange

Within the lungs, oxygen and carbon dioxide are exchanged by diffusion across a thin *alveolar membrane*. Gas exchange is affected by: by:

    (1) pulmonary ventilation;

    (2) diffusion of gases within the airways and alveoli;

    (3) diffusion of gases across the alveolar walls;

    (4) the distribution of pulmonary blood flow in a uniform manner to match to pulmonary ventilation.

In normal subjects, the rate and depth of breathing is relatively shallow in comparison to the lung volume, and the inspired air is only drawn into the most proximal air spaces. This air, rich in oxygen and free from carbon dioxide, exchanges with the alveolar gas by a rapid diffusion within the intra-pulmonary air spaces. Moreover, there are control mechanisms within the pulmonary circulation which ensure that the major portion of the pulmonary blood flow is directed to those portions of the lungs which are well ventilated, since shortage of oxygen at their surface causes narrowing of individual pulmonary blood vessels.

Diffusion of oxygen into the red blood corpuscle and carbon dioxide out of it is normally very rapid because the membrane dividing the alveolar gas and the red blood corpuscle is very thin, and the surface area for gas exchange is very large. Damage to the gas-exchanging surface of the lung may cause increased thickness of the diffusion pathway or, much more commonly, a reduction of the surface area available for gas exchange. As indicated above, the latter may be caused by reduction in the numbers of alveoli, or by failure of the inspired gas to reach some of the patent alveoli because the airways connecting them are narrowed.

The presence of these types of abnormality may most easily be detected by a reduction in the uptake in carbon monoxide under standard conditions (Chapter 11). Carbon monoxide in trace quantities has a very high affinity for haemoglobin within the red blood corpuscles, much greater than that of oxygen. This means that the uptake of carbon monoxide is limited by the amount of haemoglobin that is in close contact with the inspired gas during the test, rather than by its removal in the circulation, since the red cells do not achieve sufficiently great partial pressure of carbon monoxide during the test to limit uptake. This remains true, regardless of whether the red cells are moving or not. CO uptake is therefore "diffusion limited" rather than circulation limited, which is the case for oxygen.

Even if total pulmonary ventilation and blood flow are virtually normal, it is necessary for efficient gas exchange that they should be matched evenly within the lungs. Mismatching of ventilation and per-fusion results in two types of abnormality:

(1) alveoli having an abnormally high ventilation:perfusion ratio;
(2) alveoli with a low ventilation:perfusion ratio.

The first type of abnormality results in wasted ventilation because work has to be done to move air in and out of these alveoli without much gas exchange taking place within them.

The second type of abnormality results in lower than normal content of oxygen within the blood leaving the lungs and being distributed to the tissues, as a result of the phenomenon known as the *shunt effect*. This is most easily explained by considering the extreme case where blood reaches alveoli which are totally obstructed and have no fresh air reaching them at all during ventilation. Such blood passes straight through the lungs, taking with it haemoglobin with an excess of free oxygen receptors ("shunted" blood). Ventilation and perfusion are normally arranged so that haemoglobin is almost fully saturated in the blood leaving normal alveoli. In the presence of "shunted" blood, the mixed arterial blood has an abnormal amount of reduced haemoglobin in it. Diffusion must also be matched to blood flow for efficient gas exchange. These abnormalities may be identified by measurements of arterial blood oxygen saturation, content or partial pressure (Chapters, 5, 6).

Wagner and West (1980) have developed an elegant approach to the problem by analysing the clearance by the lungs of an intravenous infusion of gases at different solubilities.

Control of Ventilation

For any given delivery to the lungs of carbon dioxide and reduced haemoglobin the pulmonary circulation to the lungs, the pulmonary gas exchange will be determined by the rate of ventilation. Briefly, if ventilation is high in relation to perfusion, the expired air will resemble closely room air and the partial pressure of carbon dioxide in it will be low. The less the ventilation, the greater will be the partial pressure of carbon dioxide.

Blood is a buffered system and carbon dioxide in solution as carbonic acid has a pK (7.1) close to the pH of normal blood (7.4). To maintain the pH within normal limits required for optimal functioning of metabolism within the tissues, ventilatory control mechanisms have evolved which maintain Pco_2 at a level of 5.5 kPa (40 mmHg). These control mechanisms are tuned so that, as the metabolic rate increases with increasing activity, ventilation increases in proportion, thus maintaining a constant mean Pco_2 within the alveoli. Thus, Pco_2 varies very little under normal circumstances.

An elevated arterial Pco_2 therefore indicates *alveolar under-ventilation*. This may occur either because of impairment of the ventilatory mechanisms or because the control mechanisms are in some way at fault. *Alveolar hyper-ventilation*, or over-breathing, is a manifestation of a variety of states, not all abnormal:

(a) Increased *chemo-receptor* drive. There are oxygen and hydrogen ion sensors within the brain and peripheral circulation which recognize low arterial Po_2 and pH and stimulate, by a reflex, an increase in the rate and depth of breathing. These mechanisms are of great importance in normal subjects and animals at altitude where the inspired oxygen pressure is lower than at sea-level.

(b) A variety of mechanical abnormalities. Respiratory discomfort associated with certain lung diseases may stimulate hyper-ventilation even without a reduction of arterial Po_2.

(c) Other physical discomforts such as pain, external heat or cold, excitement, anxiety and prolonged talking or laughing result in a low arterial Pco_2.

SYMPTOMS OF RESPIRATORY DISEASE

Most of the patients attending for investigation in the pulmonary function laboratory will be suffering from *shortness of breath*, usually on exertion. The principal mechanisms involved are:

(1) *Respiratory discomfort.* Often, because of narrowing of the air-ways or reduction in the size of the lungs, the normal pattern of breathing during exercise is disturbed and the patient feels the sensation of discomfort. The abnormality may be chronic or it may occur transiently as a result of exercise.

(2) *Increased ventilatory requirement.* Ventilation normally increases in proportion to the increased oxygen uptake required to perform any task. This may result in a disproportionate ventilatory requirement, if a large portion of the ventilation is wasted in under-perfused parts of the lung because of ventilation perfusion mismatching, *or* if there is oxygen lack or some other stimulus to hyper-ventilation which is made worse during exercise. These may readily be identified by measurements of ventilation, Pco_2 and oxygen content or saturation during exercise (Chapter 13).

Other symptoms are of importance to physicians because they indicate the presence of bronchial or pulmonary disease. They include:

(1) *Coughing.* A cough is a paroxysm of repeated forced expirations with the vocal cords intermittently closed to produce a rapid expulsive movements of air. It is stimulated by irritation of the throat and trachea and its purpose is to expel inhaled foreign material or accumulated mucus. It is stimulated uselessly in a variety of inflammatory disorders where no foreign material is present.

(2) *Sputum production.* Sputum is excessive mucus, or pus, in the air passages. It is the result of inflammation of the airways and may occur because of infection, or irritation by cigarette smoke and other agents.

(3) *Haemoptysis or blood spitting.* This is often of no serious signi-

ficance but is important because it may be a manifestation of pulmonary tuberculosis, cancer of the lung, or other diseases. No patient with heavily infected or blood-stained sputum should have breathing tests until a chest X-ray has been taken which confirms that he is not suffering from pulmonary tuberculosis, because of the risk of infection to others.

(4) *Pain in the chest.* Pain rarely arises from the lungs but may be sensed in the heart, the digestive system, the blood vessels within the lungs, or the pleura and chest wall. It is very difficult to obtain useful measurements of pulmonary function in individuals who are suffering from chest pain at the time of the test. An electrocardiograph at the time of chest pain may be valuable to confirm or exclude a cardiac cause.

SCOPE OF THIS BOOK

This volume is concerned with describing techniques for the measurement of the overall integrity and efficiency of the ventilatory, gas exchanging and control functions of the respiratory system, employing measurements of pressure, air flow and gas analysis.

The first half of the book describes the basic equipment required for the analysis of flow rate, volume and composition of respiratory gases, and for the measurement of the respiratory properties of blood. Subsequent chapters are devoted to the various assemblies of these basic components which are used to make measurements of pulmonary function in conscious human subjects.

This is a physiological cook-book. We have assembled a distinguished team of contributors, all of whom are actively concerned in making measurements and we have asked them to describe their techniques as one might to a qualified physicist, physiologist or technician who had not previously worked in a respiratory laboratory. The contributors have concentrated most attention on those aspects which are not well covered in standard texts, in which they have made major contributions or which require skill to produce good results.

No attempt will be made to describe the radionucleide investigation of the distribution of ventilation in perfusion or lung particle clearance. The metabolic functions of the lung and its role in defence against infection will not be discussed, nor have we included a section on the deposition and clearance of inhaled particles. Sections on the clinical interpretation of the tests that we have described would have been interesting, but their inclusion would make the book far too long and the reader is referred to the volumes listed at the end of this chapter. An elementary account is given by Hughes and Empey (1981). The indispensable book by Cotes (1979) describes in detail the principles of lung function testing, with reference values for normal populations.

We have avoided lengthy discussions about the use of computers in respiratory physiology. In almost all instances, they facilitate data collection and calculation of results. The application of computers to physiological monitoring is not intrinsically difficult, though much painstaking work has to go into producing systems which are accurate and flexible. Most commercially available assemblies now operate with the aid of microprocessors. These achieve a very high level of accuracy but are only satisfactory if it remains possible to recognize the onset of mechanical or electronic failure as it was in the days when results were obtained by the painstaking analysis of polygraph traces. Moreover, the microprocessor program has to be versatile enough to permit regular calibration of the measuring instruments.

This book is mainly about equipment but we should say a word about patients. In general, lung function testing requires friendly co-operation between the operator and the patient. This is quite different from procedures such as cardiac catheterization, electorcardiography or biochemical investigations in blood and urine.

Departments of clinical respiratory physiology have always been noted for their camaraderie and the dividing lines between the functions of nurses, technicians, physicists, research fellows and the laboratory medical staff generally become blurred. There is none of the calculated risk that is involved in some cardiological studies or in anaesthesia, nor is there the sense of tragedy often found in an Intensive Care Unit. Most patients are grateful for their tests and reassured by the efforts being made to understand their condition.

Further Reading

Respiratory Physiology

Wagner, P. D. and West, J. B. (1980). *In* "Pulmonary Gas Exchange" Vol. I "Ventilation, Blood Flow and Diffusion". (Ed. J. B. West) pp. 219–262. Academic Press, New York and London.

West, J. B. (1979). "Respiratory Physiology: The Essentials", 2nd edition. Blackwell, Oxford.

West, J. B. (1978). "Pulmonary Pathophysiology: The Essentials". Blackwell, Oxford.
    These two works provide in adequate detail the basic anatomy and physiology

Pulmonary Function Tests

Cotes, J. E. (1979). "Lung Function, Principles and Practice", 4th Edition. Blackwell, Oxford.

Hughes, D. T. D., and Empey, D. W. (1981). "Clinical Pulmonary Physiology" Academic Press, London and New York.

2. DESIGN OF RESPIRATORY CIRCUITS AND SPIROMETRY

S. Freedman

Chase Farm Hospital, Enfield, U.K.

DESIGN OF RESPIRATORY CIRCUITS

This chapter is concerned with the basic "plumbing" of the respiratory laboratory. It is particularly intended for those who have never worked in respiratory physiology and are not familiar with standard pieces of equipment used for many years. Very few actual circuits are described as these are described in greater detail in appropriate chapters.

In all assemblies, equipment has to be fitted together and unfortunately much circuitry is not designed to give a particularly neat or presentable appearance. It is often possible to do this with a little care and is important where studies on patients are envisaged.

In designing and putting together a circuit, there are five factors which must be considered carefully: leaks, mixing, dead-space, compliance and resistance.

Leaks

Leaks are more critical in some situations, particularly in closed circuits and especially during rebreathing or measurement of lung volume by gas dilution. Junctions are best effected by pushing tubing over connections rather than stuffing it inside, and hoseclips or other screw clips can be used to make them absolutely gas-tight.

Leaks can be detected by putting gas in the circuit under pressure. In a closed circuit containing a spirometer, this is easily done by filling the circuit and weighting the spirometer bell. The spirometer record will show a leak. The site of the leak can then be isolated by one of two methods. First, a marker gas is introduced into the circuit and the leak detected by "sniffing" around all junctions with a sensitive fast responding detector (e.g. capnograph or mass spectrometer). Alternatively, parts of the circuit are successively isolated by disconnecting junctions and closing them with bungs or stopcocks until the spirometer record shows no leak.

Mixing

Mixing of gases is important where samples are withdrawn for analysis as in measurement of lung volumes or sampling of mixed expired gas during exercise. In open circuits, if gas is collected in bags, this is easily achieved, but otherwise, mixing chambers (Davies and Denison, 1979; Jones et al., 1975) may be interposed between the expiratory valve and the sampling point. In closed circuits where gases are recirculated, mixing can be helped by the use of sealed fans or turbines, which can also be mounted inside the bells of Tissot Spirometers.

Dead-space

This is the volume of gas in a circuit common to the inspiratory and expiratory sides. It is generally restricted to the valve-box, mouthpiece and any apparatus interposed between them. In most circuits, the aim will be to keep dead-space to a minimum—a realistic target is less than 100 ml, though for some studies a dead-space of 20 ml or less will be needed. There may be the need to compromise between the conflicting claims of low dead-space and low resistance, especially in exercise circuits. The size of the dead-space will affect a subject's total ventilation and alveolar carbon dioxide levels, and this should always be borne in mind when interpreting data from exercise studies.

Sometimes, dead-space may be added in order to increase ventilation, and methods have been devised of keeping CO_2 tension normal during voluntary hyper-ventilation using variable dead-space (Freedman, 1970) or a dead-space which is flushed at a variable rate (Eger et al., 1968). Face masks usually have a higher dead-space than a mouthpiece assembly and for this reason, and because leaks are difficult to prevent, are seldom used.

Compliance

This is determined by the volume and distensibility of tubing used in a circuit. It is important to know its value when pressure measurements are being made. When circuits are operated at pressures above or below ambient, a high compliance may vitiate the desired aims. Sometimes, compliance may deliberately be increased to smooth out big changes in flow rate.

Resistance

The resistance of circuits should be kept as low as possible. This is achieved by keeping tubing and connections as short and wide as possible. For exercise studies, 5 cm diameter tubing is required and connections should be of a comparable diameter. Resistance can also be reduced by the use of fans to help gas flow. It can be measured using a flow generator (vacuum cleaner motor), rotameter and manometer. A realistic aim in most circuits is a resistance less than 2 cm H_2O per litre per second flow.

Open Circuits

In these gas is inspired from one source (e.g. room air) and expired through another route without any mixing of inspired and expired streams or any recirculation except to a very limited extent within the valve box which clearly must be an integral part of an open circuit.

Open Circuit Reservoirs

Inspiration may be from room air or from a reservoir of a gas mixture; similarly the expirate may be collected or vented to room air. Suitable reservoirs for inspirate or expirate are Tissot Spirometers (see below) or bags. The traditional bags (Douglas) made of rubber backed with canvas, have now largely been replaced by neoprene bags. The requirements of such bags is that they are fairly light, of sufficient capacity (50–100 l) and impervious to the gas being collected. Douglas bags lose carbon dioxide quite rapidly; with a 1% error after 15 min (Shephard, 1955). Neoprene is impervious to most gases used in respiratory physiology in the short term, but will lose gas to the atmosphere over a period of hours, and only direct measurement can confirm the adequacy of a bag in this respect. An alternative which may be used if very large volumes are involved is a meteorological balloon. Such balloons are made of fine latex rubber and while occupying a small space when empty they can expand to hold 300 l or more. They are very useful in a "bag-in-box" circuit (see below).

Volume Measurement

Total inspired or expired volumes can be measured either directly (Tissot Spirometer) or by emptying the collecting bag through a gas meter or spirometer. Dry gas meters will provide an on-line measurement of inspired volume in 10 or 20 l increments. Breath by breath volume measurements in an open circuit are generally obtained using a pneumotachograph and integrator, but it is possible to arrange a spirometer to give tidal measurements in open circuit (Cunningham *et al.*, 1966).

Gas Temperature and Humidity

Cooling of the airways is a potent provoker of asthma in susceptible subjects and breathing dry gas is an unpleasant experience for all, which may provoke coughing in experiments lasting more than a few minutes. The problem is much greater in open than closed circuit and correspondingly greater where large volumes are inspired such as in exercise or voluntary hyper-ventilation.

If the gas is warmed, then humidity will increase with temperature. Warming may be achieved by passing the gas through a copper coil which is heated either by an electric coil or a water bath, but such an arrangement may not be possible in experiments with high flow rates because the extra resistance becomes unacceptable. Gas mixtures can be humidified using standard medical nebulizers.

Valve Boxes

These need to be competent, leak-free, of low dead-space and low resistance. As implied above, these requirements, especially the last two, are sometimes difficult to combine in a single design. Easy cleaning and sterilization are also desirable.

Most modern designs are based either on rubber discs or mica flaps. Rubber discs usually have a higher resistance and present more problems with cleaning but mica flaps may become sticky when wet and develop a high opening pressure.

Valve boxes which have been designed for specific purposes are: Otis–McKerrow valve with a very low resistance but a dead-space of about 250 ml which was designed specifically for studies involving hyper-ventilation (McKerrow and Otis, 1956); Lloyd flap valve with a lower dead-space and low resistance for exercise tests (Cunningham *et al.*, 1965) and the pneumatically operated taps and valve box for exercise studies described by Jones *et al.* (1975).

Closed Circuits

In these, gas is recirculated. This means either that some rebreathing takes place with a steadily rising CO_2 concentration, or else some CO_2 must be absorbed.

Rebreathing is widely employed in studies of respiratory control, to measure the ventilatory responses to oxygen and CO_2 as described later.

Carbon dioxide absorption is generally accomplished using soda-lime which can be put into a variety of containers. The commonest is a standard CO_2 absorbing canister such as is used in anaesthesia. These are difficult to make leak-proof, especially at the junctions which are of awkward size. Many spirometers were supplied with specially designed canisters which fitted in the inner jacket. With these it is important to avoid leakage of soda-lime into the water, because of its corrosive properties.

There are three consequences of CO_2 absorption. The first is that the soda-lime canister gets hot and wet. While this may be beneficial in open circuit, in closed circuits it can be a nuisance for the subject. More important, CO_2 absorption generally leads to a shrinking gas volume in the circuit because the respiratory exchange ratio is less than unity. This can either be measured and allowed for in calculation or gas can be run into the circuit at a rate sufficient to keep the volume constant (a spirometer trace is a good guide to this). The same method can be used to counteract the third problem, that of hypoxia. CO_2 absorption removes the protective hyper-ventilation of rebreathing and oxygen is progressively consumed. This becomes a problem after several minutes if the starting gas is air.

Carbon dioxide absorption need not be complete. Circuits have been designed in which gas is rebreathed and the proportion which is "scrubbed" of CO_2 is regulated by means of variable pumps to keep end-tidal PCO_2 at a constant, higher level (Laszlo et al., 1969).

Bag-in-Box Circuits

Where it is desired to keep a constant volume in an open circuit, the bag-in-box arrangement can be used, in which gas is inspired from a bag and expired back into its container. If the container has rigid walls and is not too big then tidal volume changes within it are easily measured by an attached spirometer or pneumotachograph (Donald and Christie, 1949). This method of tidal volume measurement is very conveniently used in the rebreathing method of assessing CO_2 response (Read, 1967) in which the rebreathing bag is sealed within a 20–30 l jar or perspex box which is in turn connected to a spirometer.

SPIROMETERS

The invention of the spirometer is generally attributed to Hutchinson (1846) although earlier versions did exist (Spriggs, 1978). There are two basic shapes: in both, gas is displaced in and out of a reservoir (the bell) which may be cylindrical or wedge-shaped.

Cylindrical Spirometers

These are the common traditional instruments for measuring respiratory volumes, and one ought to be in every laboratory, if only as a standard with which to compare other volumetric devices.

The bell is either made of lightweight material, (aluminium alloy; polystyrene) or is counterbalanced by a weight, and in either case is suspended by a wire over a pulley. Gas is displaced over a water seal in an outer jacket, and volume changes measured from a pen attached to the counterweight, writing on a kymograph, or on a recorder from a potentiometer attached to the pulley. If a kymograph is used, speeds from about 2–10 cm s^{-1} will be needed to record accurately during forced expiration. Electrical timing devices may be added so that the volume expired after 0.75 or 1.0 s is automatically recorded. (Gaensler, 1951).

The design of the bell spirometer changed little for a century after Hutchinson until the increasing use of tests based on forced expiration or maximum voluntary ventilation led to some reappraisal and several modifications of design, two of which deserve mention.

(a) Bernstein–Mendel Spirometer (Bernstein et al., 1952)

In this instrument the diameter of the outer jacket is increased relative to the bell so as to give a frequency response which is fairly flat up to 1.5 Hz. This instrument was designed specifically for measuring 15 s maximum voluntary ventilation.

(b) Stead–Wells Spirometer (Wells et al., 1959)

This instrument was also designed to cope with forced expiration and voluntary hyper-ventilation. The bell is a light plastic cylinder with an aluminium dome, with approximately equal diameters of the water seal within and without the bell. Suspension by wire and pulley is dispensed with and the bell has two lugs which fit around vertical plastic rods to guide it up and down without rotation. A pen is attached to one of these lugs. The frequency response is flat up to about 4 Hz, and this instrument is used as a standard in comparative studies (Gardner et al., 1980).

Tissot Spirometer (Tissot, 1904)

This instrument is used to store or receive volumes of 100 l or more and is unsuitable for measuring tidal changes. It has the same basic design as a bell spirometer but on an appropriately larger scale.

Wedge Spirometers

The design of these began with that of Krogh (1922). Basically they consist of a rectangular box as the outer jacket and another smaller one inverted as the bell. The name "wedge" derives from the sectional shape of the "bell". Originally, Krogh's machine was made of metal, had a counterweight and also contained a CO_2 absorber with gas being directed through the spirometer by valves.

In recent years the wedge shape has been employed in some dry spirometers with an extremely fast frequency response (see below) and especially by Mead (1960) in his volume displacement body plethysmograph. In this, the wedge spirometer with an extremely light metal alloy bell is situated in the "lap" of the plethysmograph to which it is connected by a very large orifice—an advantage which is due to the shape of the spirometer and its large surface area.

"Dry" Spirometers

In recent years there has been a move towards portable machines without a water seal. They were originally developed for epidemiological use; to measure indices of forced expiration in field work but have found an increasing application as standard laboratory machines. Many such machines are now available and I will mention only those which are most commonly found or which illustrate different points of design.

(a) Vitalograph

This consists essentially of a square shaped rubber bellows, mounted in a metal box. It is used solely for expiratory measurements. As expiration proceeds and the bellows expand a pen is moved vertically over a specially constructed chart while at the same time a (mains) electric motor drives the whole chart horizontally, so as to give a record of volume against time.

The newer Vitalographs have an adequate capacity of 7 l, but the chart stops moving after 6 s which may inadequate for some patients with airways obstruction. The resistance and accuracy meet the criteria described below for timed expiratory measurements.

(b) GARW Spirometer (Collins et al., 1964)

This machine also consists of a bellows, of light plastic, of 12 l capacity used similarly to the Vitalograph. The recording system is a moving dial with a battery-operated automatic timer to give expired volume at desired intervals from 0.75 to 2 s. It has proved rugged and versatile in field use and has been adapted to give a flow signal as well as volume, so that flow–volume curves can be recorded.

(c) Ohio Spirometer

This is essentially a cylinder but mounted horizontally in a box to which it is attached by a flexible cylindrical rolling seal which allows the cylinder to move as air enters. It is provided with a linear transducer and built in computer so that flow, volume, and time signals are available. Large transients of flow, e.g. peak expiratory flow rate, are not accurately recorded, probably because inertia is too great. Nevertheless, this machine is widely used for measuring indices based on forced expiration.

(d) Dry Wedge Spirometers (e.g. Med. Science, Oldelft)

These are wedge spirometers mounted vertically with rubber or plastic bellows, and linear transducers. They are extremely accurate, both in terms of volume and frequency response. They are supplied with their own computing and recording facilities so that flow–volume curves and all the indices based on forced expiration are accurately measured and immediately available. The drawback to these machines is their cost which exceeds that of some of the simpler dry spirometers by a factor of ten.

Electronic "Spirometers"

Electronic spirometers are not spirometers in the sense of the above instruments. Rather they are flow measuring devices with electronic integrators given a "volume" output. Most of them do not reliably measure volume and can be difficult to calibrate.

Calibration and Testing of Spirometers

There are two aspects to calibration; that of static volume changes and of dynamic response. The former is easily arranged and is generally a "once in a lifetime" measurement for each instrument, a spirometer usually being the independent variable against which other volume measuring devices are tested.

Dynamic performance is more difficult. Standards have been suggested by various groups, and especially carefully by the American Thoracic Society (Ferris *et al.*, 1978; Gardner *et al.*, 1979).

There is no general agreement on test methods. Some were suggested by the above group and these and some others have been critically examined by Gardner *et al.* (1980) who pointed out that there are practical and/or logistic problems with all of them. For example, if trained subjects doing forced expirations are used, there is a coefficient of variation of about $\pm 3\%$ in $FEV_{1.0}$, in the short term and a greater one in the long term. It is difficult to simulate forced expiration mechanically, and procedures such as explosive decompression of a pressurized source are an approximation. Gardner *et al.* (1980) have used a variety of tests to produce a detailed report on spirometers available in the U.S.A.

GAS METERS

There are two basic types—wet and dry.

Wet Gas Meters

These are extremely accurate but only at fairly low flow rates (up to about 30 l min^{-1}). The instrument consists of a drum-shaped container with four screw-shaped blades mounted on an axle, and which are successively immersed in a water seal. Gas flow across the blades causes rotation of the drum which is directly indicated by a pointer.

Calibration is generally done by displacing gas from a spirometer at a steady flow rate, and is very stable provided that the water level is maintained at the correct level.

Wet gas meters are most usefully used in measuring the volume of expired gas collections from Douglas bags; (the gas can be drawn through at a constant flow rate by a small pump) and also for calibrating other instruments.

Dry Gas Meters

These are the type used in the domestic gas supply system. They consist essentially of two pairs of bellows which are filled and emptied in turn and movements of which are transmitted to the pointer in a circular dial. These machines are accurate provided that they are frequently calibrated (at least twice a year) and that only whole revolutions of the pointer are counted. Within each revolution, there is a lot of alinearity such that a given volume of gas will cause different displacements of the pointer depending on what part of the clock it is moved over. It is possible to mount a potentiometer on the spindle of the pointer to get a record on a chart recorder.

Wet gas is best avoided as condensation rots the bellows but accuracy is maintained at flow rates of up to about 200 l min^{-1}, and they are of extremely low resistance, so that dry gas meters are ideal on the inspired line of open circuits, especially if connected to the inspired part of the valve box by a long length of tubing to smooth out some of the bigger flow transients.

Although the British domestic gas supply is metered in cubic feet, metric gas meters can be made to order. Formerly, two manufacturers would readily supply these machines but unfortunately this is no longer the case.

MEASUREMENT OF THORACIC DISPLACEMENT

This is of interest for its own sake but more so as a method of measuring breathing without the subject or patient having to use a mouthpiece. Accurate quantification of thoracic or abdominal movement in either antero-posterior or lateral diameters or of a circumference, can be obtained using many of the devices described below. They can all be used to get accurate records of respiratory rate and qualitative information about tidal volume and as such are widely used for long term clinical monitoring but methods of measuring tidal volume accurately, that are not critically dependent on maintenance of a constant posture or the pattern of breathing have not as yet been developed. I will discuss first the devices themselves and then some of the problems encountered in deriving volume measurements.

Stethograph or Bellows Pneumograph

This is probably the simplest device for continuously recording changes in thoracic or abdominal displacement, consisting of a length of corrugated rubber or plastic tubing tied or strapped round the chest or abdomen, with one end closed and the other connected to a tambour or to a pressure transducer. These stethographs are non-linear with reference to lung volume or circumference of the chest but give qualitative information about the depth of a breath. They are easily improvised and are valuable for monitoring phenomena such as periodic breathing or sleep apnoea.

Mercury in Silastic Strain Gauges

These are a refinement of the stethograph. The mercury is a column enclosed in a flexible plastic sheath. As the gauge is stretched the mercury column lengthens and its electrical resistance increases. The gauge is arranged in a circuit so that it is one arm of a Wheatstone Bridge and changes in thoracic and abdominal circumference cause a change in balance of the bridge. The signal is again non-linear with reference to circumference, resistance depending more on the cross-sectional area under the gauge. This problem can be partially overcome by calibrating to the square of the circumference (Shapiro and Cohen, 1965).

Linear Differential Transformer (Linearsyn)

These, as implied by their name, when suitably energized, give a signal directly related to linear displacement. They can be attached to points on the torso via wires and pulleys and were used in some of the fundamental research into how the chest and abdomen change shape with breathing (Konno and Mead, 1967; Agostoni and Mognoni, 1966), but have now largely been superseded by magnetometers.

Magnetometers (Mead et al., 1967)

Magnetometers are pairs of magnetic coils, one of which is used to generate an electromagnetic signal and the other to detect it. The coils are aligned with long axes parallel and in the transverse plane. Each pair is driven at a different, resonant frequency in the range of 500–1500 Hz. At these frequencies the influence of tissue or gas on the magnetic field is negligible. The signal varies with the cube of distance between the coils, but the displacements during breathing are so small compared with the diameters of chest and abdomen, that the signal can be treated linearly over this small range. Furthermore, equipment now commercially available has a fully linearized system capable of accepting up to four pairs of coils. Practical problems encountered with the magnetometers are first, that of fixing them to the skin satisfactorily and secondly, of arranging them so that the long axes of the coils remain parallel during breathing; any divergence will appear as linear displacement—and as the displacement during tidal breathing is of the order of 0.5 cm, this is potentially an important source of error.

Inductive Plethysmograph (See review by Sackner, 1980)

This is a recently introduced transducer, which consists of a pair of insulated wire coils attached to a close fitting vest which fits over the chest and upper abdomen. The change in mean cross-section area of the coil with breathing changes the inductance of the coil, which is measured by incorporating it as the inductive element in a resonant circuit maintained at about 1 mHz. The signal is demodulated to a DC signal which can be recorded by any conventional system.

The DC coupled system has a flat frequency response to 16 Hz and can be used to measure static and dynamic lung volumes and changes in end-expiratory level. An alternative, AC coupled system has an adequately flat frequency respone (0.5 to 8 Hz) but cannot be used to measure the absolute level of lung volume.

Cross-sectional area is measured directly rather than a diameter so that it is not affected by changes in body position in the same way as with magnetometers.

MEASUREMENT OF LUNG VOLUME FROM CHEST MOVEMENT

This has been attempted using all the instruments described above, but with reasonable results only from the magnetometers and the inductive plethysmograph. The central problem is one of calibration so as to account for changes in shape of the chest and abdomen. Konno and Mead (1967) showed that the respiratory system behaved with two degrees of freedom; volume changes could be apportioned between two compartments—the rib cage and the abdomen, with the diaphragm forming a common boundary. At any lung volume it was possible to shift volume from one compartment to another in an infinite variety of combinations between two extremes. For each compartment, antero-posterior displacement is linearly related to volume over a wide range of vital capacity. This led them to develop the "isovolume manoeuvre" to calibrate magnetometer signals.

In this, magnetometers are placed on the chest and abdomen and the subject, with a closed glottis, alternately contracts and relaxes chest and abdominal wall muscles so as to shift volume rapidly between these compartments, while the magnetometer signals are adjusted to give equal gains. A convenient way of doing this is to display the chest and abdominal signals on the x and y axes of an oscilloscope and adjust the signals until a line with a $-45°$ slope is obtained during the isovolume manoeuvre. The combined signals can then be calibrated against a spirometer or other device.

This is not always possible, especially in clinical work, and another system requiring a digital computer has been developed (Stagg et al., 1978). In this, the subject is supine and breathes into a pneumotachograph or spirometer via a mouthpiece for a few breaths. During a breath the relative motions of rib cage and abdomen vary. Magnetometer and pneumotachograph signals are recorded and the information used by the computer to set up and solve a series of simultaneous equations in which the unknowns are the calibration factors for the magnetometers.

Using this system and linearized magnetometers it is possible to get accurate volume records over a long period, provided that there are no significant changes in posture (Rees et al., 1980). Errors will be introduced by the subject breathing against a resistance, during exercise or voluntary hyper-ventilation; in all these circumstances, the phase relationship between antero-posterior and lateral chest diameters is altered.

All these considerations apply equally to the inductive plethysmograph. Although this instrument measures cross-sectional area rather than diameters, and is therefore theoretically less affected by changes in posture or the altered breathing patterns described above, in fact it appears to suffer some of the same limitations as the magnetometers. The inductive plethysomograph is calibrated by recording with the patient breathing through a pneumotachograph supine and sitting up; this is analogous to performing the isovolume manoeuvre, for either chest or abdominal motion is predominant at each posture. Other calibration techniques using digital computers, similar to that of Stagg et al., have been developed (Watson et al., 1980).

Both instruments, although calibrated against volume changes at the mouth, in fact measure changes in thoracic gas volume and will give a different volume signal from that obtained at the mouth in any circumstances in which there is significant gas compression, e.g. breathing against an expiratory obstruction, the start of a forced expiration or in patients with severe airways obstruction. A further problem in these patients which particularly affects the magnetometers is that there may be paradoxical movement of the lateral margins of the rib cage which introduces a third degree of freedom of motion into the system.

Other External Devices for Measuring Ventilation

Electric Impedance Plethysmography

The impedance across the chest increases on inspiration and falls on expiration and the changes can be measured and used to monitor ventilation. These methods are reviewed in detail by Pacela (1966). The techniques used include a bridge circuit (Hamilton *et al.*, 1965; Logic *et al.*, 1967), an impedance comparator (Kubicek *et al.*, 1964), a modulated oscillator (McCally *et al.*, 1963) and devices with a constant current source (Geddes *et al.*, 1962; Farman and Juett, 1967). This latter method is probably the one of choice for long-term monitoring.

In all these systems, electrodes are applied to the chest, generally over the lateral diameter and a high-frequency current passed between them.

Impedance plethysmography has not gained wide acceptance for measuring ventilation other than as a fairly crudely qualitative monitor for intensive care work, because of difficulties with linearity and stability.

At the root of these difficulties lies the basic uncertainty as to what causes the impedance changes. They have been attributed to change in lung tissue resistivity with aeration, to redistribution of pulmonary blood volume, modifications of the rib cage geometry, and even to small pressure changes at the skin–electrode interface (Hill *et al.*, 1967). In an analysis in experimental animals, Kira *et al.* (1971) found that the current passed through the chest in a narrow beam, the shape of which was partly determined by the shape of the electrodes, and that resistivity of lung tissue changed with aeration, so that the impedance pneumograph signal does not depend directly on changes in cross-sectional area or a linear diameter of the chest.

Ashutosh *et al.* (1974), using a constant-current source showed that volumes obtained from the pneumograph corresponded well with spirometric values over periods of up to half an hour, provided that the patients were supine, and did not have significant airways obstruction.

Jerkin Plethysmograph

This is a double layer garment which fits over the whole torso with tight seals at neck, armpits and groin (Heaf *et al.*, 1961). It is filled with air to a pressure of about 1 cm H_2O above atmospheric, and breathing movements produce pressure changes of about 1.5 cm H_2O which can be recorded. The design was adapted for use in infants (Milner, 1970). Its main disadvantages were alinearity of response and also that it affected breathing, especially reducing functional residual capacity. In a recent re-investigation, Kattan *et al.* (1978) found a logarithmic linear relationship of jerkin pressure to tidal volume over a wide range of operating pressures and concluded that it could usefully be used for long term monitoring in infants.

References

Agostoni, E. and Mognoni, P. (1966). *J. appl. Physiol.* **21**, 1827–1832.
Ashutosh, K., Gilbert, R., Auchincloss, J. H., Erletacher, J. and Peppi, D. (1974). *J. appl. Physiol.* **37**, 964–966.
Bernstein, L., D'Silva, J. L. and Mendel, D. (1952). *Thorax* **7**, 255–265.
Collins, M. M., McDermott, M. and McDermott, T. J. (1964). *J. Physiol. Lond.* **172**, 39–41P.
Cunningham, D. J. C., Elliott, D. H., Lloyd, B. B., Miller, J. P. and Young, J. M. (1965). *J. Physiol. Lond.* **179**, 498–508.
Cunningham, D. J. C., Lloyd, B. B., Miller, J. P., Spurr, D. and Young, J. M. (1966). *J. Physiol. Lond.* **18**, 17–19P.
Davies, W. J. H. and Denison, D. M. (1979). *Resp. Physiol.* **36**, 261–267.
Donald, K. W. and Christie, R. V. (1949). *Clin. Sci.* **8**, 21–30.
Eger, E. I., Kellogg, R. H., Mines, A. H., Lima-Ostos, M., Merrill, C. G. and Kent, D. W. (1968). *J. appl. Physiol.* **24**, 607–615.
Farman, J. V. and Juett, D. A. (1967). *Br. Med. J.* **4**, 2–17.
Ferris, B. G., (1978). *Am. rev. Resp. Dis.* **118**, Supp. 2, 55–88.
Freedman, S. (1970). *Resp. Physiol.* **8**, 230–244.
Gaensler, E. A. (1951). *Science* **114**, 444–446.
Gardner, R. M. and others (1979). *Am. Rev. resp. Dis.* **119**, 831–838.
Gardner, R. M., Hawkinson, J. L. and West, B. J. (1980). *Am. Rev. resp. Dis.* **121**, 73–82.
Geddes, L. A., Hoff, H. E., Hickman, D. M. and Moore, A. G. (1962). *Aerospace Med.* **32**, 28–33.
Hamilton, L. H., Beard, J. D. and Kory, R. C. (1965). *J. appl. Physiol.* **20**, 565–568.
Heaf, P. J. D., Scott, P., Smith, W. D. A. and Williams, K. G. (1961). *Lancet* **1**, 317–318.
Hill, R. V., Jansen, J. C. and Fling, J. L. (1967). *J. appl. Physiol.* **22**, 161–169.
Hutchinson, J. (1846). *Trans. Med. Chir. Soc. Lond.* **29**, 137–252.
Jones, N. L., Campbell, E. J. M., Edwards, R. H. T. and Robertson, D. G. (1975). "Clinical Exercise Testing," pp. 70–72. Saunders, Toronto.
Josenhans, W. T. and Wang, C. S. (1970). *J. appl. Physiol.* **28**, 679–684.
Kattan, M., Miyasalia, K., Volyesi, G. and Froese, A. B. (1978). *J. appl. Physiol.* **45**, 630–636.
Kira, S. (1971). *J. appl. Physiol.* **30**, 820–826.
Konno, K. and Mead, J. (1967). *J. appl. Physiol.* **22**, 407–422.
Krogh, A. (1922). *Wiener Linische Wochenschrift* **290**.
Kubicek, W., Kinnen, E. and Edin, A. (1964). *J. appl. Physiol.* **19**, 557–560.
Laszlo, G., Clark, T. J. H. and Campbell, E. J. M. (1969). *Clin. Sci.* **37**, 299–309.
Logic, J. L., Maksud, M. G. and Hamilton, L. H. (1967). *J. appl. Physiol.* **22**, 251–254.
McCally, M., Barnard, G., Robins, K. and Marlio, A. (1963). *Am. J. Med. Electron.* **2**, 322–327.
McKerrow, C. B. and Otis, A. B. (1956). *J. appl. Physiol.* **9**, 497–498.
Mead, J. (1960). *J. appl. Physiol.* **15**, 736–740.
Mead, J., Peterson, N., Grimby, G. and Mead, J. (1967). *Science* **156**, 1383–1384.
Milner, A. D. (1970). *Lancet* **2**, 80–81.
Pacela, A. F. (1966). *Med. Biol. Eng.* **4**, 1–15.
Read, D. J. C. (1967). *Australas. Ann. Med.* **16**, 20–32.
Rees, P. J., Higenbottam, T. W. and Clark, T. J. H. (1980). *Thorax* **35**, 384–388.

Sackner, M. A. (1980). "Diagnostic Techniques in Pulmonary Disease" Part I (Ed. M. A. Sackner), Marcel Dekker, New York.

Shapiro, A. and Cohen, H. D. (1965). *Trans. N.Y. Acad. Sci.* **27**, 634–639.

Shephard, R. J. (1955). *J. Physiol. Lond.* **127**, 515–524.

Spriggs, E. A. (1978). *Br. J. Tuberc. Dis. Chest*, **72**, 165–180.

Stagg, D., Goldham, M. and Newson Davis, J. (1978). *J. appl. Physiol.* **44**, 623–633.

Tissot, J. (1904). *J. Physiol. Path. gén.* **6**, 688–700.

Watson, H., Schneider, A., Friden, A. and Sackner, M. A. (1980). *Am. Rev. resp. Dis.* **121**. 203 (Abstract).

Wells, H. S., Stead, W. W., Rossing, T. D. and Oganovich, J. (1959). *J. appl. Physiol.* **14**, 451–454.

3. MEASUREMENT OF PRESSURE AND FLOW

A. R. Guyatt

Midhurst Medical Research Institute,
Midhurst, Sussex, U.K.

The pressure transducer is perhaps the most versatile instrument in respiratory physiology, since, as well as recording pressure within and outside the lung, it is used for air flow measurements, and even for the estimation of changes in volume. Most respiratory flow meters, (pneumotachographs), work by determining the differential pressure developed across a fixed mechanical resistance through which gas is flowing, the system being calibrated against a basic reference standard. Volume changes can either be obtained by electronic or digital integration of this flow signal, or be inferred from pressure changes occurring in a rigid chamber, such as the whole body plethysmograph or body box. The measurement of pressure is therefore the dominant theme in this chapter, but alternative methods of measuring flow rate are also discussed.

PRESSURE MEASUREMENT

Static Factors

The most important static factors to consider in any device are linearity of response, hysteresis, baseline drift and overall gain. In respiratory measurements, hysteresis is rarely detectable, and can be ignored, but the other factors are very relevant.

A linear response between the measured variable and the output signal is highly desirable. The use of a calibration curve is practical if only single values are to be considered, for instance the gas concentration of a static gas sample, but this process becomes very tedious with a continuous record, and impossible if two or more signals are to be compared electronically as in the loop-flattening technique of Mead and Whittenberger (1953). Most pressure and flow measuring devices give linear outputs but some depending on turbulent flow need to be linearized before analysis using electronic or digital techniques. Baseline drift is a problem with certain forms of pressure transducer, particularly when working at high amplification. Usually, pressure transducers are very stable as regards their gain, and once set up, rarely change unless mechanical damage occurs, or as a result of deterioration of the electronics. Flow measurements in contrast, are subject to the effects of changes in gas viscosity (and density in some cases), and various methods have been employed to overcome this problem.

Dynamic Factors

Since most respiratory measurements are made during normal breathing at around 0.25 Hz, or up to 2 Hz during special manoeuvres, pressure and flow measuring devices should have adequate dynamic characteristics to follow these faithfully. In an old, but still frequently quoted study, McCall et al. (1957) made Fourier analyses of flow records obtained during three breathing manoeuvres. The technique resolves the basic pattern into a spectrum of sine waves, a fundamental and a family of harmonics at higher frequencies, ignoring harmonics whose amplitude was less than 5% of that of the fundamental. Using this criterion, they concluded that the flow pattern for tidal breathing and for relaxed vital capacity manoeuvres could be adequately described by the frequencies up to 4 Hz, but for maximum voluntary ventilation it was necessary to go up to 20 Hz. An alternative rule of thumb is that a recording device should have a satisfactory dynamic range up to 10 times the fundamental frequency.

The classic theoretical treatment of pressure measurement is due to Fry (1960). He was particularly concerned with the familiar arrangement of a pressure transducer connected to the measuring site by a probe or catheter. He concluded that for most purposes the system could be adequately described by considering mass, capacitance and resistance, and this approach has been followed in this chapter. The real situation is more complex; Proulx et al. (1979) consider that the description of the behaviour of a transducer should also include inertia and an extra lag phase, but this is rarely important.

A typical pressure transducer consists of a flexible diaphragm with a strain gauge on its surface connected to an amplifying circuit. Pressure changes applied to one side of the diaphragm distort it and produce an electrical output. The mechanical characteristics of the system are determined by the diaphragm itself, by the dimensions of the transducer and by the probe connecting it to the pressure source. Figure 1 shows records of actual pressure (solid line), and the transducer output (dashed line) plotted against time for four different probes (A to D). In every case, a sudden step change of pressure is applied.

In case A, the output initially overshoots the new level, then oscillates about it with decreasing magnitude until it becomes stable. This tendency of the oscillations to decrease is due to "damping", the braking effects of viscosity and friction in the air. The frequency of vibration is the "damped natural frequency", and if no damping at all was present, the vibration would continue indefinitely at a slightly faster rate, the "natural frequency".

In case B, the same effect is seen, but the vibrations are smaller, slower and die away faster, while the overshoot is also less. The damping is greater due to the higher resistance of the connecting tube. In cases C and D, no overshoot or vibrations occur. C is the "critically damped" case, where just sufficient damping is applied to abolish overshoot, and in this case the system reaches stability in the minimum possible time. Case D is "overdamped", and the record resembles that of C but is rather more sluggish. Damping can be expressed using the ratio h, defined as the actual damping divided by that amount needed to produce the critical condition. With this definition, system C must have an h value of 1.0 while cases A, B and D have been given values of 0.2, 0.707 and 2.0, respectively.

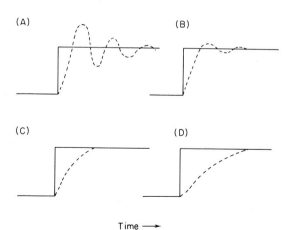

(A)   (B)

(C)   (D)

Time ⟶

FIG. 1. Response of four pressure transducers with increasing degrees of damping to a square wave pressure signal. Probe A has the largest diameter, probe D the smallest. (— — — —) transducer pressure, (————) actual output.

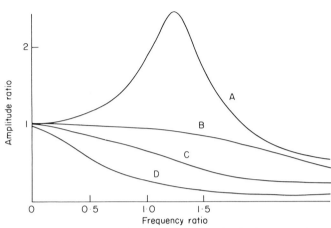

Fig. 2. Relationship of signal amplitude to frequency in the four pressure transducers considered in Fig. 1.

Consider now the response of the system to a forcing sinusoidal pressure source whose speed is variable. The amplitude of the output (peak to trough height of the sine wave), can be expressed at any speed as the ratio of the observed value to the value recorded at the lowest possible rate, where it is assumed the system is following the source faithfully. Frequency is also expressed as a ratio, in this case of the natural frequency, to facilitate comparison of different systems.

The plots of amplitude ratio against frequency ratio are shown in Fig. 2. System A shows an initial rise in amplitude as the speed increases then a sudden jump to a maximum just below 1.0, then falling away after. This maximum is produced by the device resonating at the damped natural frequency. System B shows no change in amplitude up to a value of about 0.5 (half natural frequency), then begins to fall away, the damping ratio in this case, 0.707, being the limit above which no resonance occurs. Systems C and D show falls in amplitude with all increases in frequency.

The other important dynamic characteristic is the phase relationship between the input and output signal. The phase lag of output behind input for the four systems is shown in Fig. 3, against frequency, which is again expressed as the ratio of the natural frequency. In all cases, the lag approaches 0° at the lowest rates and 90° at the frequency ratio of 1.0. In practice, the natural frequency is often measured, as the point at which the lag becomes 90°. Systems B and C show an almost linear relationship between phase lag and frequency up to the natural frequency, but A and D which are respectively, very under- and over-damped, have marked alinearity in this regard.

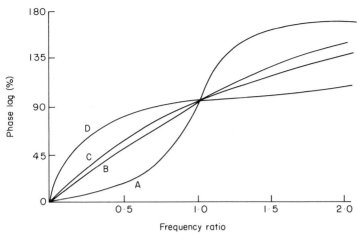

FIG. 3. Relationship of phase changes in the four pressure transducers to frequency (phase lag being measured using a reference signal).

When choosing equipment for respiratory studies, it is desirable that the natural frequency be well above that of the highest harmonic deemed necessary for accurate recording. Pressure transducers have small diaphragms with low mass, so that this condition is normally met, but difficulties may be encountered where flow is derived from a spirometer whose bell or bellows is of large mass. If an oscillating source is available, the amplitude response and phase lag should be measured over the working range, and the output should be "flat" in this case (that is the amplitude should be within 5% of the value at the lowest rate). If resonance is detected, damping should be added mechanically by increasing the tubing resistance, or better still, by electronic means by modifying the output. If the damping is too high, this should be reduced, though generally this is more difficult than increasing it, and the ideal level is somewhere between 0.707 and 1.0. When two systems are used in conjunction, they should have similar natural frequencies since they will always lag a source by the same amount and will be in synchrony with each other. The phase relationship between two systems can be checked directly by displaying the outputs on the two axes of an oscilloscope and by varying the speed of the source. If they are in phase, the resulting Lissajous figure will be a straight sloped line, but with phase difference it will become looped or distorted.

Where no oscillating source is available, the step pressure method may be substituted. If no oscillations appear on the trace, the system must be either critically- or overdamped, and the only information available is the rise time. This may be expressed as the 90% response time, that is the period needed for the signal to achieve nine-tenths of the final value. In underdamped systems, the natural frequency may be inferred, (slightly faster than observed oscillations), and the damping ratio calculated from the formula:

$$h = (z/[\pi^2 + z])^{\frac{1}{2}}$$

where $z = (\log_e x/y)^2$, x is the overshoot distance above the final level, and y the amplitude, (baseline to final level reached).

Site of Measurement

Mouth

Pressure can be measured at this site for a variety of reasons, but the most common case is in the thoracic gas estimation (DuBois *et al.*, 1956), where the subject makes panting movements against a closed shutter (Chapter 9). In these conditions of zero air flow, pressure equilibration occurs almost instaneously throughout the bronchial tree, so that the pressure actually recorded at the mouth is that acting within the alveoli. In this manoeuvre, the subject rarely develops pressures in excess of about $\pm$ 1 kPa ($\pm$ 10 cm H_2O) and since only the change in pressure is being measured, the transducer can be set to this level and overloading be ignored. Some special tests do involve measuring absolute levels, and where maximal efforts are made a range of $\pm$ 15 kPa may be necessary.

In quiet breathing, the flow rate at the mouth rarely exceeds $\pm$ 5 l s^{-1}, and a pneumotachograph limited to this range is quite adequate. In forced inspiratory and expiratory manoeuvres however, flows of $\pm$ 15 l s^{-1}, may be encountered, and a larger, low resistance pneumotachograph should be used. The differential pressure developed across the conventional pneumotachograph rarely exceeds about $\pm$ 0.1 kPa to give a low resistance to breathing.

Oesophagus

The estimation of the forces acting across the lung from pleura to airways is important for the determination of the elastic properties and air flow resistance of the whole lung. The direct measurement of pleural pressure is rarely practicable in man, but oesophageal recording provides an approximate alternative. The oesophagus is flaccid, except during swallowing, and since it lies between the lungs, the changes in intrathoracic pressure can be readily detected within it, with the subject upright.

The usual method of recording these pressures, (Milic-Emili *et al.*, 1964a and b), consists of introducing an air-filled catheter, covered at the end by a balloon, into the middle third of the oesophagus. In quiet breathing, pressure fluctuates around a level of about $\pm$ 1 kPa, but in static conditions at extreme lung volumes, a value of -3 or -4 kPa may be observed.

Two other methods of measuring oesophageal pressure have been used, a liquid-filled catheter either perfused to remove bubbles or static with just the end exposed, or a micro, *in situ*, transducer, mounted on the tip of a catheter. These methods give a more localized measurement of pressure than the 10 cm balloon, and so are more suitable for studies on neonates; they do not seem to have been used widely with adults in respiratory studies. They are however common in digestive studies for assessing the motility of the oesophagus, and several recent publications have appeared concerned with technical aspects of the methods, (Lydon *et al.*, 1975; Humphries and Castell, 1977; Klinger *et al.*, 1977 and Wallin *et al.*, 1978).

Outer Chamber

The primary example of this is the whole body plethysmograph or body box (Chapter 9). It is used in two main configurations, the constant volume or pressure box, and the flow or volume displacement box. The pressure box can record 50 to 100 ml changes in the volume of the chest while the subject is panting against a closed shutter, giving rise to pressure fluctuations of about $\pm$ 0.02 kPa. In the flow box, pressure changes are far smaller, but flow rates with a maximum of $\pm$ 0.2 l s^{-1} may need to be measured during the manoeuvres.

The system is very prone to vibration and external pressure changes, such as those produced by opening and closing doors, or on windy days. The transducers can be shock mounted, and it is generally recommended that the "neutral" side, (that is the other side from which pressure is recorded), be connected to a reservoir of air which can range in size from five litres to several hundred litres, and which has a slow leak to atmosphere. Such a device is rarely effective, probably because much of the instrumental noise comes from slight flexing of the chamber walls themselves and this problem can be overrated. The most important precaution is to prevent people using doors in the vicinity during recording, and we have been able to conduct three surveys with a body box mounted in an ordinary trailer caravan, with a floor and walls of very light construction

Types of Transducer

The primary measurement of pressure requires the use of liquid-filled manometers, but these are too sluggish to use during breathing manoeuvres, except in static tests, and for physiological measurements calibrated pressure transducers are used instead. These consist of a chamber containing a diaphragm, whose position is sensed by a variety of methods discussed by Stott (1967, pp. 23–35 and 54–56), and by Cobbold (1974, pp. 118–149).

The capacitance transducer consists of a double capacitor, that is an inner flexible metal or plastic diaphragm moving between two outer rigid metal plates. Changes in the relative capacitance between the two sides are used in the generation of an output signal.

Strain gauges are normally of the unbonded coil type. Here the diaphragm is mechanically linked to four wire coils so that the displacement in any direction stretches one pair and relaxes the other. The coils are placed in a Wheatstone bridge circuit, and as they flex, their resistance changes and produce an output. A more recent development uses silicon crystals bonded to the diaphragm as the resistive element.

Optical defocusing involves the reflection of light from a silvered membrane onto a photo-electric cell. Deformation of the diaphragm with pressure, alters the amount of light reaching the detector unit.

Variable inductance systems are variable transformers where the movement of an iron core attached to the diaphragm alters the coupling between the primary winding and a single or pair of opposed secondary coils.

Variable reluctance transducers compare the magnetic flux between a magnetically permeable diaphragm and two coils placed either side. This method is not described by the authors cited above.

All these systems are available commercially; the first two to be popular were the capacitance and unbonded strain gauge, and the latter, by virtue of its excellent construction, (Statham), was for long the instrument of choice.

The capacitance, optical defocusing and variable reluctance instruments have the great advantage of dispensing with a mechanical linkage between diaphragm and sensing element. The mass of the moving parts is small so that the frequency characteristics are excellent, and the system is insensitive to external vibration. Replacement of the diaphragm is simple if damaged, or if it is necessary to change the sensitivity. With the strain gauge the added mass of the coils and support impairs the frequency characteristics, and makes it more sensitive to vibrations and the possibility of damage, while any replacement of the diaphragm involves complete rebuilding of the instrument.

The baseline stability of the variable inductance and reluctance systems is better than that of the other systems. The capacitance and optical defocusing systems suffer by virtue of their intrinsically alinear output. This is overcome by restricting the range of movement of the diaphragm with greater amplification of the signal which leads to electronic drifting. The output of the unbonded strain gauge is low, and is very temperature dependent, so that this system is also inherently unstable; the silicon bonded system has a much higher output, but since this is also very alinear and affected by temperature, the same baseline problems occur.

Most systems consist of a transducer joined to a separate preamplifier by a cable, which allows considerable freedom in assembling equipment and reducing the lengths of catheters. The capacitance and optical defocusing systems are often built as a single unit in a box, and this can cause problems of assembly.

Differential Pressure Measuring Systems

The components of a differential pressure measuring system are shown in Fig. 4. Pressure is detected at two points a and b, which may be sited in a tube or chamber. The sampling port is normally just a side arm, but if there is risk of considerable airflow past it, precautions may be necessary to avoid Venturi effects. Care must be taken to prevent any liquid, which could form bubbles, entering the tube, since the resultant surface tension effects produce severe instability and alinearity.

Fry (1960), has described the probe, transducer system in considerable detail, but to a first approximation it can be treated as a resistance, capacitance network, if the inertia of the system is disregarded. The tube acts as the resistive element and the capacitance is the volume of air contained in the tube and more importantly in the diaphragm chamber. The performance of such a system can be described using the time

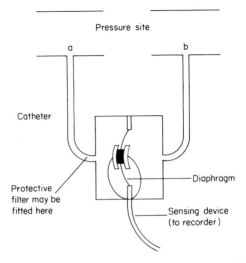

FIG. 4. Configuration of differential pressure transducer.

constant, the product of resistance and capacitance, which is inversely related to the dynamic performance.

For minimum resistance, the tubing should be as short as possible, and of as large a bore. The inclusion of even a short connector of narrow bore, such as a Luer fitting can have disastrous effects on the response, since laminar air flow resistance varies as the fourth power of the radius. Some transducers, intended for industrial use, incorporate a metal filter in the input tubing to protect the diaphragm against dust, and this will also tend to increase the resistance. The capacitance of the system can be kept low by employing the minimum possible chamber volume, and the most rigid connecting tubing which are convenient.

In flow measurements, it is very important that the time constants of both probe chamber systems, on the two sides of the diaphragm are identical. In most modern systems, care is taken to make the system as symmetrical as possible, but this does not obtain with some older designs. Kafer (1973), found that the Statham PM15, a very commonly used strain gauge, had chamber volumes of 6.67 and 35.5 ml, while the Sanborn 270, a variable inductance device, had volumes of 4.7 and 3.42 ml.

Kafer's method of testing for asymmetry is shown in Fig. 5, where the transducer is connected to a pneumotachograph, the ends of which are joined with a loop of wide-bore tubing. Air injected into this closed system produced a pressure wave, which should have affected both sides of the transducer equally. Asymmetry results in a transient signal

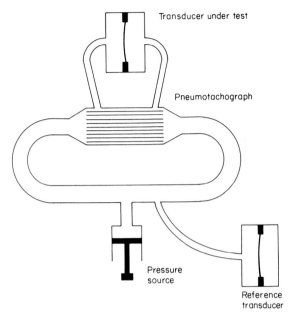

Transducer under test

Pneumotachograph

Pressure source

Reference transducer

FIG. 5. System for "tuning" differential pressure transducer. The length of tubing on either side of the transducer is varied to minimize the signal recorded during a step pressure change.

because the side of the diaphragm with the smallest volume, and hence the lower time constant, responds much more rapidly. This effect can be reduced by shortening the length of tubing on the side with the larger chamber. Grossly asymetric transducers should not be used for differential pressure measurements. All systems should be tested for this effect and most can be satisfactorily "tuned" by slight adjustment of the tube lengths.

The final stage in pressure measurement is the preamplifier, which produces the electrical output, and its link to the recording device such as an oscilloscope, pen recorder or magnetic tape unit. The input impedance of these devices should be matched to the characteristics of the transducer preamplifier, and while with most modern recording devices, the impedance is high, Stott (1967, pp. 1 and 2), has shown that some reduction in signal strength is likely even with oscilloscopes. More serious problems can occur with low impedance galvanometers such as those used in ultraviolet photographic systems, and some modern pen recorders. Sometimes it may be necessary to mix signals from two preamplifiers, as in the loop-flattening techniques, and if the outputs are connected directly to a potentiometer, rather than through an extra buffer amplifier first, this may also result in a low impedance input of variable characteristics. Mismatch of the impedances may, in extreme cases, damage the preamplifier, output device or both together, or drastically reduce or distort the output signal. It is also advisable in calibration, to use the same output configuration, as for the measurements proper, since otherwise differences in the impedance loading may cause large changes in gain.

Oesophageal Pressure

While many of the same principles apply to this measurement, the actual technique is more complicated, and will therefore be described in some detail. The probe is, in this case, a narrow catheter, about 70 cm long, with a 1 mm bore. The proximal 10 cm are perforated and enclosed in a cylindrical balloon, 3.5 cm in circumference, with a wall thickness of 0.06 mm, and containing about 0.2 ml of air, the design of this is critical (Milic-Emili et al., 1964a and b).

Cotes, (1979, pp. 118–120), has summarized the usual methods of introducing the catheter into the oesophagus. The most patent nostril is first selected, and the nasopharynx anaesthetized at the front and back. The balloon is lubricated with a suitable gel, before insertion into the nostril. When it reaches the back of the throat, the subject starts sipping water through a straw until the balloon reaches the stomach (this is indicated by a reversal in the polarity of the pressure swings during breathing). Care must be taken to avoid the tube coiling in the back of the nasopharynx during swallowing. The catheter is then withdrawn about 20 cm into the operating position; if it is withdrawn too far, pressure artefacts will be produced when the subject strains, flexes his neck, or has pressure applied to his supersternal notch.

In practice, this procedure can be simplified. Many experienced subjects, prefer to dispense with local anaesthetic and like the balloon to be moistened with water. The subject sips cold water to numb the throat. The balloon can be positioned by swallowing it to a predetermined mark on the catheter, 40 or 42 cm from the tip. The proper siting can be checked as described above, alternatively the measurement site can be inferred from the form of the cardiogenic oscillations, (Trop et al., 1970). It is important to anchor the tube properly to prevent it being swallowed further, and this can be done by taping the tube to the nostril or forehead, and checking the position of reference marks on the tube at frequent intervals.

The balloon must be correctly inflated and this can be conveniently done if the system is first emptied completely, then 0.2 to 0.4 ml of air is introduced until the cardiogenic oscillations appear. Trop *et al.* conclude that the pressure actually recorded with this degree of inflation is the most negative acting over the length of the balloon, and that the cardiogenic oscillations are sensed at the same point.

Allowance can be made for cardiogenic oscillations in static conditions, by always making the reading at a fixed point such as mid-way between the extremes, (Turner *et al.*, 1968), or this can be averaged using a damped recording system. Paper records made during tidal breathing can be smoothed by eye before measurement or digital techniques can be applied to the outputs, (Rabin and Lewis, 1968). No correction can be made for the effect of swallowing; the pressure becomes very positive instead of negative for at least two seconds, and measurement is impossible in this period. It is advisable to monitor oesophageal pressure continuously during recording, so that all records marred by this effect can be repeated whilst the balloon is still in position.

The catheter has a high resistance, and it is particularly important to ensure that the diaphragm chamber is kept as small as possible to achieve the lowest possible time constant, (Schilder *et al.*, 1959). If the catheter is connected to a conventional transducer with a large chamber the pressure output may not adequtely follow the fundamental breathing frequency, let alone describe the higher harmonics.

Normally, the oesophageal pressure is used in the estimation of transpulmonary forces, so that the reference side of the transducer is connected to the tubing at the mouth.

Static Calibration

The mouth and oesophageal pressure systems described above, work over a range of at least $\pm$ 1 kPa, and can be readily compared with a water or aneroid manometer to examine the various static characteristics discussed above. A simple design of water manometer is shown in Fig. 6. A large flask of 5 l or more acts as a gas reservoir, and as one limb of the manometer. The flask is pressurized using a sphygmomanometer bulb, allowing time for the system to stabilize. It can be repeatedly connected to the transducer system under test with only a small loss of pressure each time. The surface area of the air–liquid interface in the flask is very large compared with that of the other limb, which is contained within a 0.5 cm tube, so that almost all the differential movement of the two sides occurs within the tube, and can be read using a mirrored scale to reduce parallax errors. For most purposes, a pressure up to 10 kPa (about 100 cm H_2O) is adequate.

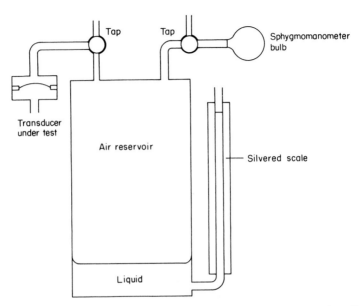

Fig. 6. Water manometer used for calibrating pressure transducer (as described by Dr. Ivor Gabe).

Alternatively, anaeroid systems are available commercially. They are much more expensive, and since they are a secondary standard, errors can easily occur through maladjustment or damage to the equipment.

Transducers working over these ranges normally give linear responses, and the gain is unlikely to change over a period of months or years. The baseline position should be checked fairly regularly during a session of use, particularly when capacitance or strain gauge devices are being used.

The transducers used for the body box or differential pressure across a pneumotachograph are normally used at a ten times more sensitive level and cannot be calibrated accurately by these systems, unless the gain of the amplifier is reduced. Special water manometers are available with inclined tubes to increase the sensitivity or using a micrometer to sense the meniscus position. A simple alternative is shown in Fig. 7. One side of the transducer is connected to a large bottle of known volume, for example ten litres. Measured volumes of air are injected into this from a syringe, to produce an estimated pressure rise, which can be compared with the resultant electrical output. The pressure change will be adiabatic, but this can be converted to an isothermal change if the container is packed with metal foil to act as a heat sink, or if

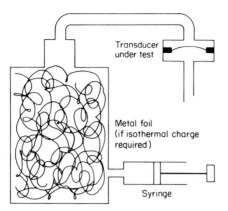

FIG. 7. Static system for calibrating transducer at low pressure levels.

sufficient time is allowed for the temperature to return to ambient after each injection. It is of course crucial that the system is leak-free, and the room temperature is constant over the period of calibration.

An improvement to the system is to use the quasi-static technique. The position of the syringe plunger is sensed by a linear potientiometer, and the outputs of transducer and potentiometer are displayed on the two axes of an oscilloscope. The syringe is pumped slowly in and out, and the slope of the resultant Lissajous figure yields the gain of the amplifier multiplied by the adiabatic factor of 1.41 unless the system is rendered isothermal using the metal foil. Any non-linearity or hysteresis of the system is immediately obvious from the form of the trace, though this is very uncommon in practice.

Dynamic Calibration

The step pressure or square wave pressure test can be performed by connecting the transducer to a chamber within which a balloon is burst, using a sharp point or hot wire, or a membrane, stretched over a tube and pressurized, is substituted. Proulx et al. (1979) have however expressed reservations regarding these simple devices and prefer a more complex system which involves release of compressed air from a specially designed cylinder.

Oscillating pressures can be readily produced by a large loudspeaker such as a 15 inch "woofer", driven via a power amplifier by a sine wave generator, (Mead, 1960; Grimby et al., 1968). This can test almost the whole frequency range, but the actual output, that is volume displacement, varies with rate, being approximately at a maximum at 1 Hz with a 1 1 displacement, but falling rapidly at higher frequencies. Below about1 Hz, leakage through the cone becomes an important factor and the system is less effective. The position of the loudspeaker can be inferred from the driving signal or, better still from a linear transducer mounted on the cone, and this is compared with the pressure output to establish the phase relationships.

An alternative source is a motor-driven pump, either specially constructed such as that of Reynolds and Hyett (1974), or a 500 cc motor cycle engine driven by an electric motor with a speed control. The output will not be sinusoidal, although this condition will be approached if the stroke is very short compared with the length of the connecting rod. The frequency range is much less than for the loudspeaker, the highest speed being about 15 Hz, but it will run at much lower rates, and since the output does not vary with frequency, the amplitude changes can be readily examined. The system should again incorporate a linear transducer to sense the position of the piston, and so provide the necessary information for phase studies. A smaller version of this with a stroke about 50 ml, is very useful for the routine calibration of the body plethysmograph.

Both dynamic systems have their own particular value. The loudspeaker enables the phase relationships to be examined over the full dynamic range including the estimation of the natural frequency, which may for a pressure transducer be very high. The pump allows the amplitude ratio to be measured unambiguously. With these systems single transducers can be evaluated, two can be compared by displaying their respective outputs on the axes of an oscilloscope and examining the resultant Lissajous figures at different frequencies, or a differential transducer can be "tuned".

FLOW MEASUREMENT

Differential Pressure Systems

These systems rely on two different patterns of air flow through the device, laminar or turbulent. The theoretical derivation of the methods have been given by Linford (1961, pp. 62–78), but these can be summarized by the two formulae:

$$dP = \dot{V}k \text{ (laminar)}$$
$$dP = \dot{V}^2K \text{ (turbulent)}$$

where dP is the differential pressure, $\dot{V}$ the flow rate, $k = [(8l)/r^4] \times \mu$, where l and r are the tube length and radius, and μ the viscosity of the gas, and k is a factor which incorporates both viscosity and density of the gas. Laminar devices produce a signal which is proportional to flow and turbulent ones proportional to the square root of flow.

Capillary

This is one of the most popular of all designs and is shown diagramatically in Fig. 8A. As originally described by Fleisch (1925), it consisted of a bundle of parallel capillary tubes, 20 cm long within a pipe through which the subject breathed. As air flowed through the capillaries, the flow profile became parabolic and the differential pressure was recorded across a 9 cm gap at the centre where the flow was almost laminar. Fry *et al.* (1957) compared two other designs, where the tubes were concentric or parallel plates were employed, and preferred the latter system,

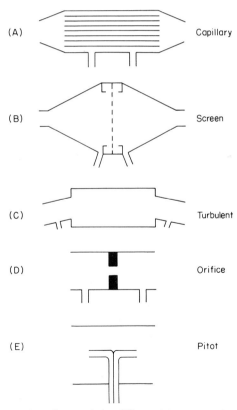

FIG. 8. Various forms of the differential pressure flow meter.

since there was less chance of blockage with condensation. Modern commercial designs use a corrugated plate wound round an axial spindle to simulate the capillary tubes. A wide range of sizes is available to cover requirements ranging from small animals to forced expiratory manoeuvres in healthy man.

Screen

In this design, Fig. 8B, which is again extremely popular, laminar flow is also used, but the resistive element is a metallic screen, usually of 400 gauge mesh, (400 strands to the inch in either direction). The principle was simultaneously described by Silverman and Whittenberger (1954) and Lilley (1954). In Lilley's design the screen is about 5 or 6 cm in diameter and surrounded on each side by an annular ring from which the pressures are recorded. Two conical sections, one on each side, reduce the diameter to about 3 cm for connection to the ordinary breathing tube. This expansion will reduce the velocity of air to about a quarter of the rate in the tubing and will thus help to produce laminar flow.

Turbulent Flow

Linford (1961, pp. 62–148) has described several industrial applications of turbulent flow meters employing the Bernoulli principle, such as the Venturi and Dall tubes, the orifice and Dall orifice and nozzle designs, but these have found little place in the respiratory studies, particularly since most of them are unidirectional. Elliot et al. (1977) described a system, (Fig. 8C), for use in patient ventilator circuits where considerable condensation occurred; turbulence was produced within a chamber by the use of offset entry and exit tubing. Orifice plates can also be useful (Fig. 8D); for instance, in the measurement of cigarette smoke where they can be incorporated in a small cigarette holder for studies during smoking, presenting a small dead space, being insensitive to blockage with tar and easy to clean.

Osbourne (1978) attempted to combine the advantages of laminar and turbulent flow devices with a variable orifice device for ventilator circuits. The orifice was bounded by an elastically hinged flap which opened as flow increased, so that this turbulent device gave a linear relationship between flow and pressure without running the risk of being blocked by condensate. The performance of this device is however critically dependent on its construction and the properties of the flap.

Pitot Tube

This device, (Fig. 8E), records velocity at a point, rather than total flow, but within a system of fixed geometry can function as an ordinary flow meter. Linford (1961) has shown its wide use in industrial contexts, where considerable expertise has been developed, and Brackenbury (1972) has discussed at length its use in physiological work. In this field, it usually consists of a double probe ending in holes facing directly up and down the breathing tube; the pressure gradient between the holes is proportional to the square root of flow, as in the turbulent devices. It is of particular value where space is limited; for instance, Brackenbury described its use within the airways of birds.

We have recently examined the use of this principle to measure nasal air flow (Guyatt *et al.*, 1982). Pressure at the nose is recorded using a transducer connected to a nasal oxygen cannula, and calibrated by simultaneously recording air flow through a face mask. The relationship between pressure and flow signals is more complex than with the simple pitot tube, but can be readily computed digitally, to allow non-invasive measurement of nasal ventilation over periods of 5 or 10 minutes.

Comparison of Methods

The capillary and screen types are by far the most widely used flow meters in respiratory studies. They have the great advantage of producing linear output with flow, though at the expense of a larger deadspace than some other types; the turbulent and Pitot designs suffer from a lack of sensitivity at the low end of the range and turbulent devices may also produce intolerable resistance to breathing at high flow rates. These systems do however have the advantage of a large cross-sectional area, which makes them much less likely to be blocked, for example by water; the laminar devices are less satisfactory in this regard, particularly the screen devices. This latter system is also susceptible to long term increases of resistance through blockage of the gauze and corrosion.

Fry *et al.* (1957), found that the screen pneumotachograph had a less linear relationship with a reference flow measurement than the capillary type, an observation also confirmed by Finucane *et al.* (1972). These latter workers however found that the capillary device was much less sensitive to the geometry of the circuit within which it was placed, since the parabolic profiles within the capillaries could be distorted more by the flow patterns entering the system than within the holes of the screen design. They recommended that the calibration of a capillary device should be done with the instrument *in situ*, and that flow should be passed in both directions. They also found an alinear relationship between flow and pressure drop across the two ends of the capillary device, and thought that in consequence it would be unsatisfactory for use with a body plethysmograph, but this system is however used in one commercially available instrument.

They also investigated the dynamic characteristics of both designs. The screen pneumotachograph showed no measurable phase lag or amplitude up to 10 Hz, but at this frequency the capillary device showed a phase lag of 8° on air, and on the dense gas sulphur hexafluoride, 29° with measured amplitude 15% down. They attributed this effect to inertia of the gas within the cylindrical elements.

Spirometry

Flow can be estimated directly from a volume record as the rate of change of volume with time (an account of mechanical spirometers is given in Chapter 2).

Any spirometer which gives an electrical output can be used for providing a flow signal, though of course the dynamic characteristics of the instrument must be adequate. Farmer and Portnoy (1974) described an electrical circuit which differentiated a volume signal by comparing the current volume with one which had been electronically delayed. Commercially available designs of spirometer, such as the wedge and rolling seal piston types record flow directly as the velocity of the sensing element, that is the bellows or piston.

The principle has the advantage of being independent of gas viscosity and density, so that it is ideal for comparative studies involving various gases. It does however suffer from the problems of inferior dynamic response and instrumental noise. The mass of the sensing element, bell, bellows or piston is much greater than that of the pressure transducer diaphragm, so that while with pressure techniques, the dynamic problems are largely those of the tubing connections, here it is a function of the detector itself. The signal can often be corrected electronically, as explained below, but much attention has been paid to improving the basic instrument. This usually involves increasing the surface area of the bellow or piston, to respond to the slightest change in pressure, at the price of decreasing the distance the elements have to travel for a given volume change. This renders the measurements of the velocity more difficult.

Differentiation of an electrical signal will itself accentuate noise. Random vibrations or electrical noise may be of small amplitude but be of high frequency, yielding enormous flow signals. A volume signal may show a barely discernable ripple, but give rise to a flow output whose fine detail is buried by noise. Electronic filtering can be used, but this will degrade the dynamic characteristics of the system still further. An alternative approach is to produce a better primary source; Cumming (1966) described a Krogh spirometer whose position was sensed in the usual way by a rotary potentiometer, but which had a separate coil moving within the shaped pole pieces of a powerful permanent magnet. The EMF obtained from the coil which corresponds to flow gave a very clean signal which enabled even quiet breathing to be recorded accurately. In general, however, the spirometric approach is more satisfactory with the higher flow rates in forced respiratory manoeuvres where noise is less important.

Miscellaneous Electronically Sensed Methods

Hot Wire Anemometer

When a wire is heated by a current flowing through it, its final temperature, and hence its electrical resistance is reached when the rate of heat production is matched by the loss to the surroundings. This flux depends both on the velocity of the gas about the wire, and on the gas thermal conductivity. The response to gas velocity is non-directional and some other device must be added if the phases of respiration are to be distinguished (Scheid and Piiper, 1971).

This system is very useful where a non-invasive probe is required, for instance in making determinations at the nostril. The thermal inertia of a small wire is very low so that it has excellent dynamic characteristics and can be used for instance to sense the timing of zero flow, (Guyatt et al., 1975). Its use as a quantitative device is less satisfactory; Fitzgerald et al. (1973) in their unfavourable examination of electronic spirometers, considered two instruments based on this principle and deemed neither to be sufficiently accurate.

Bentley (1980), overcame these problems by placing the anemometer behind an orifice which produced a vortex during gas flow. This in turn caused rapid pressure fluctuations, the frequency of which vary with the flow rate and could be detected by the hot wire as a ripple over the standing signal.

Rotating Vane

These instruments developed for medical use by Wright are used in anaesthetic circuits. Originally measuring minute ventilation, they have been adapted to determine flow using a digital signal from the rotating vane (Wright, 1955; Smith, 1972). A tendency to under-read at low flows may be corrected by microprocessor techniques. These instruments now achieve a high degree of accuracy and linearity.

Ultrasonic

This approach has been developed for ventilator systems, where the minimum resistance to breathing and insensitivity to blockage are of paramount importance. The subject breathes through a tube, across which pulses of ultrasound, at 100 kHz, are beamed to and fro, at an angle of 45° to the air flow. The transit time for the pulse is recorded in both directions; if pulse and flow are in the same direction the time is reduced, if they oppose each other the time is increased, and from the difference the actual flow rate may be determined. Blumenfeld *et al.* (1974), showed that the results were considerably affected by gas composition, humidity, temperature and pressure, all of which affect the speed of sound in the gas. This system is too expensive for routine use.

Gap Velocity

This device, described by West (1960), was intended to record velocity in confined spaces, in particular the bronchi. A pair of capillary tubes are inserted into the desired part of the bronchial tree at bronchoscopy; one carries a stream of tracer gas, in this case an argon–air mixture, and the other is a sample line connected to a mass spectrometer. At the sample area, protected by a cage, the two tubes are bent at right angles to face each other with a narrow gap between the open ends. If the gas is at rest within the bronchus, most of the argon leaving the first tube will blow directly into the second, but when the flow occurs in the airway, some of it will be deflected. The resultant argon signal will be inversely related to the gas flow inside the bronchus, although the signal will be unidirectional. It has the attraction of employing the gas analyser as the detector unit, and this can be of value where a comparison of flow and gas concentrations is needed, since all the readings are in synchrony.

Measurement of Peak Expiratory Flow Rate

The measurement of the peak flow which can be achieved in a forced expiration has become a valuable clinical tool. Although the test is very effort-dependent, requiring motivation on the part of the subject, it has the advantage of requiring simple, portable and cheap equipment which does not use a power source. Three systems have been described. Two of them, the orifice (Hadorn, 1942) and a mechanical version of the turbine (Friedman and Walker, 1975; Poppius and Mattson, 1977) are inaccurate and not in general use.

Wright and McKerrow (1959), described a variable aperture device, (defined by Linford (1961), as a "spring controlled, hinged gate" type). This has become the standard instrument for measuring peak flows in the field. The subject breathes forcibly through a tube entering a cylindrical chamber tangentially. One side of the chamber, away from the inlet is blocked off, the other has a rectangular vane. The vane is pivoted at one end to the chamber centre. Blowing on this vane, it rotates against a spring, uncovering an orifice through which the air escapes, (the area of the orifice increases as the vane moves). The vane is connected to a pointer on a scale, and it reaches a stable position when the torque produced by the air flow is matched by that of the spring which is now under compression. The vane is held in its highest position by a ratchet so that the reading can be made at leisure before resetting the device for the next test; the standard instrument will read up to 1000 1 min^{-1}, (16.67 1 s^{-1}). Altman et al. (1977) found that individual instruments gave results that agreed to 5%. Bushman et al. (1978), have suggested that the reproducibility of the measurement can be improved by using a flanged mouthpiece, and have described a calibrating device which gave repeated readings on the instrument with a standard deviation of only about 1 1 min^{-1}. The instrument records the maximum expiratory flow rate sustained for 10 ms and this has become the accepted definition of peak expiratory flow rate.

More recently, cheaper plastic versions of the instrument have appeared, where the vane is replaced by a piston moving within a cylinder, the wall of which has a rectangular slot cut in it to allow the air the escape. These instruments are cheap enough to distribute to individual patients, who can then monitor themselves at home or work, and record diurnal or daily changes for later analysis. Satisfactory comparisons have been made between these devices and the standard peak flow meter, (Campbell et al., 1974, Haydu et al., 1976 and Perks et al., 1979).

Influence of Changes in Gas Composition

Expired air is warmer and more humid than inspired air, and normally contains about 5% carbon dioxide. Grenvik *et al.* (1966), calculated that a 1°C rise in temperature would increase the gas volume by 0.17% (for comparison, a 1 mm Hg change in barometric pressure makes less than 0.1% difference). The presence of carbon dioxide would reduce the signal by about 1%.

Several methods of minimizing these effects have been described.

Heated pneumotachograph heads. Heating of the pneumotachograph not only prevents condensation, but by warming the inspired air minimizes the differences between the two phases. Grenvik *et al.* (1966), Blumenfeld *et al.* (1973) and Hardt and Zywietz (1976) all consider the residual differences in a properly adjusted system to be 1.2% or less. If the flow signals are being used to generate volume records via an integrator, this discrepancy can be readily corrected for, by adjusting the instrumental baseline setting.

Rebreathing humidified warmed air. For certain techniques, the differences can be minimized by allowing the subject to rebreath air which is fully saturated with water at 37°C, from a bag which is connected to the other end of the pneumotachograph, (Jaeger and Otis, 1964 and Sackner *et al.*, 1964). This process is not very comfortable, but is sometimes used in measuring airways resistance by body plethysmography.

Spirometery. If the subject breathes into a spirometer of the kind already discussed, the expired air will be cooled due to the high thermal capacity of the device, so that the temperature effect will be minimal. Measurements made with this system are independent of gas density and viscosity but may suffer from problems of poor frequency response and noisy signals.

Bag in box systems. The subject breathes from or into bags placed within a rigid box, flow being measured by a pneumotachograph placed in an outlet of the box to the atmosphere. The system can record both phases of respiration equally well since the gas is cooled to ambient level before recording, while the actual gas monitored is room air whose viscosity and density remains constant. The system has the advantages of the spirometer, and yields a better flow signal, but again the frequency response may be impaired due to the damping effect of the volume of gas in the rigid box.

Mathematical correction. With modern computational methods, the flow signal can be corrected for these effects, but to take full advantage of the approach, the temperature and gas composition should be monitored simultaneously and the final calculations are liable to be complex.

Certain experiments require changes in inspired gas composition, such as the use of helium/oxygen for forced expiratory manoeuvres, or the washout of nitrogen from the lung using oxygen or argon/oxygen mixtures. The same correction methods may be applied, the most useful devices being the spirometer or bag in box. The worst problems will arise from the use of turbulent flow detectors where changes in both viscosity and density must be corrected for. Sodal *et al.* (1977) have described a complex computer-based calibration system to evaluate these factors.

Effects of Gas Compression

The box bag system, and to a greater extent the flow displacement body plethysmograph, suffer from impaired frequency characteristics due to gas compression. This problem is illustrated in Fig. 9, where a rigid box has two ports, inlet (A) and outlet (B), to the first of which is connected a sinusoidal air flow source, while the second leads to atmosphere. The flow oscillations recorded at (B) will lag those at (A), and at high frequencies will have a smaller amplitude. To a first approximation the system acts as a capacitance/resistance network, the capacitance being the box volume, the resistance being that of port (B) and the connected flow meter.

A correction may be made in one of two ways. If a pressure transducer is connected between the box (C) and atmosphere, it will record

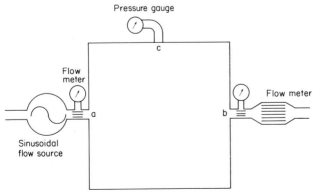

Fig. 9. System for correcting flow, as measured by box bag or body plethysmography, for gas compression.

pressure swings whose amplitude increases with frequency. If outlet port (B) were occluded, these swings would represent the adiabatic compression and rarefaction of the whole gas entering and leaving port (A), the magnitude of the swings being a function of the volume change, box size and transducer sensitivity. If the outlet port (B) is now opened, the pressure swings will decrease, and will now represent at any instant the imbalance between the volume of gas entering the box and leaving. If the time constant of the box is low (small size box and/or low resistance pneumotachograph at outlet (B)), the pressure swings will be very small as the flows recorded at (A) and (B) will be nearly in phase.

If the apparent volume changes at (B) are obtained by electronic integration of the flow signal, the record can be corrected by adding an appropriate proportion of the pressure signal from within the chamber (C). In practice the integrated flows from A and B are compared on the two axes of an oscilloscope and the resultant loop is flattened by tuning in the pressure signal. This pressure correction technique is used in body plethysmography (Ingram and Schilder, 1966; Grimby et al., 1968); for a detailed discussion see Woestijne and Bouhuys (1969). It can give a flat response and phase synchrony up to at least 8 Hz.

A similar approach comes from the realization that the pressure measured between the box and atmosphere is equivalent to the driving head across the pneumotachograph at outlet (B), so that the profiles of the two signals are essentially identical if the flow meter is operating over a linear range. Pressure itself need not be measured at all, and the flow signal be substituted for it in the "tuning" process just described. Bargeton and Barres (1969) have considered this process in detail, but Stanescu et al., (1972) found it less satisfactory than separate pressure correction, possibly because their plethysmograph used a capillary rather than a screen pneumotachograph.

In practice, these corrections can easily be applied electronically to the body plethysmograph or bag in box, and even, if necessary, to a spirometer. The second method, using the flow signal itself, can be applied to data already stored on magnetic tape if the appropriate "tuning" factor is known.

Steady State Calibration

Volume Change With Time

This is the primary method where flow is estimated from the volume of gas passing through the system is a known time. The collection can be a

Douglas bag, whose volume is measured subsequently, or a direct recording spirometer such as a Tissot of 100 l capacity or more. To produce very small flows, a gas cylinder may be adequate, but normally a domestic vacuum cleaner with a blower attachment is recommended. The speed can be varied using a large variable voltage transformer, though at low rates an appreciable time must be allowed for the blower motor to reach a steady speed. The gas flow is likely to be very turbulent, particularly at high rates, and this can be smoothed by passing air first into a reservoir such as a large empty oil can, and then through a partly occluded respiratory tap; the can and tap together acting as a capacitance resistance system to help smooth the flow. The transducer output may still be very noisy at high flow rates, and can be damped electronically to give a steady reading; it should be monitored continuously throughout gas collection to ensure the flow rate remains steady.

Rotameter

A rotameter is a variable aperture device by Linford (1961, pp. 235–256), consisting of a vertical tube whose bore increases steadily from bottom to top, containing a float (Fig. 10). If air flows through the tube

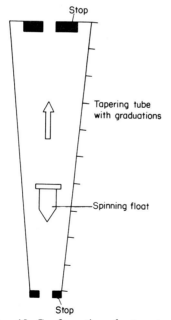

Stop

Tapering tube
with graduations

Spinning float

Stop

FIG. 10. Configuration of rotameter.

from the base, the float rises and begins spinning, (this latter effect stabilizes the reading and in fact accounts for the name rotameter). As the flow rate increases, the float rises up the tube, and in so doing allows more space round it for the air to escape because of the taper in the tube. Flow is measured from the position of the float, taking as a reference level the top rim, and comparing this to graduations on the tube itself, or a separate scale. The range of flows which can be read on any one instrument is normally one to ten, hence to cover the range of 1 to 1000 l min^{-1} three different tubes would be required with limits of 1–10, 10–100 and 100–1000 l min^{-1}. However, the range of any device is a product not only of tube size but also of float size and mass, gas density and viscosity. The usefulness of any tube can therefore be extended by changing the float type, (which will have the same diameter but will have a different shape and mass), so that a system reading from 10–100 l min^{-1} might be converted to read from 30–300 l min^{-1}. For most purposes, the gas measured will be air, but it should be noted that if, for example, pure oxygen is used, the calibration will be in error, and that if the temperature changes again the observations will need to be modified. Full information is generally available of these factors, based on formulae of the kind presented by Linford, and available for each instrument from the manufacturers.

The rotameter can be used with the blower circuit described above, but this system is obviously much quicker, since a reading can be taken as soon as the float is steady. A number of precautions are necessary, the tube must be vertical with any external scale properly aligned, and stops in position at either end of the tube to prevent the float being displaced. The float should not be allowed to become dirty, or its mass will increase, and the output resistance between the top of the tube and atmosphere should be as low as possible, or the pressure in the rotameter will increase, altering its density and calibration factor.

Integration

Where flow is to be integrated electronically, the calibration technique can be augmented using this system. If a pump of known stroke is worked to and fro at various rates, the resulting flows will vary, but if the system is linear, the final estimated volumes should be the same. If the pump is mechanically driven at a known rate, the gain of the system can be estimated from the volume signal over a given time, and this method can also be used with digital analysis.

Dynamic Calibration

The step change method is very useful particularly for devices used in forced expiratory manoeuvres. Petusevsky *et al.* (1980), described an explosive decompression device, where a 4 l metal cylinder containing copper mesh to avoid adiabatic effects is charged to two atmospheres, then discharged into the instrument under test through one of four mechanical resistors. A variation on this device, tested by Glindmeyer *et al.* (1980), uses a standard cartridge of liquid carbon dioxide as a volume source. Both devices were claimed to be very reproducible, but the second is likely to be more expensive to run, and since it does not use air, will need a calibration factor for use with non-spirometric systems.

The continuous forms of dynamic calibration have all been discussed above. In summary, three stages are involved; "tuning" the differential transducer where this is used in order to maximize the common mode rejection, establishing the amplitude and phase relationships with the flow source and with other units, and where gas compression is a serious problem in box bag or body box, adding in some differential signal.

Acknowledgement

I wish to thank Mr. C. J. Mills of this Institute for considerable help in the preparation of this chapter.

References

Altman, D. G., Irwig, L. M. and Jagdish, V. (1977). *Bull. Europ. Physiopath. Resp.* **13**, 281–284.

American Thoracic Society (1979). *Amer. Rev. resp. Dis.* **119**, 831–838.

Bargeton, D. and Barres, G. (1969). *In* "International Symposium on Body Plethysomography, Nijmegen 1968" (Eds, A. B. Dubois and K. P. Woestijne), pp. 2–23. S. Kager Basel, New York.

Bentley, J. P. (1980). *Transducer Tech.* **2**, 29–34.

Blumenfeld, W., Turney, S. and Cowley, R. A. (1973). *Med. Biol. Eng.* **11**, 546–551.

Blumenfeld, W., Wilson, P. D. and Turney, S. (1974). *Med. Biol. Eng.* **12**, 621–625.

Brackenbury, J. H. (1972). *Med. Biol. Eng.* **10**, 241–252.

Bushman, J. A., Ali, A., Perry, I. R. and Williams, G. M. E. (1978). *Brit. J. Anaesth.* **50**, 551–554.

Campbell, I. A., Smith, I., Johnson, A., Prescott, R. J., Anderson, C. and Campbell, J. (1974). *Lancet* **2**, 199.

Clement, J. and Woestijne, K. P. van de (1969). *J. appl. Physiol.* **27**, 895–897.

Cobbold, R. S. C. (1974). "Transducers for Biomedical Measurements: Principles and Applications". John Wiley and Sons, Chichester and New York.

Cotes, J. E. (1979). "Lung Function, Assessment and Application in Medicine", 4th edn. Blackwell Scientific Publications, Oxford.

Cumming, G. (1966). *J. appl. Physiol.* **21**, 291–292.
DuBois, A. B., Botelho, S. Y., Bedell, G. N., Marshall, R. and Comroe, J. H. (1956). *J. clin. Invest.* **35**, 322–326.
Elliot, S. E., Shore, J. H., Barnes, C. W., Lindauer, J. and Osbourne, J. E. (1977). *J. appl. Physiol.* **42**, 456–460.
Farmer, F. G. and Portnoy, W. M. (1974). *Med. Biol. Eng.* **12**, 873–874.
Finucane, K. E., Egan, B. A. and Dawson, S. V. (1972). *J. appl. Physiol.* **32**, 121–126.
Fitzgerald, M. X., Smith, A. A. and Gaensler, E. A. (1973). *New Engl. J. Med.* **289**, 1283–1288.
Fleisch, A. (1925). *Archiv. ges. Physiol.* **209**, 713–722.
Friedman, M. and Walker, S. (1975). *Lancet* **1**, 310–311.
Fry, D. L. (1960). *Physiol. Rev.* **40**, 753–788.
Fry, D. L., Hyatt, R. E., McCall, C. B. and Mallos, A. J. (1957). *J. appl. Physiol.* **10**, 210–214.
Glindmeyer, H. W., Anderson, S. T., Kern, R. G. and Hughes, J. (1980). *Amer. Rev. respirat. Dis.* **121**, 599–603.
Grenvik, A., Hedstrand, V. and Sjogren, H. (1966). *Acta. Anaesth. Scand.* **10**, 147–155.
Grimby, G., Takishima, T., Graham, W., Macklem, P. and Mead, J. (1968). *J. clin. Invest.* **47**, 1455–1456.
Guyatt, A. R., Parker, S. P. and McBride, M. J. (1982). *Am. Rev. resp. Dis.* **126**, 434–438.
Guyatt, A. R., Siddorn, J. A., Brash, H. M. and Flenley, D. C. (1975). *J. appl. Physiol.* **39**, 341–348.
Hadorn, W. von (1942). *Schweiz. med. Wschr.* **23**, 946–950.
Hardt, H. van der and Zywietz, Ch. (1976). *Respiration* **33**, 416–424.
Haydu, S. P., Chapman, T. T. and Hughes, D. T. D. (1976). *Lancet* **2**, 1225–1226.
Humphries, T. J. and Castell, D. O. (1977). *Digest. Dis.* **22**, 641–645.
Ingram, R. H. and Schilder, D. P. (1966). *J. appl. Physiol.* **21**, 1821–1826.
Jaeger, M. J. and Otis, A. B. (1964). *J. appl. Physiol.* **19**, 813–820.
Kafer, E. R. (1973). *Anaesthesiology* **38**, 275–279.
Klinger, D. R., Harell, G. S. and Zboralski, F. F. (1977). *Invest. Radiol.* **12**, 515–519.
Lilley, J. C. (1954). In "Methods in Medical Research", Vol. 2 (Eds, J. H. Comroe *et al.*), pp. 113–121. Year Book Publishers Inc., Chicago.
Linford, A. (1961). "Flow Measurement and Meters", 2nd ed. E. and F. N. Spon Ltd., London.
Lydon, S. B., Dodds, W. J., Hogan, W. J. and Arndorfer, R. C. (1975). *Digest. Dis.* **20**, 968–970.
McCall, C. B., Hyatt, R. E., Nobel, F. W. and Fry, D. L. (1957). *J. appl. Physiol.* **10**, 215–218.
Mead, J. (1960). *J. appl. Physiol.* **15**, 736–740.
Mead, J. and Whittenberger, J. L. (1953). *J. appl. Physiol.* **5** (1952–3), 779–796.
Milic-Emili, J., Mead, J., Turner, J. M. and Glauser, E. M. (1964a). *J. appl. Physiol.* **19**, 207–211.
Milic-Emili, J., Mead, J. and Turner, J. M. (1964b). *J. appl. Physiol.* **19**, 212–216.
Osbourne, J. J. (1978). *Critical Care Med.* **6**, 349–351.
Perks, W. H., Tams, I. P., Thompson, D. A. and Prowse, K. (1979). *Thorax* **34**, 79–81.
Petusevsky, M. L., Lyons, L. D., Smith, A. A., Epler, G. R. and Gaensler, E. A. (1980). *Amer. Rev. respirat. Dis.* **121**, 343–350.

Poppius, H. and Mattson, K. (1977). *Scand. J. respirat. Dis.* **58**, 269–272.
Proulx, P. A., Harf, A., Lorino, H., Altan, G. and Laurent, D. (1979). *J. appl. Physiol.* **46**, 608–614.
Rabin, S. and Lewis, F. J. (1968). *J. appl. Physiol.* **25**, 433–438.
Reynolds, J. A. and Hyett, A. W. (1974). *J. Phys. E. Sci. Instrum.* **7**, 166–167.
Sackner, M. A., Feisal, K. A. and DuBois, A. B. (1964). *J. appl. Physiol.* **19**, 534–535.
Scheid, P. and Piiper, J. (1971). *Respirat. Physiol.* **11**, 308–314.
Schilder, D. P., Hyatt, R. E. and Fry, D. L. (1959). *J. appl. Physiol.* **14**, 1057–1058.
Silverman, L. and Whittenberger, J. L. (1954). *In* "Methods in Medical Research" (Eds, J. H. Comroe *et al.*), pp. 104–112. Year Book Publishers Inc., Chicago.
Smith, C. L. (1972). *In* "Novel Types of Transducers". IEEE Colloquium, London.
Sodal, I. E., Adamson, H. P. and Kibler, S. K. (1977). *Biomed. Sci. Instrument* **13**, 69–72.
Stanescu, D. C., Sutter, P. de and Woestijne, K. P. van de (1972). *Amer. Rev. respirat. Dis.* **105**, 304–305.
Stott, F. D. (1967). "Instruments in Clinical Medicine". Blackwell Scientific Publications, Oxford.
Trop, D., Peeters, R. and Woestijne, K. P. van de (1970). *J. appl. Physiol.* **29**, 283–287.
Turner, J. M., Mead, J. and Wohl, M. E. (1968). *J. appl. Physiol.* **25**, 664–671.
Wallin, L., Boesby, S. and Madsen, T. (1978). *Scand. J. clin. Invest.* **38**, 375–381.
West, J. B. (1960). *J. appl. Physiol.* **15**, 976–978.
Woestijne, K. P. van de and Bouhuys, A. (1969). *In* "International Symposium on Body Plethysmography, Nijmegen 1968". (Eds, A. B. DuBois and K. P. Woestijne) pp. 64–74. S. Kager Basel, New York.
Wright, B. M. (1955). *J. Physiol. Lond.* **127**, 25 p.
Wright, B. M. and McKerrow, C. B. (1959). *Brit. med. J.* **2**, 1041–1047.

C

4. RESPIRATORY GAS ANALYSIS AND BLOOD pH

Patricia M. Tweeddale

City Hospital, Edinburgh, U.K.

PHYSIOLOGY

Oxygen and carbon dioxide are transported in the blood both in simple solution and in chemical combination. The partial pressure of the gas and its solubility in blood determine the amount which is carried in solution, although reference to Table I shows that this amount is a small

TABLE I
Normal values for blood O_2, CO_2 and pH[a]

Measurement	Arterial blood	Mixed venous blood
Partial pressure O_2, mmHg (kPa)	100(13.30)	40(5.33)
O_2 saturation, %	98	73
Total O_2 content, ml per 100 ml (mmol^{-1})	20.0(8.93)	14.8(6.61)
O_2 dissolved, ml per 100 ml (mmol^{-1})	0.3(0.13)	0.1(0.05)
O_2 in the form of oxyhaemoglobin, ml per 100 ml (mmol^{-1})	19.7(8.80)	14.7(6.56)
Partial pressure CO_2, mmHg (kPa)	40(5.33)	46(6.12)
Total CO_2 content, ml per 100 ml (mmol l^{-1})	48.5(21.6)	53.0(23.6)
CO_2 dissolved, ml per 100 ml (mmol l^{-1})	2.5(1.1)	2.8(1.25)
CO_2 in the form of bicarbonate (mmol l^{-1})	(19.5)	(21.0)
CO_2 in the form of carbamino-haemoglobin (mmol l^{-1})	(1.0)	(1.4)
pH	7.40	7.38
Hydrogen ion concentration (nmol l^{-1})	40	42

[a] Values relate to a blood haemoglobin concentration of 14.8 gm per 100 ml. To convert from mmHg to kPa multiply by 0.133; to convert from ml O_2 per 100 ml blood to mmol l^{-1}: multiply by 0.449; to convert from ml CO_2 per 100 ml blood to mmol l^{-1}: multiply by 0.446.

contribution compared to that which is carried in chemical combination.

Oxygen combines with haemoglobin in the red blood cells (erythrocytes) to form oxyhaemoglobin, this being a rapid and reversible process called oxygenation. One gram of haemoglobin can combine with 1.34–1.39 ml O_2 (Hufner, 1894, Bernhart and Skeggs, 1943, Braunitzer, 1963); thus, the normal capacity of blood for oxygen is about 20 ml per 100 ml blood. If this capacity is achieved the blood is said to be fully saturated. In healthy young adults, blood passing through the lungs becomes about 98% saturated. On passage through the tissues, oxygen is released from the blood so that Po_2 and saturation fall again. The relationship between Po_2 and saturation is not linear but follows a curve which is an expression of the affinity of haemoglobin for oxygen (Fig. 1). The shape and position of the curve can alter, if it shifts to the left the affinity is said to increase, if to the right it is said to decrease. The major factors affecting the curve *in vivo* are blood pH, body temperature and the level of carbon monoxide. An increase in either acidity or temperature shifts the curve to the right and an increase in carbon monoxide concentration makes the curve more hyperbolic.

Although some CO_2 can be transported in combination with haemoglobin as carbamino-haemoglobin, this, like the contribution of dissolved CO_2, is small in comparison to CO_2 in the form of bicarbonate. The hydration of CO_2:

$$CO_2 + H_2O \rightleftharpoons H_2CO_3 \rightleftharpoons H^+ + HCO_3^-$$

is catalysed by carbonic anhydrase in the erythrocytes. CO_2 is added to

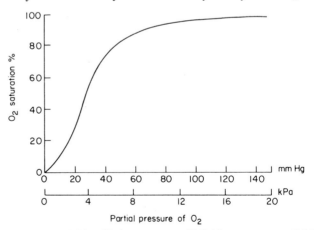

FIG. 1. Oxygen-haemoglobin affinity curve, at pH 7.40, temperature 37°C, carboxy-haemoglobin 0.

the blood as it passes through the tissues and removed as it passes through the lungs. For clinical purposes the relationship between total carbon dioxide concentration and P_{CO_2} can be considered as linear. The relative concentrations of bicarbonate and of carbonic acid in the blood determine the acidity of the blood as described by the Henderson–Hasselbalch equation which simplifies to:

$$pH = pK + \log([\text{Bicarbonate}]/[\text{Carbonic acid}])$$

where pK is the dissociation constant, bicarbonate and carbonic acid are in mmol l^{-1} and carbonic acid is taken as the product of P_{CO_2} and the solubility coefficient. Perhaps simpler to handle is a derivation of the original Henderson equation:

$$[H^+] = P_{CO_2} \times 24/[\text{Bicarbonate}]$$

where 24 incorporates the solubility of CO_2 and the dissociation constant, bicarbonate is in mmol l^{-1} and P_{CO_2} is in mmHg. Measurement of arterial P_{CO_2} and hydrogen ion concentration enables the nature of the acid-base disturbance to be determined.

The Pco in blood is very small (less than 0.1 mmHg) and therefore negligible quantities are carried in solution. Carbon monoxide can however combine with haemoglobin at the same site as O_2, forming carboxyhaemoglobin. Haemoglobin in this form cannot carry O_2. The affinity of Hb for CO is some 250 times greater than that for O_2 and therefore significant saturations can be achieved at very low Pco. The half-life of HbCO *in vivo*, when breathing air, is about 4 h. The normal HbCO level of non-smokers is about 1% (Cole, 1975) but in heavy smokers may rise to 20% which has a significant effect on blood oxygenation.

It can be seen that O_2, CO_2 and CO can be considered in terms of the partial pressure or the concentration in the blood, but additionally for O_2 and CO, in terms of haemoglobin saturation. Technical and clinical considerations come into the decision as to which measurements are actually made.

BLOOD GAS AND pH ELECTRODES

Over the past two decades electrode systems for measuring P_{O_2}, P_{CO_2} and pH have been developed to such an extent that even blood samples of 0.1 ml can be analysed with accuracy. Use of blood gas equipment has therefore become a routine part of clinical laboratory procedure.

Chapter 5 begins with a description of the principle of construction of electrodes sensitive to P_{CO_2} and P_{O_2}, to which the reader is referred.

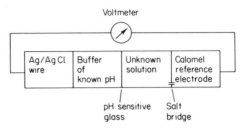

Fɪɢ. 2. Schematic diagram of a pH electrode system.

Many commercial systems expose blood samples to all three electrodes simultaneously, and some general comments on the use of combined electrode assemblies follow.

pH electrodes can take many forms but all have an area of so-called "pH-sensitive" glass at the electrode tip or in the form of a capillary tube. Blood is brought into contact with this surface. On the inner side of the pH sensitive glass, contained in the pH electrode is a buffer solution of known hydrogen ion concentration into which a silver wire is sealed. The electrode is connected by a saturated KCl salt-bridge to a reference calomel electrode. The potential developed across the glass membrane because of the difference in pH between the blood and buffer can then be measured. The system is represented schematically in Fig. 2.

Calibration of Electrodes and Quality Control

To obtain reliable results with blood gas equipment, careful attention to calibration, cleanliness and quality control are necessary. Blood gas electrodes are generally calibrated with two gas mixtures of known concentrations of O_2 and CO_2 (balance N_2). Typical concentrations would be 0% and 10% O_2 and 5% and 10% CO_2. These special mixtures can be produced by gas mixing pumps with adjustable settings or by preset mixing pumps. Mixtures using flow meters to regulate the concentrations are not accurate enough for calibration purposes. Frequently, laboratories use gas cylinders made up with the required concentrations. O_2 and CO_2 concentrations can be confirmed by Haldane analysis (see below). Alternatively, certificates of analysis can be paid for in which case it is advisable to enquire how the analyses are performed. If large cylinders are used, care must be taken to ensure that settling of the gases does not take place within the cylinder over time. Laying the cylinders on their sides helps to counteract this.*

* Free-standing gas cylinders are dangerous: they should always be adequately supported. Cylinders on their sides are also a potential hazard to feet if allowed to roll.

Since gas introduced directly from a cylinder into an electrode system thermostatically controlled at 37°C both cools and dries the membranes to an extent dependent on the flow rate of the gas, gases are usually humidified and heated and the flow rate controlled to ensure optimal and reproducible conditions for calibration. Attention must be paid to the tubing connecting cylinders and instrument to ensure that it is resistant to gaseous diffusion, e.g. neoprene. The response of the electrodes can vary both between days and within a day, for example, because of protein build-up, changes in electrolyte composition, membrane function and, in the case of Po_2 electrodes, build-up of silver ions at the cathode. Calibration must therefore be carried out at least twice in any one day. A single point check with a gas mixture near physiological levels, e.g. 12% O_2, 5% CO_2 is useful in between calibrations. Linearity of the Po_2 electrode cannot be assumed over the range 0–760 mmHg when calibration is only over the range 0–100 mmHg. This is of importance when samples are to be analysed for patients breathing high oxygen and applies particularly to older manual assemblies. In such cases, it is desirable to confirm Po_2 accuracy at high oxygen concentrations.

For calibration of pH electrodes, phosphate buffers of known pH are used. These are supplied in bottles or in small vials with values in the region of 6.840 and 7.380. Although they are buffers, contact with air or CO_2 affects the pH. Vials therefore tend to be more accurate for calibration purposes, providing they are used immediately on opening and then discarded.

Electrode systems tend to be more stable if used frequently but, equally, contamination with fat or protein deposits then becomes a more significant problem. Adequate rinsing of the electrode chamber and, if necessary, the use of special cleaning agents (as recommended by the manufacturers) are important.

Even when Po_2 and Pco_2 electrodes·are working well they can demonstrate a so-called blood gas difference., i.e. lower values are registered for blood than for a gas mixture with the same Po_2 and Pco_2 (see section on tonometry). This factor is more noticeable for Po_2 since there is a gradual build-up of silver ions at the cathode which increases the oxygen "consumption" of the electrode itself and so increases the blood gas difference. A 3–4 mmHg difference at Po_2 100 mmHg is quite common, particularly with early blood gas equipment. The difference increases the longer the Po_2 electrode is in use. Manufacturers have improved electrode performance by such means as making blood move slowly past the electrodes during analysis, using liquid calibration and by utilizing correction factors for Po_2 readings.

As membranes deteriorate and contamination builds up, so electrode response can become slow and erratic with blood even when calibration with gas and buffers seems satisfactory. Clearly some form of quality control is necessary to determine if electrode function has deteriorated to an extent that electrodes need cleaning and replacement of membranes.

Calibration errors in Po_2 and Pco_2 can be identified by the use of a third gas mixture but this is not easy with all designs of blood gas analyser. Of greater value are the gas-equilibrated buffer controls which are now available with high, normal and low levels of Po_2 and Pco_2 and acid, alkaline and normal pH. These vials are rapidly contaminated by air, the Po_2 being the most unstable and for this reason they cannot be used for more than one analysis and must be presented to the electrodes in as anaerobic a way as possible. Since electrode systems differ in design, the measured values will vary with different makes of machine. However, they are still very useful if the standard error of readings with a particular analyser is determined with one batch of buffer controls when electrodes appear to be functioning well. This gives a comparison for electrode behaviour when buffer controls are used on other occasions.

Since gas-equilibrated buffer controls have different characteristics, notably viscosity and temperature coefficients from blood, the ideal quality control system should involve the use of blood. Blood control vials are now available but have the disadvantage of expense and limited shelf-life. It is therefore advocated that tonometry of blood should become a routine part of laboratory practice to assess electrode function. The number of times that tonometry should be performed per week will obviously depend on the workload of the laboratory. For busy units daily tonometry may be necessary, for others it may be more appropriate once a week or less frequently (see p. 65).

Automated blood gas analysers are now in common use. Programming ensures that automatically the analyses are printed out, the measuring chamber is flushed out and the electrodes are regularly calibrated. There are good facilities for diagnosis and therefore correction of many technical problems. However, if these analysers are to produce accurate results, proper handling of the blood and daily supervision by trained staff, including quality control measures, are still essential.

ANALYSIS OF CO_2 AND OXYGEN IN GAS MACHINES

The Lloyd–Haldane apparatus (Haldane, 1912; Lloyd, 1958) provide a method for the determination of O_2 and CO_2 concentrations in gases, to an accuracy of 0.02%. The method is based on the change in volume of a gas sample when first the CO_2 and then the O_2 is absorbed chemically. The apparatus is largely enclosed in a water jacket into which air is bubbled to equalize the temperature. The gas burette has a capacity of 10 ml and the level of mercury, and therefore of gas, in the burette can be raised or lowered by moving the mercury reservoir appropriately (Fig. 3). At the top of the burette there is a five-way tap which can be turned to allow admission of the gas sample into the burette or disposal of residual gas, or connection of the burette with either the CO_2 or O_2 absorbing chambers. These chambers are connected to the burette by a vertical glass capillary tube, on each of which is a mark. Each time the burette is read the level of the absorbent fluids are adjusted precisely to these marks. The absorption chambers are connected to twin connected reservoirs containing atmospheric air. These chambers can be shut off to room air and the common air space in the reservoirs then provides a compensating volume when absorbent fluid levels are brought to the marks. The air in the compensatory

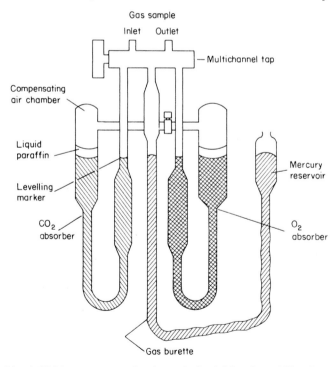

FIG. 3. Lloyd–Haldane apparatus for the analysis of CO_2, O_2 and N_2 (diagrammatic).

reservoirs is prevented from contaminating the absorbent fluids by a layer of liquid paraffin. The design of the equipment means that the volume in the burette is unaffected by changes in temperature and atmospheric pressure during an analysis.

Before making an analysis the apparatus must be filled with N_2. This is effected by drawing in a sample of room air and absorbing first the CO_2 and then the O_2 by appropriate movements of the tap and mercury reservoir. The residual N_2 in the burette is then expelled to atmosphere and the equipment is ready for use. Air samples should be analysed before any unknown gas mixture, to ensure that the apparatus is working satisfactorily. Burette readings are made with the aid of a hand lens to three decimal places. All analyses must be done in duplicate and these should agree within 0.02%. Attention to the following details is helpful:

(a) The burrette and mercury must be clean and the connecting tubing to the mercury reservoir in good condition and of a material resistant to gaseous diffusion.

(b) Absorbent fluids must be active. This can be tested by confirming that no further O_2 or CO_2 is taken up when a gas has the absorption procedure carried out a second time.

(c) The sides of the burette must be moistened frequently with acidulated water. If the burette becomes dry the volume of an air sample will apparently increase following CO_2 absorption instead of decreasing as expected, and the readings will increase steadily for a minute or two after CO_2 absorption instead of being stable.

(d) Good quality tap grease must be used on the tap which should be treated with great care so that it does not get scratched or chipped. If the seal is good the grease will look clear, there will be no air trapped and the tap will turn smoothly and easily. Grease should be applied sparingly since an excess clogs up the orifices and interferes with analysis. Too little grease allows leaks to occur. If the grease becomes contaminated with absorbent fluid, it must be changed.

(e) Care must be taken to prevent absorbents reaching the tap and running into the burette, or mercury being pushed over into the absorbent. This occurs when the mercury reservoir is lowered or raised too far or too quickly. The mercury level, when passing gas in and out of the absorbers, should be kept in the upper half of the burette but below the tap. Mercury movement can be slowed by partial clamping of the mercury tubing with a screw-clip.

TONOMETRY

Tonometry is the name given to the process of equilibrating liquid with a gas mixture of known concentration. For blood gas quality control, whole blood is used and the gas and the blood are both presented to the electrode system so that the accuracy of response to blood can be assessed. Where gas samples cannot be analyzed in the same way as blood samples, Po_2 and Pco_2 are calculated from the gas concentrations and used for comparison with the blood values.

The design of blood tonometers varies a great deal, but all aim to expose the blood over a large surface area to a continuous gas flow to bring about rapid equilibration. Glass vessels are used most commonly, these are either mechanically shaken or rotated within a water bath or thermostatically controlled chamber. Static bubble tonometers are also available. The following are points to consider in the design and use of tonometry systems.

(a) The tonometer is an appropriate size for the volumes of blood to be equilibrated.

(b) It is easy to remove and clean.

(c) The system does not bring about significant changes in the blood, e.g. frothing, haemolysis of erythrocytes or change in blood volume during equilibration. A disadvantage of bubble tonometers is that the likelihood of haemolysis is increased and an antifoam agent has to be added to the blood to prevent frothing. It has yet to be established whether the antifoam has any long-term effect on the electrodes. Condensation problems may have to be dealt with in other tonometry systems.

(d) The gas flow must be adequate and the gas warm and humidified before contact with the blood.

(e) Tonometry time is adequate to bring about complete equilibration with the gas.

(f) The temperature of blood in the tonometer is the same as the temperature of the electrode system. Blood equilibrated at a lower temperature than the measuring system, when heated anaerobically in the analyser, will show a higher Po_2 and Pco_2 than expected. Conversely, blood equilibrated at a higher temperature will, on cooling in the analyser, record lower values.

BLOOD GAS CONCENTRATIONS

Manometry

A classic reference technique is that of Van Slyke and Neill (1924).

Skilled operators can achieve results with a high degree of accuracy but, because of the skill involved and the fact that a single analysis requires ten minutes or more, this is not now in routine use. Readers are referred for detailed instructions to the description of methods by Peters and Van Slyke (1932).

The principle of operation is that the gas to be measured is extracted from a known volume of blood in an extraction chamber at low pressure. The volume of the gas is then reduced to an arbitrary level by admission of mercury from a levelling bulb. The pressure exerted by the gas on the manometer is noted. The gas is then absorbed and, after relevelling, the new pressure noted. The volume which the gas would occupy at 0°C and 760 mmHg is calculated by multiplying the pressure fall by a single factor which is a function of temperature. A correction for any gas present in the reagents and for the fall in the manometer reading caused by introduction of reagents, is determined by performing an analysis in which the blood is omitted. This correction is then subtracted from the pressure fall seen during blood analysis.

Blood oxygen, carbon dioxide and carbon monoxide concentrations can be determined in this way to an accuracy of 0.05 volumes per cent on blood samples of 0.5–2.0 ml, although considerable skill is required to achieve this. O_2 and CO_2 can be measured in the same blood sample by extracting the gases with an acidified ferricyanide and saponin solution, absorbing CO_2 with sodium hydroxide and O_2 with anthrahydroquinone beta sulphonate and sodium hyposulphite solution. CO analysis starts in the same way with extraction of gases then, with the adaptation of Sendroy and Liu (1930), the gases are passed into a Hempel pipette where O_2 and CO_2 is absorbed. The remains of the blood in the chamber are replaced with water, CO and N_2 are then returned to the chamber from the pipette and the pressure measured before and after the removal of CO with Winkler's cuprous chloride.

Attention to small details and total concentration is the secret of success with Van Slyke and Neill apparatus but, as with Haldane analysis, good lubrication of the taps is essential. The tubing must be resistant to gaseous diffusion and the manometer free of water vapour. The extraction chamber should be washed well between analyses, reagents must be fresh and the pipettes clean and accurate.

The Lloyd–Haldane and Van Slyke and Neill apparatus both contain large volumes of mercury. Technicians should be aware of the hazards of mercury poisoning. The apparatus should stand on a solid-based tray with a rim and be used under conditions of good ventilation. The mercury reservoir should be kept covered and any spillages dealt with immediately.

Techniques Involving Gas Release from Blood with Subsequent Change in the Surrounding Gas or Liquid Phase

These techniques are fairly simple to use but, since the equipment required for the different gases is so varied, the blood concentrations have to be determined separately. The accuracy of all these methods depends upon the precise measurement of the blood volume and the calibration of the analyser used.

OXYGEN

Polarography

This method depends upon the quantitative conversion of the oxyhaemoglobin in the blood sample to physically dissolved oxygen. The resulting increase in Po_2 of the lysing and releasing solution is measured and the volume of oxygen which was present in the blood is calculated from the change in Po_2, the solubility coefficient of oxygen and the volumes of solution and blood which are used.

Either standard oxygen electrode systems can be used (Hedden, 1970) or a specially constructed cell into which a Po_2 electrode is fitted (Tucker, 1967). The method of Hedden (1970) is typical in using nitrogen gas to zero the Po_2 electrode. A sample of ferricyanide solution, reduced with N_2, is then presented to the electrode and the Po_2 recorded. A further sample of reduced ferricyanide is then mixed with 0.1 ml blood in a syringe and the Po_2 of this solution measured. The calibration of the electrode is checked with air-equilibrated water. Calculation of the oxygen content of the blood is made using the change in Po_2 recorded. The reproducibility of the method is within 0.12 ml O_2 per 100 ml blood. It is dependent, however, on the maintenance of anaerobic conditions during the mixing procedure and precise ferricyanide and blood volumes.

Oxygen Content Analyser

This method depends on the electrical output of a detector comprising a cadmium anode and carbon cathode separated by a porous material soaked in potassium hydroxide. The equipment consists of a glass assembly containing distilled water and the detector unit. A gas mixture of CO, Helium and N_2 flows through the circuit. 20 μl blood is injected into the distilled water, oxygen is released from the blood and carried by the gas through the circuit to the detector. The subsequent reduction of

O_2 at the cathode surface causes an increase in electrical output which registers as a direct readout of oxygen content on the display. The analyser can be used both for gas samples and blood. Reproducibility is within 0.20 ml O_2 per 100 ml blood (Selman et al., 1975). The equipment is calibrated with air and its accuracy depends on the patency of the injection port, the rate of flow of gas through the circuit and the stability of the detector.

The techniques, described above, of measuring O_2 content are easy to learn and quick to perform. They require only small samples of blood and, providing the blood is handled properly, they given an accuracy which is adequate for clinical purposes.

CARBON DIOXIDE

Infra-Red Absorption

This technique depends upon the release of carbon dioxide from the blood sample and its subsequent measurement by infra-red analysis (Chapter 4). A basic method is described by Ortega et al. (1966) although adaptations can be made according to need and equipment available (Van Kempen and Kreuzer, 1972). CO_2-free air is bubbled through a cuvette containing a given volume of 0.1 mol CO_2-free lactic acid and an antifoam agent. The cuvette is part of a closed circuit including the infra-red analyser and a compartment containing a drying agent for the gas before it passes through the analyser. 0.25 ml blood is then injected into the cuvette, CO_2 is released and is circulated to the analyser. The final steady CO_2 reading is referred to a calibration chart determined with standard sodium bicarbonate solutions and so the CO_2 concentration of the blood sample is determined. The method should be accurate to within 0.1 mmol l^{-1}. The response of the analyser can be affected by changes in temperature and barometric pressure and also by the presence of water vapour in the gas passing through the analyser, and so the daily calibration with bicarbonate solutions is advised. Any tubing in the circuit should be resistant to CO_2 diffusion or replaced by copper tubing.

Automated Analysis

These techniques are also based on the reversibility of the hydration of CO_2. Acid is used to release CO_2 into solution. The CO_2 then diffuses across a membrane into an aqueous solution where the hydration of the CO_2 causes release of hydrogen ions. The presence of an indicator in the aqueous medium enables the concentration of CO_2 to be determined colorimetrically. This is the basis of the automated analysis systems used in many clinical chemistry departments. Typical reagents would be dilute sulphuric acid and bicarbonate buffer containing phenolphthalein. The concentration of CO_2 is related to the loss of pink colouration in the buffer. Such methods have a coefficient of variation of about 6%.

Now available is a CO_2 analyser based on the release of CO_2 from the blood by acid with its subsequent measurement by a simple gas chromatographic detector comparing the conductivity of room air and a mixture of the unknown CO_2 and room air. The equipment is easy to use and displays the answer directly. It is calibrated with bicarbonate solutions and has a coefficient of variation of 1.7% at a CO_2 concentration of 30 mmol l^{-1}.

BLOOD SATURATION FOR O_2 AND CO

O_2 Saturation Derived from PO_2, PCO_2 and pH

This applies to O_2 saturation only and makes use of standard oxygen–haemoglobin affinity curves. It is assumed that the O_2-carrying characteristics of the blood are normal and the saturation is read off the curves at the appropriate PO_2 and pH. Curves have been converted into numerical form in a blood gas calculator, which operates like a slide rule and makes calculations of saturation easy (Severinghaus, 1966). The newer blood gas analysers compute saturation from the measured blood gases and pH using similar equations to the calculator. It must be emphasized that the assumption of normal affinity of the haemoglobin for O_2 in the sample leads to misleading results in the case of patients with haemoglobinopathies or large concentrations of methaemoglobin, or more commonly, increased CO levels. However, as a general indicator, derivation of saturation is helpful.

O_2 or CO Saturation Derived from Content

In order to calculate the saturation it is necessary to have a capacity value for the sample. The capacity is the same for O_2 and CO. It can be calculated or measured directly. Where capacity is calculated, the haemoglobin concentration of the blood is multiplied by the oxygen combining power (Braunitzer, 1963) of haemoglobin. The content expressed as a percentage of the capacity gives the saturation. Where capacity is to be measured directly, blood is usually equilibrated with room air. Although Po_2 levels of 300–400 mmHg are required to ensure total saturation, the Po_2 of 140–150 mmHg present in room air is adequate to produce 99% saturation, and this is sufficiently near for clinical purposes. The O_2 content of the sample is then measured by the normal technique. The value so obtained includes O_2 in simple solution (approximately 0.45 ml O_2 per 100 ml blood) which must be subtracted from it, leaving the actual capacity. The higher the O_2 concentration above air value which is used to achieve saturation, the more significant the contribution of O_2 in simple solution to the O_2 content of the sample. The capacity of the sample can also be determined by equilibrating it with pure CO and then measuring the CO concentration. Although this is an efficient method, it has the disadvantage of utilizing a toxic gas.

Optical Methods of Measuring Saturation

These methods depend on the difference in spectral absorption between different haemoglobin species. They have the advantage of assessing saturation directly, so that no correction has to be made for O_2 in simple solution. Values are, however, affected by the presence of abnormal haemoglobin derivatives or other light absorbing substances. To allow absorbance readings to be made, blood usually has to be diluted and often lysed as well. In the case of measurements, contamination of the sample with oxygen from the diluent is a possibility, as is also the change from one haemoglobin species to another during treatment.

Manual Methods

The measurement of O_2 saturation depends on the preparation of fully reduced and oxygenated samples for comparison with the unknown. Original methods utilized sodium hyposulphite as a reducing agent and pure O_2 for oxygenation. Haemolysis was achieved by freezing and thawing or by addition of saponin and dilution was carried out with ammoniated solutions. Wade *et al.* (1953) measured the absorbance of the samples at one wavelength only, Holling *et al.* (1955) at two wavelengths. Subsequent developments speeded up the procedure (Nahas, 1958; Venel *et al.*, 1960) but also showed that reading at one wavelength only led to inaccuracies. In those methods utilizing reducing agents there is some question as to the validity of using this chemically altered haemoglobin molecule for zero saturation instead of haemoglobin physiologically reduced with nitrogen.

The measurement of CO saturation is carried out following dilution of the blood with ammonia solution and reading at four wavelengths. The technique of Commins and Lawther (1965) required that half the blood sample was oxygenated for comparison with the unknown, which made the procedure time consuming. However, a later modification of Small *et al.* (1971) and utilizing a more stable spectrophotometer removed this necessity, making the method more acceptable.

The major problem with these techniques is the spectrophotometer used. Accuracy is markedly reduced if there is machine variation in absorbance readings or drift in wavelength calibration. Small *et al.* (1971) showed that a drift of 0.15 nm in wavelength caused a shift in CO saturation of 0.14%. In addition, cleanliness of cuvettes and the maintenance of constant temperature during analysis are essential.

Purpose Designed Equipment

Oximeters for measuring O_2 saturation have been on the market for some years. They are of two sorts, reflection and transmission oximeters. Earlier models were of the reflection variety and involved treating a blood sample with diluent, placing it in a light path and measuring the quantity of reflected light. The wavelength used in the machine differed with make, as did the use of one or two wavelengths. O_2 saturation was displayed directly. The stability of these oximeters and their accuracy at low saturations was not impressive and they have largely given way to transmission oximeters. The recent models are more automated and, following injection, the blood is diluted and lysed automatically. Light is passed through the sample to a photodetector, interference filters sometimes being used to select the wavelengths, and the readings obtained at the three or four wavelengths are computed and displayed as concentration of haemoglobin, percentage O_2 and CO saturation, and methaemoglobin.

These instruments are quite stable and quick and easy to use. They are accurate over a wide range of saturations. As with the manual methods, cleanliness of the measuring cuvette is essential, the presence of small clots or air bubbles interfering with the results. Accuracy over time also depends on the lamp intensity and stability of filters so periodic checks of calibration are necessary for all channels. Minor adjustments for haemoglobin concentration may be necessary more frequently.

When considering O_2 saturation in patients, there are two points to bear in mind. First, although the saturation may be high, if the haemoglobin is very low the patient can still be hypoxic. Second, if there is a high concentration of HbCO in the blood, the capacity for O_2 falls and so the O_2 content of the blood, when expressed as a percentage of measured capacity, i.e. haemoglobin available for combination with oxygen, will be higher than that expressed as a percentage of theoretical capacity, i.e. total haemoglobin. With automated oximeters, it is important to confirm which mode of expression has been used in the computation of results.

HANDLING OF BLOOD

However comprehensive the maintenance of equipment and attention to detail during analysis, the result can be ruined by bad handling of the blood. The following points are noteworthy.

(1) Of prime importance is the adequate anticoagulation of the blood. For syringe samples using liquid heparin, it is necessary only to fill the dead-space after drawing the heparin down the syringe and pushing it back out again. Excessive heparin acts like air contamination of the blood and, in addition, causes slight acidification. The weakest heparin preparation (1000 units ml^{-1}) is preferable.

(2) If any air has entered the syringe following withdrawal of the blood from the patient, as soon as possible the syringe nozzle must be pointed upwards, without shaking the blood, and the air expelled.

(3) The sample must be mixed immediately after being taken, to ensure that small clots do not form in it. Hand rotation is adequate, frothing should not be induced.

(4) The needle should be removed and replaced by a syringe cap to keep the sample under as anaerobic conditions as possible.

(5) If more than ten to fifteen minutes is to elapse before the sample is to be analysed, the sample should be put in a refrigerator at $4°C$ or in icy water. This slows down the rate of metabolism of the cells in the sample and so reduces the fall in P_{O_2}, rise in P_{CO_2} and acidity that occurs.

(6) The degree of sedimentation of erythrocytes from the plasma with time is a very variable phenomenon, and therefore mixing of the sample prior to presenting it to the machine for analysis is important.

(7) The blood at the tip of the syringe must be discarded before analysis since this is contaminated with air. This gives the chance to see if there are any clots in the sample, as well as improving accuracy. More blood than is required should be injected into the

machine (excess goes to waste line) so that the blood in contact with the electrodes is representative of the main bulk in the syringe. Alternatively, for those machines sucking in the sample, the probe should be pushed right into the syringe.

(8) When blood is taken from a patient with hypothermia and put into a measuring chamber at 37°C, the gas pressures and hydrogen ion activity will increase, thus the machine values will be higher than those which exist in the patient. In the case of blood from a patient with fever, the machine values will be lower than the *in vivo* values. Temperature correction factors have been determined so that *in vivo* values can be derived (reviewed by Andritsch *et al.*, 1981). The factors have been incorporated into the blood gas calculator (Severinghaus, 1966) and are available at the press of a button for automatic blood gas analysers. Since the clinical value of correcting the blood gas measurements to the patient temperature is still under debate, hospitals adopt different practices (Hansen and Sue, 1980), but the facility for temperature correction should always be available.

References

Andritsch, R. F., Muravchick, S. and Gold, M. I. (1981). *Anesthesiology* **55**, 311–316.
Bernhart, F. W. and Skeggs, L. (1943). *J. biol. Chem.* **147**, 19–22.
Braunitzer, G. (1963). *Nova Acta Leopold* **26**, 113–125.
Cole, P. V. (1975). *Nature* **255**, 699–700.
Commins, B. T. and Lawther, P. J. (1965). *Br. J. ind. Med.* **22**, 139–143.
Haldane, J. S. (1912). *In* "Methods of Air Analysis". Griffin, London.
Hansen, J. E. and Sue, D. Y. (1980). *New Engl. J. Med.* **303**, 341.
Hedden, M. (1970). *Br. J. Anesth.* **42**, 15–18.
Holling, H. E., McDonald, I., O'Halloran, J. A. and Venner, A. (1955). *J. appl. Phys.* **8**, 249–254.
Hufner, G. (1894). *Arch. Anat. Physiol.* **1894S**, 130–176.
Lloyd, B. B. (1958). *J. Physiol. Lond.* **143**, 5–6.
Nahas, G. G. (1958). *J. appl. Physiol.* **13**, 147–152.
Ortega, F. G., Orie, S. A. M. and Tammeling, G. J. (1966). *J. appl. Physiol.* **21**, 1377–1380.
Peters, J. R. and Van Slyke, D. D. (1932). *In* "Quantitative Clinical Chemistry", Vol. II. Baillière, Tindall & Cox, London.
Selman, B. J., White, Y. S. and Tait, A. R. (1975). *Anaesthesiology* **30**, 206–212.
Sendroy, J. and Liu, S. (1930). *J. biol. Chem.* **89**, 133–152.
Severinghaus, J. W. (1966). *J. appl. Physiol.* **21**, 1108–1116.
Small, K. A., Radford, E. P., Frazer, J. M., Rodkey, F. L. and Collison, H. A. (1971). *J. appl. Physiol.* **31**, 154–160.
Tucker, V. (1967). *J. appl. Physiol.* **23**, 410–414.
Van Kempen, L. H. J. and Kreuzer, F. (1972). *In* "Alfred Benzon Symposium IV.

Oxygen affinity of Haemoglobin and red cell acid-base status". (Eds M. Rorth and R. Astrup). Munksgaard, Copenhagen.

Van Slyke, D. D. and Neill, J. M. (1924). *J. biol Chem.* **61**, 523–573.

Venel, D., Saynor, R. and Kesteven, A. B. (1960). *J. clin. Path.* **13**, 361–363.

Wade, O. L., Bishop, J. M., Cumming, G. and Donald, K. W. (1953). *Br. med. J.* **2**, 902–907.

5. BLOOD GAS ANALYSIS BY INVASIVE AND NON-INVASIVE TECHNIQUES

D. Parker and D. T. Delpy

University College Hospital, London, U.K.

Since the development of the membrane-covered polarographic oxygen electrode by Clark in 1956 and the carbon dioxide electrode by Stow (Stow *et al*., 1954) and Severinghaus (Severinghaus and Bradley, 1958), shortly afterwards *in vitro* measurement of the partial pressures of oxygen and carbon dioxide (Po_2, Pco_2) and pH of blood samples has become a routine procedure in many hospitals and biological research laboratories. More recently, the oxygen saturation (S) of blood has regained interest either as a value derived from other measured blood variables or as a measurement made directly by spectrophotometric analysis. This chapter discusses current techniques available for the measurement of the partial pressures of gases in blood by electrochemical sensors, mass spectrometry and gas chromatography as well as the measurement of blood oxygen saturation by optical techniques, and their adaptation to achieve the measurements continuously by invasive and non-invasive methods.

The principles of construction of blood gas electrodes are given here; further advice on their use in the routine analysis of blood samples in the chemical laboratory is given in Chapter 4.

The concept of the partial pressure of carbon dioxide in blood is well understood and needs no further definition. Although the measurement of blood Po_2 and oxygen saturation is also well established, some discussion of the distinction between these two variables may be useful in order to assess more clearly the relevance of these measurements in the management of the patient. In this regard, three variables need to be considered: oxygen content, oxygen saturation and Po_2.

Oxygen content (Co_2) is the volume of oxygen at standard temperature and pressure contained in 100 ml of blood and is expressed in volumes per cent. It is the sum of the volume of oxygen physically dissolved in the blood and the volume chemically combined with haemoglobin. According to the Fick principle the rate of oxygen delivery to the tissues (Vo_2) is directly proportional to the blood flow (Q) and to the difference between the oxygen content of the arterial and venous blood.

$$Vo_2 = Q \ (C_a \ o_2 - C_v \ o_2)$$

For all tissues, at a given blood flow, the total potential oxygen availability is measured by the arterial oxygen content.

Blood oxygen saturation (S) is the ratio of the amount of oxygenated haemoglobin to the total amount of haemoglobin present expressed as a percentage

$$\left(S = \frac{HbO_2}{HbO_2 + Hb} \times 100 \right).$$

Since the volume of oxygen physically dissolved in blood is relatively small, oxygen content is approximately equal to the product of haemoglobin concentration, oxygen saturation and the oxygen-carrying capacity of haemoglobin. That is, oxygen content is approximately directly proportional to S for any given haemoglobin concentration.

Po_2 of blood is that partial pressure of oxygen in equilibrium with the blood (expressed in kPa or mmHg.) The amount of oxygen physically dissolved in blood is directly related to Po_2. The tendency of oxygen to combine with haemoglobin is related to partial pressure. The rate of diffusion of oxygen from one part of the body to another is proportional to Po_2 difference between compartments. Po_2 can be related to oxygen saturation and to oxygen content by means of the oxygen haemoglobin dissociation curve. However, in the normal physiological range, Po_2 estimates oxygen content less directly than oxygen saturation. Therefore, if oxygen saturation is required it is clearly preferable to measure it directly rather than to measure Po_2 and then calculate oxygen saturation from the oxygen dissociation curve.

MEASUREMENT OF Po_2

The measurement of the Po_2 of blood is made in almost all analysers by a polarographic oxygen sensor. Such a sensor, shown in Fig. 1, consists of an electrolyte, a cathode and a reference electrode (the anode) with an external voltage source and a current meter. When the cathode (made of platinum, gold or silver) is made a few tenths of a volt negative with respect to the anode, oxygen molecules dissolved in the

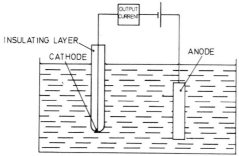

FIG. 1. Basic polarographic system for the measurement of the partial pressure of dissolved oxygen.

electrolyte are reduced at the cathode surface. This causes a current in the external circuit which is measured by the ammeter. If the voltage is made more negative, the current increases until a current limit is reached as shown in Fig. 2. This current limit (the plateau) is determined by the rate at which oxygen is supplied to the cathode by diffusion from the electrolyte. In practice, a constant applied voltage, which falls within the plateau region, is chosen so that the heights of the plateau will be proportional only to the concentration of dissolved oxygen (or Po_2).

This polarographic technique was modified by Clark for medical applications by separating the cathode, anode and electrolyte from the

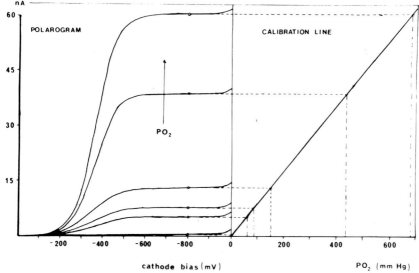

FIG. 2. Polarograms and calibration line for a polarographic oxygen electrode.

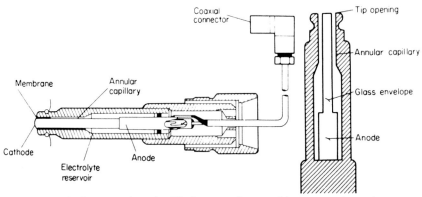

FIG. 3. Construction of a Clark type polarographic oxygen electrode.

blood sample by means of a diffusion membrane permeable to oxygen but impermeable to water, ions, proteins or blood cells. Such a sensor is shown in Fig. 3. The most commonly used membranes are teflon, polypropylene and polyethylene. All these membranes are also good electrical insulators. Generally, the cathode of a Po_2 sensor is platinum, the reference electrode is silver coated with silver chloride (Ag/AgCl) and the electrolyte solution usually contains potassium chloride together with a buffering agent. The electrolyte pH is generally about 7 although higher pH values are also used.

Theory of Electrochemical Po_2 Measurement

The electrochemistry of the reduction of oxygen at the cathode is complicated and as a consequence many reaction schemes have been suggested. The simplest and commonly used model assumes that at the cathode, the following reaction occurs:

$$O_2 + 2H_2O + 4e^- \rightarrow 4OH^-$$

These hydroxyl ions created are buffered by the electrolyte. The anode accepts negative charge from the solution and maintains a constant potential with respect to the solution. At the Ag/AgCl reference the reaction is

$$Ag \rightleftharpoons Ag^+ + e^-$$

and since the electrolyte solution contains chloride ions,

$$Ag^+ + Cl^- \rightleftharpoons AgCl$$

Thus there is a continuous flow of charge between the cathode and anode the rate of which is determined by the supply of oxygen to the

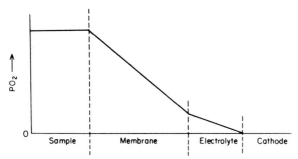

FIG. 4. P_{O_2} gradient across the sample, membrane and cathode of a working oxygen electrode.

cathode. This results in a current in the external circuit. The diffusion membrane of a P_{O_2} sensor is so chosen that the supply of oxygen to the cathode is limited only by the diffusion resistance of the membrane. Under operating conditions the reaction above ensures that the P_{O_2} at the cathode is zero. Thus, the fall in P_{O_2} between the sample and the cathode surface is as shown in Fig. 4. The sensor output current reflects the partial pressure of oxygen at the outer membrane surface and, in the case illustrated in Fig. 4, this is equal to the P_{O_2} in the bulk medium. In most practical sensors, however, this is only the case when measuring in the gas phase where the oxygen diffusion coefficient is very high. In solution, the sensor will record a P_{O_2} value slightly below the actual P_{O_2} (normally 2 to 3%) unless the sample is stirred.

In a simplified model the current output from the sensor is proportional to the number of molecules reaching the cathode in unit time. Applying the Fick Law of diffusion for a quantity of oxygen, Q, diffusing through a distance x, then

$$\frac{dQ}{dt} = -DA \frac{dc}{dx}$$

where D is the diffusion coefficient of oxygen, A is the surface area of the membrane across which Q diffuses and $\frac{dc}{dx}$ is the concentration gradient. (We assume here that A equals the surface area of the cathode. This is true only where the diameter of the cathode is large compared with the membrane thickness as is usually the case in the design of, for example, intravascular P_{O_2} electrodes.) According to Faraday's Law the current, i, produced in the reduction of oxygen is:

$$i = \frac{nF}{V} \frac{dQ}{dt}$$

where F is Faraday's constant, V is the molar volume and n is the number of electrons involved in reducing each oxygen molecule. Combining these two expression, we obtain the following expression for current,

$$i = \frac{nF}{V} A \frac{Po_2}{\frac{d_e}{P_e} + \frac{d_m}{P_m}}$$

where d_e, d_m and P_e, P_m are the electrolyte and membrane thicknesses and oxygen permeabilities, respectively. Since the permeability of oxygen in the electrolyte (P_e) is very much greater than in the diffusion membrane (P_m)

$$\frac{d_e}{P_e} << \frac{d_m}{P_m}$$

so that we can write

$$i = \frac{nF}{V} A \frac{P_m}{d_m} Po_2$$

or
$$i = \text{constant} \times Po_2$$

Oxygen cathodes are usually polarized at about -700 mV with respect to the reference electrode so that the current in this diffusion-limited region will be directly proportional to the Po_2 of the sample, as shown above.

Measurement of Blood Oxygen Saturation (S)

The oxygen saturation of blood (S) is the ratio of the amount of oxygenated haemoglobin to the total amount of haemoglobin present expressed as a percentage.

$$S = \frac{HbO_2}{HbO_2 + Hb} \times 100 = \frac{HbO_2}{C} \times 100$$

where C is the concentration of haemoglobin. Thus, when blood is fully reduced, $S = 0\%$ and when fully oxygenated $S = 100\%$.

Oxygen saturation can also be expressed in terms of the difference between the oxygen content and the physically dissolved oxygen in blood.

$$S = \frac{\text{oxygen content} - \text{dissolved oxygen}}{\text{oxygen capacity} - \text{dissolved oxygen}} \times 100$$

Since the volume of oxygen physically dissolved in blood is relatively small (at $20°C$, 0.70 ml oxygen is dissolved in every 100 ml of blood) oxygen content is approximately equal to the product of oxygen saturation and the oxygen capacity of the blood. That is, oxygen content is approximately equal to the product of oxygen saturation, haemoglobin concentration and the oxygen-carrying capacity of haemoglobin. Therefore, for any given haemoglobin concentration, content can be regarded as directly proportional to oxygen saturation.

Theory of Oxygen Saturation Measurement

When light passes through a solution in a test cell, some of the light is absorbed by the solution. The intensity of the emergent light depends on several factors, including the length of the cell, the concentration of the substance in solution and the wavelength of the light.

According to the Lambert–Beer Law:

$$I_t = I_0 e^{-Ecd}$$

where I_t is the intensity of the light after transmission through the cell, I_0 is the intensity of the light impinging on the cell, e is the base of natural logarithm, c is the concentration of the substance in solution, d is the length of the cell. E is a proportionality constant known as the extinction coefficient. It varies as a function of the substance and the wavelength of the light. Its dimensions depend on the units selected for the concentration; if c is not mol l^{-1}, then E is the molar extinction coefficient.

The term Ecd is called the absorbance or optical density, D, of the solution. Therefore, for a given cell length and for a light of a particular wavelength, the absorbance is a function of the (molar) concentration c, of the substance in solution. The concentration of a coloured substance in a solution may be determined by measurements, made at a given wavelength, of either the absorbance or the amount of light transmitted through the solution.

The absorbance or optical density, D, can be expressed as:

$$D = Ecd = 2.303 \log \left(\frac{I_o}{I_t} \right)$$

The measurement of blood oxygen saturation is achieved by the use of transmission or reflection oximeters. Oximeters measure absorbances by detecting the light transmitted through or reflected from a layer of blood at known wavelengths. These spectrophotometric methods for measuring oxygen saturation are based on the difference in light absorption between haemoglobin and oxyhaemoglobin. At 650 nm (Fig. 5) there is a large difference in optical absorption between

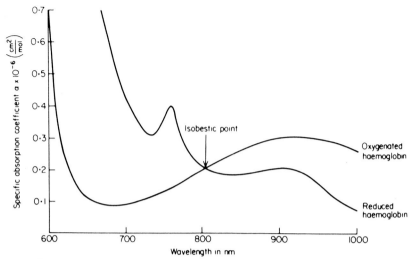

FIG. 5. Absorption curves for oxygenated and reduced haemoglobin.

reduced haemoglobin and oxyhaemoglobin. In the near infra-red region of the spectrum, at 805 nm, the optical absorption of fully reduced haemoglobin and fully oxygenated haemoglobin are equal. Such a wavelength is called an isobestic point. Hence, a measurement at this wavelength gives the total amount of haemoglobin present, and the difference between the measurements at 650 nm and 805 nm is an index of the oxygen saturation of the blood. There are, in fact, several of these isobestic points and their existence is vital to the principle of operation of oximeters.

Thus the oxygen saturation of haemoglobin

$$S = a\frac{D^{650}}{D^{805}} - b$$

where a and b are constants, and D is the absorbance at the wavelengths indicated.

MEASUREMENT OF P_{CO_2}

P_{CO_2} is most commonly measured by the Stow–Severinghaus technique. Stow first conceived the possibility of determining the partial pressure of CO_2 in either liquids or gases by measuring the pH of a thin film of distilled water separated from the sample by a thin rubber membrane. Rubber is freely permeable to CO_2, but not to water, H^+ or HCO_3^-. Severinghaus improved the sensitivity of these sensors by replacing the distilled water by a bicarbonate solution.

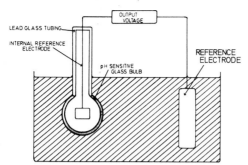

FIG. 6. The principles of measurement of carbon dioxide in solution.

The P_{CO_2} sensor is, in effect, a glass pH electrode covered by a membrane permeable to carbon dioxide molecules, with a bicarbonate layer placed between the pH electrode and the membrane. Such a sensor is shown schematically in Fig. 6. CO_2 molecules diffuse through the membrane into the bicarbonate solution thus changing its pH. This change in pH is measured as a change in voltage between the pH electrode and the Ag/AgCl reference electrode. The P_{CO_2} sensor is an equilibrium device (no CO_2 is consumed during measurement) and to minimize the time taken by the sensor to reach a new equilibrium, the layer of bicarbonate between pH glass and membrane is kept very thin.

Theory of Electrochemical P_{CO_2} Measurement

When CO_2 molecules diffuse through the membrane to equilibrate with the electrolyte, carbonic acid is formed and a second reaction can take place which results in the formation of hydrogen ions (H^+) and bicarbonate ions (HCO_3^-):

$$CO_2 + H_2O \underset{}{\overset{K_1}{\rightleftharpoons}} H_2CO_3 \underset{}{\overset{K_2}{\rightleftharpoons}} H^+ + HCO_3^-$$

K_1, K_2 are equilibrium constants.

The equilibrium between carbonic acid and bicarbonate can be expressed as

$$K_2 = \frac{[H^+][HCO_3^-]}{[H_2CO_3]}$$

therefore

$$[H^+] = K_2 \frac{[H_2CO_3]}{[HCO_3^-]}$$

Because P_{CO_2} is in equilibrium with carbonic acid concentration

$$[H_2CO_3] = \alpha\, P_{CO_2}$$

where α is the solubility coefficient of CO_2. Therefore,

$$[H^+] = K_2 \frac{\alpha \, Pco_2}{[HCO_3^-]}$$

Since pH is the negative logarithm (base 10) of the hydrogen ion concentration

$$pH = -Log \, [H^+] = \log \frac{1}{[H^+]}$$

Thus by taking logarithms of both sides, the Henderson–Hasselbalch equation is derived

$$pH = pK_2 + \log \frac{[HCO_3^-]}{\alpha \, Pco_2}$$

(pK_2 is the negative logarithm (base 10) of the dissociation constant). This can be rewritten as:

$$pH = pK_2 + \log \, [HCO_3^-] - \log \alpha - \log Pco_2$$

therefore $pH = \text{constant} + \log \, [HCO_3^-] - \log Pco_2$

Since the electrolyte of the Pco_2 sensor already has a large concentration of bicarbonate ions, the increase in this concentration due to the dissociation of carbonic acid can be neglected. Thus $\log \, [HCO_3^-]$ can be regarded as a constant.

The relationship between the measured pH and Pco_2 can therefore be written as:

$$pH = \text{constant} - \log Pco_2$$

i.e. the output voltage measured between the glass pH and reference electrode is proportional to the negative logarithm of the Pco_2 of the sample.

A plot of pH (or voltage output) against $\log Pco_2$ will give a straight line and the sensitivity of a Pco_2 sensor is defined as the slope of this line.

$$\text{Therefore, Sensitivity} = \frac{\Delta \, pH}{\Delta \log Pco_2}$$

If the concentration of the sodium bicarbonate is between 0.001 and 0.1 mol l^{-1}, the sensitivity will have values close to -1.00. Thus, a ten-fold increase in Pco_2 will result in a change in pH of one pH unit in the thin bicarbonate layer. Under these conditions, an ideal glass pH electrode will give a change in output of 61.5 millivolts at 37°C.

CONTINUOUS MEASUREMENT OF BLOOD GASES

The impetus for the development of continuous blood gas measurements has been the need to monitor arterial gas levels in new-born infants suffering from respiratory distress. The reasons for measuring arterial Po_2 in the new-born relate to the frequent need to administer oxygen to these infants and to the particular phenomenon that a high arterial Po_2 can, in preterm infants, be followed by retrolental fibroplasia and blindness. Low P_ao_2, on the other hand, may be fatal or cause permanent brain damage. The effects of arterial oxygen and carbon dioxide on the brain and its blood flow are also important. Respiratory illnesses, usually accompanied by cerebral haemorrhage or infarction are the commonest causes of early neonatal death in infants born in this country. Recent evidence points strongly to the conclusion that rupture of vessels in the germinal layer can happen as a consequence of fluctuations in cerebral blood flow, caused partly or largely by alterations in the level of oxygen and carbon dioxide in the blood.

Because respiratory illnesses are so common and because of the profound effects on the brain of abnormalities of arterial oxygen and carbon dioxide levels, neonatal paediatricians have been seeking ways of measuring and controlling the amount of oxygen and carbon dioxide in the blood. For many years the only way of measuring arterial oxygen and carbon dioxide was to pass a catheter through the baby's umbilical artery and into the aorta, so that samples of blood could be taken and analysed in a blood gas analyser. Alternatively, samples were obtained through minute catheters sited in peripheral arteries—or by the repeated needling of arteries. The problem with all these methods is that they deplete the baby of blood and, more important, they only give information about how much oxygen or carbon dioxide there is in the blood at the time of sampling. It has now become clear that large variations can occur over the course of a few minutes—or even seconds. Continuous measurement of oxygen and carbon dioxide—without the need for repeated blood sampling—is clearly preferable. There are essentially two approaches to continuous blood gas measurement—invasive and non-invasive monitoring.

INVASIVE BLOOD GAS MONITORING

Po_2 and Pco_2

Both Po_2 and Pco_2 catheter-tip sensors have been developed but the continuous measurement of Po_2 has become by far the more widespread. This may partly reflect clinical need but also indicates the technical difficulties inherent in incorporating a Severinghaus Pco_2 sensor in the tip of a catheter. In this respect the potential fragility of the pH glass bulb, the very high electrical impedance of the sensor and the requirement of a two point, sterile *in vitro* calibration, have left the development of a clinically usable catheter-tip Pco_2 sensor essentially unrealized.

The most widely used catheter-tip Po_2 sensor for neonatal monitoring is shown in Fig. 7 (Parker and Soutter, 1975). The cathode is the tip of a 180 μm diameter Trimel-coated silver wire. The reference electrode is a silver cap, and the contact to the reference electrode is a Trimel-coated silver wire sealed to it with conducting epoxy resin. The silver cap is held onto the catheter with epoxy resin, while the space between the cathode and the reference electrode and the space behind are filled with epoxy resin of negligible water absorption.

The catheter is a 1.65 or 1.33 mm diameter (5F) or (4F) polyvinyl chloride tube of bilumen cross-section. An entry port in the catheter wall enables blood samples to be drawn through one lumen for compa-

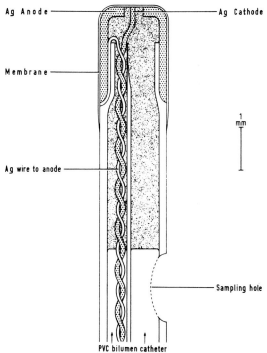

FIG. 7. Schematic diagram of a catheter tip oxygen electrode (G. D. Searle Ltd.).

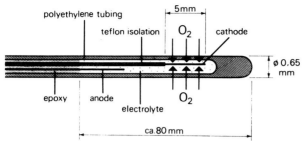

FIG. 8. Cross-section of an intravascular Po_2 sensor (Hoffman La Roche Ltd.).

rative Po_2 analysis as well as Pco_2, pH measurements and other studies. The second lumen carries the cathode and reference electrode connecting wires.

After shaping the tip, it is dipped in a mainly KCl electrolyte (Po_2 electrolyte, Instrumentation Laboratories) and hot-air dried. The tip is then dipped in a solution of rubber modified polystyrene in toluene and left to dry in air. At this stage the sensor is completely dry and inactive and in this condition has a long shelf life. The sensor is sterilized by gamma-irradiation at a dose of 2.5×10^6 rad.

These catheter-tip sensors are introduced into the aorta of the newborn baby via an umbilical artery. A solution of sodium bicarbonate, dextrose and heparin is infused through the catheter at about 65 ml per kg per day. On contact with blood, water vapour diffuses through the diffusion membrane, dissolves the KCl crystals and a conventional polarographic Po_2 sensor is formed. The time taken for the output current to stabilize can vary from 10 to 45 minutes. The zero current of the sensor is assumed to be negligible so that the device can be calibrated against an arterial blood sample. The response time of these sensors varies depending on the membrane thickness but typically is in the range 20–50 s (for a 95% change).

A more conventional catheter-tip Po_2 sensor has been developed in which the electrolyte is incorporated in the form of a gel (Eberhard, 1975). This device is shown in Fig. 8. In this case, the polyethylene catheter wall is used as the diffusion membrane.

An alternative structure for a polarographic Po_2 sensor is the monopolar device in which the cathode is covered with a hydrophilic diffusion membrane and the anode is placed on the opposite side of the membrane—usually on the skin (Fig.9). The advantage of this approach is the small physical size which is achievable because of the simplified construction. Monopolar sensors as small as 0.3 mm diameter have been reported for insertion in the radial artery of critically ill patients (Watanabe, 1973).

D

Monopolar Catheter-Tip PO_2 Electrode

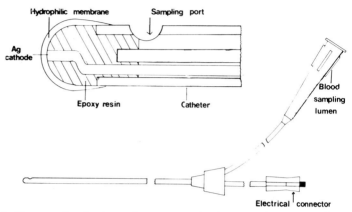

FIG. 9. Constructional scheme for a monopolar intravascular oxygen electrode.

Continuous monitoring of Po_2 in the newborn is particularly useful during periods of short-term clinically significant changes of oxygenation which may go unnoticed in the time between blood sample analyses. Such a situation is shown in Fig. 10. The recording shows that the baby was initially able to maintain an adequate P_aO_2 of 50 mmHg while breathing spontaneously in pure oxygen. The baby's condition then deteriorated and he became restless and began to gasp eventually becoming apnoeic. The catheter-tip sensor enabled continuous monitoring of the P_aO_2 so that ventilation could be commenced before the baby was seriously compromised. Mechanical ventilation was associated with an immediate improvement of the baby's condition as reflected by the dramatic increase in P_aO_2 shown by the sensor. Adjustments of the fractional concentration of oxygen in the inspired gas were then necessary to keep P_aO_2 below the level likely to cause retrolental fibroplasia. Finally, the recording shows a second dramatic fall in P_aO_2 when the baby's endotracheal tube was aspirated, a simple nursing procedure necessary at regular intervals during mechanical ventilation.

A catheter-tip sensor has been reported (Coon et al., 1976) which measures Pco_2 and pH simultaneously in vivo. The sensor consists of a PdO (palladium oxide) hydrogen ion-sensitive electrode and an Ag/AgCl reference electrode surrounded by a thin layer of bicarbonate solution and enclosed with a gas-permeable silicone polycarbonate copolymer membrane, the tip of which is pH sensitive. For Pco_2 measurement, the Severinghaus technique is used with the PdO surface being used to detect the change in the pH of the bicarbonate solution.

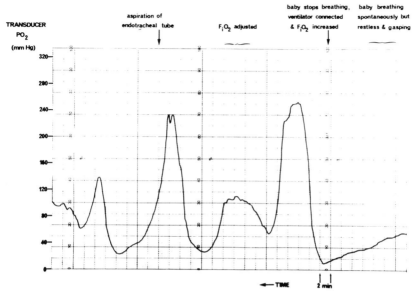

FIG. 10. P_aO_2 recorded in a neonate using an intravascular oxygen electrode (G. D. Searle Ltd.). P_aO_2 decreases as the infant becomes distressed and eventually stops breathing. Resuscitation by mechanical ventilation and increase in inspired oxygen concentration (F_iO_2) brings about an increase in P_aO_2 which can then be quickly restored to a suitable level by observation of the transducer output.

For pH measurement, an additional reference electrode outside the sensor but in contact with the blood is required. The measured voltage potential between the Pd/PdO wire and the external reference is a linear function of the pH of the solution.

The pH-sensitive membrane is made up of copolymer elastomers containing about 60% polysiloxane and 40% poly (bis-phenol-A) carbonate. A mobile H^+ "carrier", p-octadecyloxy-m-chlorophenylhydrazone $meso$-oxalonitrile (OCPH), is added to provide the H^+ selectivity. These catheter-tip Pco_2 sensors are commercially available* and are approximately 0.6 mm in diameter.

Blood Oxygen Saturation

Continuous measurement of blood oxygen saturation has been achieved by the use of light-conducting plastic fibres incorporated into a bilumen catheter for insertion in a vein or artery. These measurements are made by reflection spectrophotometry in which blood flowing past

* Biochem International, Wauwatosa, Wisconsin, U.S.A.

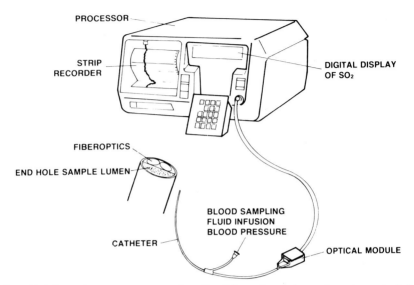

FIG. 11. The catheter tip oximeter. Details of the catheter tip can be seen on the left.

the tip of the catheter is illuminated by some of the optical fibres while the remaining fibres convey the reflected light to the measuring system.

One of the more recent *in vivo* oximeters (Wilkinson *et al.*, 1978)* has optical fibres incorporated in sterile 4F, 5F or 6F bilumen polyurethane catheters. These catheters have an end-hole lumen for blood sampling, fluid administration and pressure measurements. Custom LEDs are used as light sources. The light intensities at various wavelengths, reflected from the blood, are measured and stored a few thousand times a second. At one second intervals these measurements are processed to compute blood oxygen saturation using experimentally determined equations. Such a system is shown in Fig. 11.

The advantages of *in vivo* oximetry are its rapid response time (10 s) and stability (<0.5% saturation in 24 h).

In clinical situations where blood oxygen content is the variable of interest, the continuous measurement of oxygen saturation at a known haemoglobin concentration will give a reasonable estimate of the total amount of oxygen in blood.

NON-INVASIVE BLOOD GAS MONITORING

Although intravascular monitoring of arterial Po_2 remains an important part of new-born intensive care, catheterization of the umbilical artery

* Oximetrix Inc., Mountain View, California, U.S.A.

is not without risk. Further, this method of monitoring is available only for the first few days of life while the umbilical artery remains patent.

These are some of the reasons which have led to the advent and rapid growth of non-invasive blood gas analysis. Electrochemical sensors are now commercially available which measure the oxygen and carbon dioxide diffusing through intact skin and allow a continuous estimation to be made of arterial Po_2 and Pco_2. This method is called the transcutaneous technique.

Transcutaneous PO$_2$ Monitoring

The Po_2 at the surface of skin at normal temperature is near zero. However, if skin temperature is increased the Po_2 measured at the surface of the skin can approach the arterial value quite closely. This was demonstrated as early as 1951 when Baumberger and Goodfriend showed that when a finger was immersed in an electrolyte at 45°C, the Po_2 of the solution approached that of arterial blood. The vasodilation which accompanies this temperature increase is a crucial factor in ensuring good correlation between the skin surface Po_2 and arterial Po_2 (Huch et al., 1969).

The estimation of arterial Po_2 by the transcutaneous technique (Huch et al., 1972; Eberhard et al., 1972) relies on the correct choice of skin temperature. At this temperature, a fortuitous cancellation of errors occurs resulting in a measurement of Po_2 at the surface of the skin which reliably reflects arterial Po_2. Heating the skin causes several effects.

(1) Vasodilatation of the dermal capillaries, thereby "arterializing" the capillary blood.
(2) A rightwards shift of the oxyhaemoglobin dissociation curve, i.e. Po_2 increases at the electrode site.
(3) An increase of oxygen diffusion through the stratum corneum of the skin.

What happens is that heating causes vasodilatation, and by effect (2) above, results in a capillary Po_2 below the electrode, which is greater than arterial Po_2. However, by a judicious choice of temperature, this over-reading can be arranged to balance the reduction in Po_2 caused by tissue metabolism. Thus, on the further condition that the consumption of oxygen by the transcutaneous sensor is low, the Po_2 measured at the skin surface will reflect arterial Po_2. In new-born infants a sensor temperature of 44°C has been found to be optimal for reliable monitoring of arterial Po_2. (It is estimated that at this sensor temperature the skin itself will be about 43°C.)

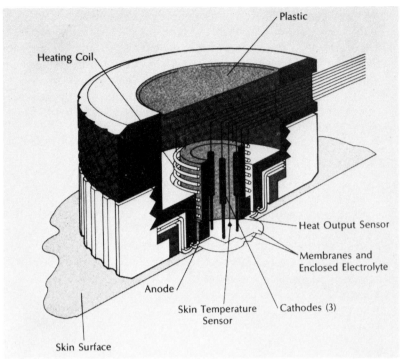

Fɪɢ. 12. Transcutaneous Po_2 electrode: schematic (Huch *et al.* (1974). Reproduced by permission.)

A transcutaneous Po_2 sensor is shown in Fig. 12. Essentially, it is a polarographic oxygen sensor of low oxygen consumption in which is incorporated an electrical heater to maintain the skin at the necessary temperature. Typically, the cathode is 20 μm diameter platinum fused in glass and surrounded by a silver anode. The electrolyte is contained by a 25 μm Teflon diffusion membrane. The current output of such a sensor at 44°C is in the range 3–4 $\times$ 10^{-9} A at a Po_2 of 150 mmHg. A thermistor is used to indicate sensor temperature and a second thermistor acts as a safety cut-out to prevent overheating of the sensor in case of a primary thermistor malfunction.

In the new-born and adult patients attachment of the transcutaneous sensor to the skin is achieved by the use of a double-sided adhesive disc similar to those employed in ECG electrodes. It is important to achieve a gas-tight seal around the circumference of the sensor. Calibration of the sensor is undertaken in air (20.9% oxygen) and the zero of the system determined by exposure of the sensor to nitrogen.

Figure 13 shows the results of a comparison of transcutaneous Po_2

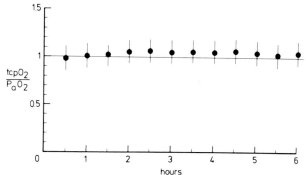

FIG. 13. Correlation between a transcutaneous (Dräger) and an intravascular (Searle) oxygen sensor over a six hour monitoring period. The measurements were made on 10 neonates of mean gestation age 33 weeks. The full line displays the standard deviation.

(tcP_{O_2}) and $P_{a}O_2$ in new-born infants over a period of six hours. tcP_{O_2} was measured with a Dräger* transcutaneous sensor and $P_{a}O_2$ with a Searle† intravascular P_{O_2} sensor. The ratio of $\dfrac{tcP_{O_2}}{P_{a}O_2}$ against time, is shown for the transcutaneous sensor calibrated *in vitro* (Pollitzer *et al.*, 1979).

In order to minimize the possibility of skin damage the monitoring period in practice is now generally limited to four hours.

Transcutaneous P_{CO_2} Monitoring

The non-invasive estimation of arterial P_{CO_2} is similarly achieved by the use of a transcutaneous P_{CO_2} sensor attached to the skin of the patient. The sensor is based on the Stow–Severinghaus principle, as described earlier, and incorporates a heater for raising the skin temperature (Fig. 14).

The transcutaneous measurement of P_{CO_2}·(tcP_{CO_2}) differs in theory from the non-invasive P_{O_2} measurement, although the measurement technique is very similar. In the case of tcP_{CO_2} measurement, there is no balance-of-errors equation. In this case, heating the sensor has the following effects on the tcP_{CO_2} readings:

(1) Heating decreases the solubility of CO_2 thus increasing P_{CO_2}.
(2) It will increase metabolism of tissue beneath the sensor site and cause an increase in CO_2 production.
(3) Heating increases the diffusion of CO_2 through the stratum corneum.

* Manufacturer: Dräger GmBH, Lubeck, W. Germany.
† Manufacturer: G. D. Searle and Co. Ltd., High Wycombe, Bucks., England.

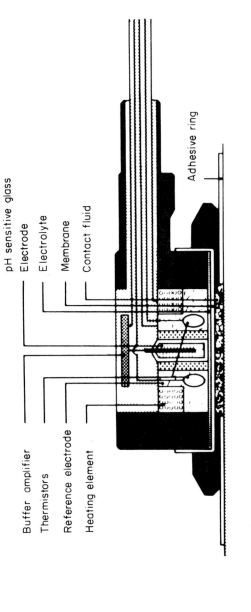

pH sensitive glass

Electrode

Electrolyte

Membrane

Contact fluid

Buffer amplifier

Thermistors

Reference electrode

Heating element

Adhesive ring

lcm

FIG. 14. The cross-section of a transcutaneous CO_2 sensor (Hoffman La Roche Ltd.).

All these effects give positive errors and since the P_{CO_2} sensor does not consume gas the tcP_{CO_2} measurement at the skin surface will be higher than arterial P_{CO_2}. tcP_{CO_2} measurements in the new-born infant are made at 44°C, as is the case with oxygen monitoring.

The relationship between tcP_{CO_2} measured at a sensor temperature of 44°C and arterial P_{CO_2} (P_aCO_2) can be expressed as

$$tcP_{CO_2} = mP_aCO_2 + c.$$

Many differing values have been reported for m and c, but the values reported by Eberhard of $m = 1.22$ and $c = 6.6$ appear to have gained general acceptance (Eberhard and Schäfer, 1981). However, it is likely that the relationship above is dependent on the temperature profile in the skin and may therefore be dependent on the geometry of the particular sensor.

A combined tcP_{O_2}/P_{CO_2} sensor has been developed (Parker *et al.*, 1979), which is capable of measuring both gases at the surface of the skin. The single sensor is essentially a tcP_{CO_2} device with a cathode incorporated in it to measure P_{O_2}. Since the current output of a tcP_{O_2} sensor is necessarily small, the production of hydroxyl ions by the cathode is small resulting in a correspondingly small change in the pH of the electrolyte. The sensor thus uses a common electrolyte for both P_{O_2} and P_{CO_2} measurement in addition to a common diffusion membrane and anode. The sensor is shown in Fig. 15. The main advantages

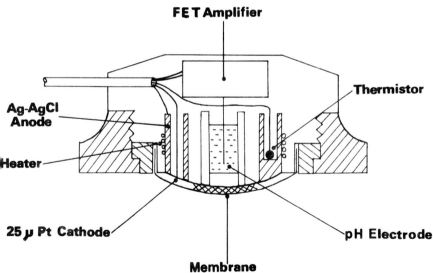

FIG. 15. Schematic diagram of a combined O_2/CO_2 transcutaneous sensor.

of this sensor are its convenience of use, potentially lower cost and the minimizing of skin damage by monitoring on a single skin site.

Clinical Experience with Transcutaneous Monitoring

Continuous $tcPo_2$ measurements as an estimation of arterial Po_2 have been found to be generally satisfactory at a sensor temperature of 44°C in the case of healthy and sick new-born infants (Huch *et al.*, 1974; Le Souëf *et al.*, 1978). Good correlation is obtained on condition that the infants are not in shock and that the core temperature is not low. In the case of $tcPco_2$ monitoring, clinical experience with these devices has been much more limited but again indications are that at 44°C the correlation with P_aco_2 in the new-born infant follows the relationship described earlier. In both cases, clinical practice now limits the monitoring period 4 h to minimize the possibility of skin damage.

In adult monitoring, $tcPo_2$ has generally not been found to reflect P_ao_2 reliably even at a sensor temperature of 45°C. This may be attributed to the greater skin thickness requiring an intolerably high sensor temperature to offset the greater effect of metabolism. However, it has been suggested that $tcPo_2$ accurately represents tissue oxygen delivery during shock and is thus a useful indicator of peripheral perfusion (Tremper *et al.*, 1981). It may well be that with further clinical experience, $tcPo_2$ measurements in the adult may be found to be more useful as a measurement of some intrinsic importance rather than as an estimation of arterial Po_2.

Continuous $tcPco_2$ measurements are currently undergoing similar assessment.

Results in neonates and adults (Eberhard *et al.*, 1980) have confirmed that at a sensor temperature of 44°C $tcPco_2$ values were higher than P_aco_2. The regression line was shown to be described by:

$$tcPco_2 = m\ P_aco_2 + C$$

where   for *neonates* $m = 1.22$, $C = 6.6$ mmHg ($r = 0.958$)
        for *adults* $m = 1.30$, $C = 8.2$ mmHg ($r = 0.963$)

These results would appear to support the belief that transcutaneous Pco_2 values are likely to estimate arterial values reliably in both neonates and adults. It is also likely that the measurement will be less dependent on peripheral flow than is the case with non-invasive oxygen monitoring.

Oxygen Saturation

Blood oxygen saturation has been measured non-invasively by the use of an ear oximeter (Merrick, 1975). The ear oximeter, shown in Fig. 16, consists of a fibre-optic earprobe and associated instrumentation. The optical attenuation of light by the ear at eight selected wavelengths is measured. Transmission through the ear is a function of both saturation and skin pigmentation. There are, however, other absorbers in skin which make the determination of oxygen saturation by this technique a complex matter. These absorbers include melanin (skin pigment) and carboxyhaemoglobin (haemoglobin combined with carbon monoxide).

The oxygen saturation equation derived for the instrument uses a model of the ear based on the Beer–Lambert Law. This model assumes that the absorbers act independently and additively and that the effects of light scattering by the ear tissue can be minimized by proper source and detector geometry. The instrument measures ear transmittance at eight wavelengths 20 times a second, performs the necessary calculations and displays the results.

Arterialization of the ear is maintained by a thick film heater circuit contained in the ear proble. The heater is controlled to 41 ± 0.5°C. Calibration of the system is performed *in vitro* and need be repeated only every 24 hours.

A limitation with this technique as with transcutaneous Po_2 monitoring, is the unreliability of the measurement during shock when the perfusion of the ear is reduced. Nevertheless, the ear oximeter has

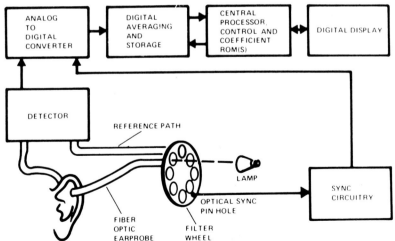

FIG. 16. Simplified block diagram of the ear oximeter (Hewlett Packard Ltd.).

proved to be useful in the care and treatment of patients with impaired lung function and during exercise studies.

BLOOD GAS ANALYSIS BY MASS SPECTROMETRY

The theory of operation of mass spectrometers is dealt with in Chapter 7, to which the interested reader is referred. The application of mass spectrometry to blood gas analysis (invasive or non-invasive) is an attractive one. The ability of the mass spectrometer to analyse quantitatively virtually any gas presented to it is its great strength. Further, the fact that the analysis is performed at a point removed from the sensor, means that this element, whether catheter or transcutaneous probe, can be greatly simplified, since it merely becomes a gas collection device. This simplification is however accompanied by more stringent requirements on the mass spectrometer inlet line design, than is the case in respiratory gas analysis.

In the measurement of blood gases, extremely small amounts of gas (typically 10^{-5} to 10^{-7} ml s^{-1}) are collected for analysis. These are then fed directly into the ion source of the mass spectrometer. Since the gas levels involved are low, the leak rate into the tubing and valving connecting the probe to the mass spectrometer must be correspondingly low. To achieve this, metal connecting cannulae are employed. In order to retain some degree of flexibility, metal tubing of relatively small diameter and wall thickness is used. Typical cannulae are two to three metres long and 0.5 to 2 mm ID. The usual material employed is annealed stainless steel. The use of such long thin connecting cannulae does lead to considerable delay times for the gas travelling along its length. Typically, a 2 m cannula will add a delay to the signal of 20 to 30 s (Delpy *et al.*, 1980). The response times of these inlet systems is also poor, mainly because of the need to have one or more valves in the inlet line to protect the vacuum system from catastrophic leaks. Most valves have an appreciable dead-space, and, this combined with the poor pumping speed along the thin cannula limits the response time in general to 5 s or more (63% response). Woldring (1970) covers many aspects of inlet line characteristics.

In vivo Analysis

Continuous *in vivo* monitoring of blood gases is extremely important in many clinical areas. Oxygen and carbon dioxide are the gases most commonly monitored, but many others e.g. nitrous oxide, halothane argon, xenon can be used to provide useful clinical data. At present, only oxygen is routinely monitored in a continuous manner using catheter tip sensors (Parker *et al.*, 1975; Eberhard *et al.*, 1975). Since the mass spectrometer can monitor all the gases of clinical interest, it would appear to be an obvious choice for this purpose. In 1966, Woldring *et al.* described the first mass spectrometer blood gas catheter, yet since that time, this type of measurement has rarely left the research laboratory. The reason for this is probably that the present designs of commercially available catheters are too stiff for routine insertion into a vein or artery.

Catheter Designs

The first reported catheter (Woldring *et al.*, 1966) consisted of a latex rubber membrane tied onto the tip of a standard polyethylene catheter. Gases diffusing through the latex membrane passed along the connecting cannula to the mass spectrometer for analysis. Unfortunately, the walls of the catheter were also gas permeable, and approximately half of the signal received came from such "leakage". In 1970, Brantigan *et al.*, reported a catheter design which consisted of a fine stainless steel tube covered with a thin silicone rubber sheath. Gases diffused through this membrane and entered the tube by means of small perforations machined into the tube near the tip. This catheter is illustrated schematically in Fig. 17. The use of the stainless steel tube eliminates wall diffusion but leads to a less flexible catheter. A similar design of catheter was later described (Brantigan *et al.*, 1972) which employed a Teflon membrane. This later catheter* had a lower gas consumption per unit area, and could therefore be used to measure gas levels in tissue. The response time was however long (>3 minutes). In a later communication (Brantigan *et al.*, 1976) a similar design of catheter was described

* Chemetron Medical Products, St. Louis, Missouri 63110, U.S.A.

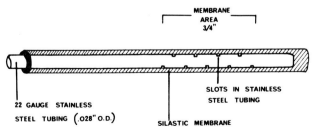

FIG. 17. Schematic diagram of a mass spectrometer blood gas catheter (Brantigan, 1970).

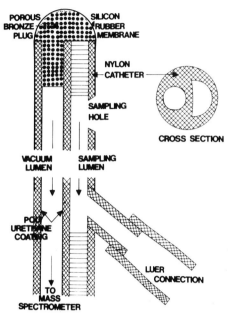

FIG. 18. Schematic diagram of a flexible bilumen mass spectrometer blood gas catheter (Delpy and Parker, 1976).

in which the perforated section of steel tube was replaced by a spiral slot. This catheter claimed a faster response time, 63% change for oxygen in 40 s and 65 s for carbon dioxide.*

In order to overcome the problem of stiffness in these catheters, several workers have described plastic based catheters, though none of these is commercially available. Wald *et al.* (1970) described the use of a nylon catheter with a silicone rubber membrane at the tip. This design was modified by Key (1975) and ourselves (Delpy and Parker, 1976) in order to reduce the problem of water vapour diffusion through the catheter walls. This was achieved by coating the inside of the catheter with polyurethane. Figure 18 is a schematic diagram of one of these catheters. This design incorporates a blood sampling lumen and a porous metallic support for the diffusion membrane. This support allows relatively thin membranes to be employed, and response times of less than seven seconds have been achieved. Figure 19 shows the output of such a catheter compared with that from a catheter tip oxygen sensor. Further designs of flexible catheters have been described by Seylaz *et al.* (1974) and Middleton *et al.* (1980).

* Sorenson Research Corp., P.O. Box 15588, Salt Lake City, Utah 84115, U.S.A.

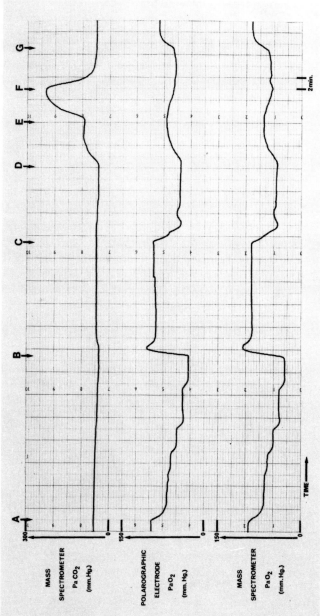

FIG. 19. Tracings obtained from a catheter tip polarographic O_2 electrode and a mass spectrometer blood gas catheter in the aorta of a rabbit. Between points A and B the inspired O_2 concentration ($F_{I}O_2$) was lowered then returned to air at point B. The $F_{I}O_2$ was again lowered at C, and extra CO_2 added at E and F. Air breathing was resumed at G.

All the catheters described are capable of being used to analyse most of the gases of clinical interest. The only gas which presents particular problems is halothane, since it can cause swelling of plastic materials. This could alter the permeability of the gas diffusion membrane on the catheter. However, Roberts *et al.* (1975) have reported that low halothane concentrations (<3%) do not significantly affect the permeability of silicone rubber for periods up to seven hours.

Transcutaneous Analysis

The theory of transcutaneous analysis has been dealt with in pp. 91–96. It is however important to note the problems associated with the application of mass spectrometry to this field. The major problem is that of low signal level. The amount of gas that can be removed from the skin by a sensor without disturbing the gas profile in the tissues is around 10^{-7} ml cm^{-2} s^{-1} (Eberhard, 1975). The collection area of a clinically useful transcutaneous sensor is typically less than 1 cm^2, therefore the signal levels available are limited. In practice, this means that even when using a steel inlet cannula to minimize background leakage the signal to background ratio is unlikely to exceed 50:1.

(i) Sensor designs

The transcutaneous probe is essentially a heated gas collection chamber, and a typical design is illustrated schematically in Fig. 20. It is essentially similar in design to that first described by ourselves in 1975 (Delpy and Parker, 1975). The probe consists of a plastic body

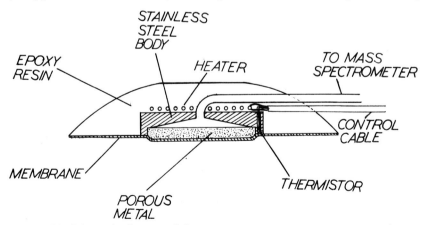

FIG. 20. Schematic diagram of the transcutaneous mass spectrometer probe.

TABLE I

Gas	Membrane response time (63%) (s)	Sensor response time (s) at end of 2.0 m long 0.5 mm diameter cannula
O_2	8	17
N_2	10	22
CO_2	12	22

enclosing an inner stainless steel chamber. The open side of the chamber has a porous metallic plug inserted which acts as a support for the gas permeable membrane. The membrane used is a high density polyethylene "Bartuff 3",* 25 μm thick. The membrane is bonded onto the probe body using a contact adhesive tape.

The inside of the vacuum chamber is tapered so as to present minimal resistance to gas flow. This is extremely important since the pumping speed at the end of the 2 m connecting cannula is low, and the chamber volume relatively high. Even with these provisions, the response time of the complete sensor/cannula assembly is considerably slower than the inherent membrane response time (see Table I). Goodwin and Makin (1980) have also described a transcutaneous sensor using a plastic moulded body.†

In clinical use these sensors have been used to monitor oxygen, carbon dioxide, nitrogen and nitrous oxide at one site. Detection of halothane transcutaneously is extremely difficult due to the low concentrations of gas diffusing through the skin. Figure 21 shows a recording obtained with a transcutaneous sensor on a neonate.

BLOOD GAS ANALYSIS BY GAS CHROMATOGRAPHY

The gas chromatograph, like the mass spectrometer, is an instrument capable of separating and analysing most of the gases of clinical interest using very small samples. Its primary disadvantage lies in the fact that it does not provide continuous analysis. Discrete samples are instead injected into the analyser at regular intervals. This may be a disadvantage in some clinical applications but gas chromatographs are considerably less costly than mass spectrometers.

The principle of operation of the gas chromatography is simple (Fig. 22). The crucial component of the analyser is the chromatograph

* Manufacturer: The American Can Co. Ltd., Greenwich, Conneticutt 06130.
† Manufactured by Cyprane Ltd., Keithley, Yorkshire.

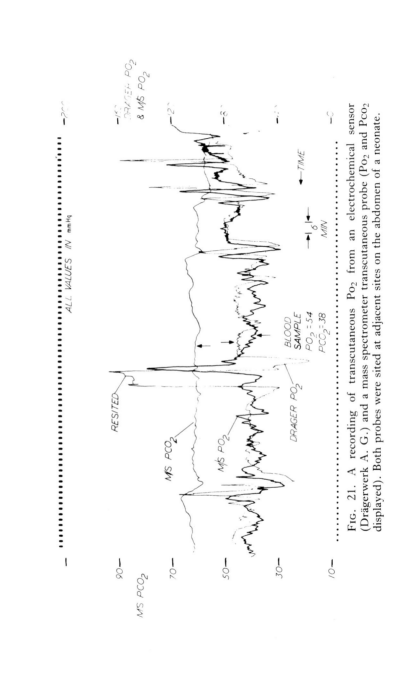

Fig. 21. A recording of transcutaneous Po₂ from an electrochemical sensor (Drägerwerk A. G.) and a mass spectrometer transcutaneous probe (Po₂ and Pco₂ displayed). Both probes were sited at adjacent sites on the abdomen of a neonate.

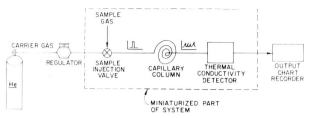

FIG. 22. Principles of operation of a gas chromatograph.

column. This consists of a length of steel or glass tubing through which a carrier gas flows at a fixed rate. Typical carrier gases are helium, hydrogen, nitrogen and argon. At the start of the column is a motorized valve which, when operated, injects a small volume of sample gas (often < 100 μL) into the carrier gas stream. The column is usually packed with a molecular sieve material (artificial zeolite) or cross linked polymer beads (Poropak). Bead sizes are usually 80–100 mesh. In certain applications a fine bore unpacked column is used; its inside wall coated with a suitable stationary phase (often a silicone fluid), which separates the component gases in the injected sample by exploiting the difference in the molecular forces between the components in the sample and the column packing or stationary phase. Gases with a high affinity for the column materials will tend to be held by these materials and therefore take longer to be flushed from the column. The result is that at the end of the column the original injected sample has been separated into a series of boli each separated by intervals of carrier gas. These are most frequently sensed by a thermal conductivity detector or katharometer. This will typically consist of a fine wire placed in the gas stream. The wire is heated by a constant current, and the voltage across it (and hence its temperature) is sensed by suitable circuitry. When one of the separated gas components passes over the wire, the difference in thermal conductivity between it and the carrier gas causes the wire temperature to alter and thus the gas is detected. The output of the chromatograph is therefore a series of pulses or "peaks" one from each component gas in the original sample. Each column has a characteristic "clearance time" for a given gas and therefore by measuring the time between sample injection and peak detection the gas can be identified. The area of the peak is proportional to the amount of the gas present. The size of gas chromatographs has decreased considerably in the last two decades (Wilhite, 1966). This has led to a reduction in sample volume size and column clearance times. The latest developments in this field are now being made by the application of microelectronic etching techniques to the production of columns and valves. Terry and

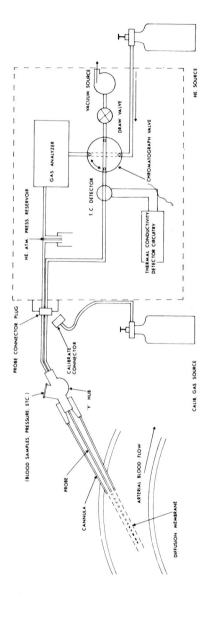

in vivo BLOOD GAS CHROMATOGRAPH SYSTEM

FIG. 23. Schematic diagram of the "Sentorr" gas chromatograph based blood gas monitor. (Ohio Medical Products Inc.).

Angell (1978) have recently reported the construction of a micro-miniature gas chromatograph etched on a single 2″ slice of silicon. This chromatograph requires a sample volume of less than 50 nl. Gas volumes of this size can be collected rapidly from blood or tissue. Such miniature chromatographs may therefore have a useful application in the future of blood gas analysis.

Invasive Blood Gas Analysis by Gas Chromatography

Gas chromatography has been used in the past for analysis of a whole range of gases dissolved in blood. This has normally been achieved by extracting the gases from a blood sample and then analysing them in the chromatograph (Hamilton, 1962).

Recently, a blood gas analysis system became available* employing a purpose designed catheter and a micro gas chromatograph (Massaro and Behrens-Tepper, 1976). The system is illustrated schematically in Fig. 23. The miniature gas chromatograph used is of conventional design, employing a thermal conductivity detector. The catheter however, employs a novel sampling system. Its tip consists of a gas collection chamber 7.5 cm long, covered by a 50 μm thick silicone rubber membrane. The membrane is supported by a spiral spring. In operation, helium is flushed through the chamber and then the flow stopped. Gas diffuses through the silicone rubber into the chamber until an equilibrium is reached with the gas partial pressures outside (this takes approximately 3½ min). The sample is then flushed out of the chamber and into the analyser. A detector senses the sample in the transport line and switches the injection valve so that only the sample enters the analysis column. By using this technique, connecting lines which are relatively permeable to gases can be used, since only the equilibrated sample enters the gas chromatograph. Since the system operates in an equilibrium mode, the gas levels measured are relatively independent of diffusion membrane permeability. Fibrin deposition on the diffusion membrane should not, within certain limits, affect the readings obtained with the catheter.

Transcutaneous Gas Analysis by Gas Chromatography

In transcutaneous monitoring, the amount of gas available for sampling is much smaller than that for *in vivo* monitoring. It is therefore not practical to employ the "equilibrium mode" of analysis described in the previous section, since the equilibration time would be excessive. We

* Sentorr: Manufacturer Ohio Medical Products, Madison, Wisconsin.

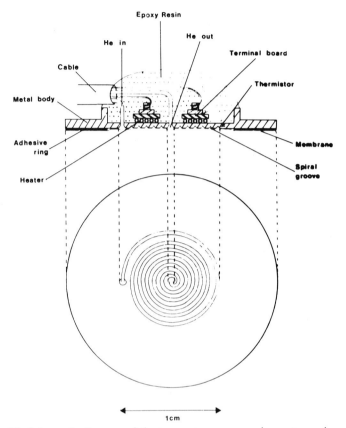

FIG. 24. Schematic diagram of the transcutaneous gas chromatograph probe.

therefore developed a transcutaneous probe in which helium carrier gas
flowed around a spiral channel machined into the probe head (Delpy *et
al.*, 1979) (Fig. 24). A diffusion membrane over the channel allows gas
to diffuse from the skin into the helium. The carrier gas is then collected
in a sample loop having a volume of 100 μl. This sample is injected into
the chromatograph at one minute intervals. In order to minimize
leakage into the carrier gas, the tubes connecting the probe head to the
chromatograph are made of stainless steel (0.25 mm OD; 0.1 mm ID).
The system produces readings for the partial pressures of O_2, CO_2, N_2,
and H_2O at one minute intervals. Oxygen channel drift is less than
0.4% per hour, and carbon dioxide less than 0.2% per hour. System
resolution on the nitrogen channel was however poor ($\sim$ 20 mmHg).

FUTURE TRENDS

Two developments still confined to the research laboratory ought to be mentioned for the sake of completeness. First, micro-electronic semiconductor manufacturing techniques are being applied to the assembly of miniature sensors. Of these, the development of ion-sensitive field effect transistors is perhaps the most advanced. Using these developments, it is possible to foresee the manufacture on a very small slice of silicon of a range of sensors for the detection of CO_2, pH, K^+, Ca^{++} etc. The second field of development is that of optical sensing techniques. These advances have been spurred by the developments in the telecommunication field of semiconductor laser diodes and detectors, together with associated glass fibre links. These developments, in conjunction with gas and ion-responsive dyes, offer exciting possibilities for clinical monitoring.

Continuous gas monitoring using transcutaneous sensors has, in the few years since its introduction, become established as a routine way of monitoring P_aO_2 in neonates. In adults, correlation with P_aO_2 is poorer. Considerable effort is, however, being made to understand the reasons for this. If these reasons can be quantified, accurate non-invasive P_aO_2 monitoring in adults may prove to be possible. However, even without this proviso, it may prove that transcutaneous O_2 and CO_2 are of themselves clinically useful indicators, especially in the assessment of tissue oxygen supply, peripheral perfusion and systemic shock.

It is apparent that continuous blood gas monitoring is a rapidly expanding field of clinical interest. In a little over a decade, instrumentation and techniques have been developed which allow these measurements to be made on a routine basis. This trend is likely to continue and accelerate in the next decade.

Acknowledgements

We would like to thank Hewlett Packard Ltd, Wokingham, U.K., Instrumentation Laboratory (UK) Ltd, Warring, U.K., Kontron Instruments Ltd, St Albans, U.K. and Oximetrix Inc., California, U.S.A. for permission to reproduce figures; also the American Academy of Pediatrics and Butterworths and Co Ltd for reproducing copyrighted material.

References

Baumberger, J. P. and Goodfriend, R. B. (1951). *Fed. Proc. Fedn. Am. Socs exp. Biol* **10**, 10–11.

Brantigan, J. W., Gott, V. L., Vestal, M. L., Ferguson, G. J. and Johnston, W. H. (1970). *J. appl. Physiol.* **28**(3), 375–377.

Brantigan, J. W., Gott, V. L. and Martz, M. N. (1972). *J. appl. Physiol.* **32**(2), 276–282.

Brantigan, J. W., Dunn, K. L. and Albo, D. (1976). *J. appl. Physiol* **40**(3), 443–446.

Clark, L. C. Jnr. (1956). *Trans. Am. Soc. Art. Int. Organs* **2**, 41.

Coon, R. L., Lai, N. C. J. and Kampine, J. P. (1976). *J. appl. Physiol.* **40**, 625–629.

Delpy, D. T. and Parker, D. (1975). *Lancet*, 1016.

Delpy, D. T. and Parker, D. (1976). *Proc. 11th Int. Conf. on Biomed. Engng.*, Ottowa, 60–61.

Delpy, D. T., Parker, D., Reynolds, E. O. R. and Wilhite, F. (1979). *In* "Continuous Transcutaneous Blood Gas Monitoring". Birth Defects: Original Articles Series, Vol. XV, No. 4, pp. 91–101. A. R. Liss, New York.

Delpy, D. T., Parker, D., Halsall, D. N., Whitehead, M. D., Pollitzer, M. J. and Reynolds, E. O. R. (1980). *In* "Fetal and Neonatal Physiological Measurements". (Ed. P. Rolfe), pp. 430–434. Academic Press, London and New York.

Eberhard, P., Hammacher, K. and Mindt, W. (1972). *Proc. Medezin-Technik 1972, Stuttgard*, 26.

Eberhard, P. (1975). *Proc. Biocapt. 75, Paris*, 57–62.

Eberhard, P. (1976). PhD. Thesis, University of Nijmegen.

Eberhard, P. and Schäfer, R. (1981). *J. Clin. Engg.* **6**, 35–39.

Goodwin, B. and Makin, R. P. (1980). *In* "Fetal and Neonatal Physiological Measurements" (Ed P. Rolfe), pp. 435–441. Academic Press, London and New York.

Hamilton, L. H. (1962). *Ann. N.Y. Acad. Sci.* **102**, 15–28.

Huch, A., Huch, R. and Lübbers, D. W. (1969). *Arch. Gynaekol.* **207**, 443–451.

Huch, R., Lübbers, D. W. and Huch, A. (1972). *Pflügers Arch. Ges. Physiol.* **337**, 185–198.

Huch, R., Lübbers, D. W. and Huch, A. (1974). *Arch. Dis. Childh.* **49**, 213–218.

Key, A. (1975). *Med. and Biol. Engng.* **13**, 583.

LeSouëf, P. N., Morgan, A. K., Soutter, L. P., Reynolds, E. O. R. and Parker, D. (1978). *Acta Anaesth. Scand., Suppl.* **68**, 91–97.

Massaro, T. A. and Behrens-Tepper, J. (1976). *Biomat., Med. Dev., Art. Org.* **4**(3 and 4), 385–396.

Merrick, E. (1975). *Proc. Biocapt. 75, Paris*, 185–190.

Middleton, P., Goodwin, B., Watt, J. W. H. and Harris, F. (1980). *In* "Recent Developments in Mass Spectrometry in Biochemistry and Medicine", Vol. 6. (Ed. Frigerio, A. and McHamish, M.) pp. 477–482.

Parker, D. and Soutter, L. P. (1975). *In* "Oxygen Measurements in Biology and Medicine". (Eds Payne, J. P. and Hill, D. W.) pp. 269–283. Butterworths.

Parker, D., Delpy, D. T. and Reynolds, E. O. R. (1979). *In* "Continuous Transcutaneous Blood Gas Monitoring". Birth Defects: Original Article Series, Vol. XV, No. 4, pp. 109–116. A. R. Liss, New York.

Pollitzer, M. J., Reynolds, E. O. R., Morgan, A. K., Soutter, L. P., Parker, D., Delpy, D. T. and Whitehead, M. D. (1979). *In* "Continuous Transcutaneous Blood Monitoring". Birth Defects: Original Article Series, Vol. XV, No. 4, pp. 295–304. A. R. Liss, New York.

Roberts, M., Cotton, E. T., Owens, G., Thomas, D. D. and Watkins, G. M. (1975). *Med. Biol. Engng.* **13**(4), 535–538.

Severinghaus, J. W. and Bradley, A. F. (1958). *J. appl. Physiol.* **30**, 515–520.

Seylaz, J., Pinard, E., Correze, J. L., Aubineau, P. F. and Mamo, H. (1974). *J. appl. Physiol.* **37**(6), 937–941.

Stow, R. W. and Randall, B. F. (1954). *Am. J. Physiol.* **179**, 678.

Terry, S. C., Angell, J. B. (1978). *In* "Theory, Design and Biomedical Applications of Solid State Chemical Sensors". (Ed. Cheung, P. W. *et al.*) pp. 207–218. CRC Press.

Tremper, K., Waxman, K., Bowman, R. and Shoemaker, W. (1980). *Crit. Care Med.* **7**, 377–381.

Wald, A., Hass, W. K., Siew, F. P. and Wood, D. H. (1970). *Med. Biol. Engng.* **8**, 111–128.

Watanabe, H. (1973). *Proc. 8th Meeting A.A.A.M.I.*

Wilhite, W. F. (1966). *J. Gas Chromat.*, Feb., 47–50.

Wilkinson, A. R., Phibbs, R. H. and Gregory, G. A. (1978). *J. Pediat.* **93**(6), 1016–1019.

Woldring, S., Owens, G. and Woolford, D. C. (1966). *Science* **153**, 885–887.

Woldring, S. (1970). *J. Assn. Advan. Med. Instr.* **4**, 43–56.

6. PHYSICAL GAS ANALYSERS

Philip Morgan

P. K. Morgan Ltd., Rainham, Kent, U.K.

THERMAL CONDUCTIVITY ANALYSERS

Helium concentrations are commonly estimated by thermal conductivity. The thermal conductive property of gases was investigated extensively in the mid-19th century in an effort to establish a relationship between molecular activity, conductivity and viscosity. In 1840, T. Andrews used a hot wire method to compare the conductivity of different gases and changes of conductivity of a gas at different temperatures. Experimental results vary a great deal, however, due to the interaction of physical properties and the practical difficulties of the available methods.

An intense interest in thermal conductivity analysis arose during the first world war in an effort to provide a reliable method to measure the purity of hydrogen gas used in balloons and as a leak detector for the flotation vessels in airships. The design of these instruments changed very little and identical devices were used 30 years later on barrage balloons during the London blitz. After the war the same instruments appeared on the Government surplus market and were used in lung function laboratories to measure concentrations of hydrogen in lung volume determinations by dilution; a rather hazardous and unreliable procedure. When helium gas became available from America in 1950 and lung volume measurement commenced in earnest, the hot wire analyser was improved and redeveloped. The modern medical katharometer thermal conductivity analyser dates from this period.

Principle

The electrical resistance of a length of wire is inversely related to the temperature, i.e. the higher the temperature of the wire, the greater the resistance. If the current through the wire is controlled then the

TABLE 1

Thermal conductivity of gases with respect to air

	At 0°C	At 100°C
Air	1.00	1.00
Argon	0.68	0.70
Carbon Dioxide	0.61	0.70
Carbon Monoxide	0.96	0.96
Helium	5.97	5.55
Hydrogen	7.15	6.90
Nitrogen	0.995	1.996
Oxygen	1.013	1.014
Water Vapour	—	0.78

temperature and resistance remain constant but dependent on the conductive properties of the ambient gas.

From Table 1 it will be seen that there are wide variations in gaseous thermal conductivity and, therefore, a wire surrounded by helium with a thermal conductivity constant of 5.97 will assume a lower temperature than it would when surrounded by air which has a conductivity constant of 1.

The sensing element of a thermal conductivity analyser may take the form of (1) a straight wire, usually platinum, or (2) a thermistor of low mass or thermal equivalent. In a flowing stream of gas the temperature of the wire will also be dependent on the flow rate of the sample. This can be minimized by mounting the detector element in a side arm of the conduit where changes of gas concentrations will be effected by diffusion (Fig. 1).

The use of the diffusion cell greatly reduces the flow sensitivity of the katharometer gas analyser but the response time is increased. Some

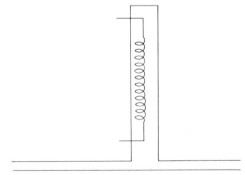

Fɪɢ. 1. Thermal conductivity analyser. Arrangement of wire in side arm.

diffusion cell instruments are fitted with a sintered glass filter to isolate the sensing element from the flowing stream, increasing the time required for full scale response still further. The design of a respiratory gas analyser must, therefore, accommodate reasonable response time with sufficient insensitivity to changes in flow rate.

A variety of cell configurations have been designed to make use of the more rapid flow through the cell to reduce flow sensitivity yet retain speed of response. A diffusion type cell where changes of sample flow rate varying between 0.5 l min^{-1} and 3 l min^{-1} have little or no effect on the reading, might require from 15–25 s for full scale deflection.

A "flow-through" cell will respond in 3–6 s. This can be a great advantage when observing dilution changes in lung volume determination. The sample pump flow rate must be stabilized and the cell protected from pressure differentials in the circuit.

It is common practice in katharometer design to make use of one sensing element for measurement and another for reference of comparison. Normally an electrical bridge circuit is used and the system balanced to zero potential difference across the bridge when the sample cell and the reference cell are exposed to the same conditions of ambient gas and flow rate.

A separate pump for the sample and reference gas is required and some means of observing and regulating the respective flow rates to eliminate the effect of differentials (see Fig. 2.)

To reduce the complexity of equipment and to construct a practical compact unit for use in lung function laboratories a double diaphragm electromagnetic pump has been used to convey both sample and reference gases at equal and constant velocity. It is advisable to present the pump output at a flow that produces the best cell clearance time commensurate with good stability and leave the operator only two controls: a zero balance and a sensitivity potentiometer (Fig. 3.)

When using helium for lung volume measurements the concentration of the gas used in the spirometer used to be kept as low as possible to maintain physiologically normal conditions and to economize on a very expensive laboratory commodity. Helium is comparatively cheap now but when originally introduced it was precious. Early instruments were calibrated with a full scale deflection of 0–0.5% He, and while this might be considered admirable for economy and natural background gas conditions it did exacerbate other interfering influences.

From the table it can be seen that all gases conduct heat to some degree and the katharometer is, therefore, a non-specific instrument which can only be calibrated for a binary change. It is a very simple device but it has this great disadvantage when used in respiratory work

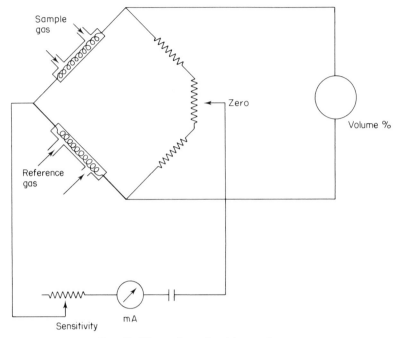

FIG. 2. Thermal conductivity analyser.

where complex mixtures naturally occur. On the other hand its sensibility to all gases identifies it as the detector to be used in gas chromatography where because of the principle involved, it is able to deal with one gas at a time as they emerge from the separating column.

When the thermal conductivity method is used for respiratory analysers steps must be taken to eliminate the effect of interfering gases. In lung volume measurements, the spirometer will contain volumes of nitrogen, oxygen, water vapour, carbon dioxide and helium. Since most measurements are made against a background of ambient oxygen concentration and oxygen is fed into the spirometer to maintain constant volume during the dilution test this interfering effect is stabilized. Carbon dioxide and water vapour can be removed by absorber tubes containing calsoda and calcium chloride and the katharometer left to deal with the relationship of air versus helium—a binary change.

The highly sensitive flow-through cell is affected by the inclusion of impurities in the balancing stream of oxygen. Thus, oxygen produced by electrolysis of water or by imperfect liquefaction techniques has inclusions of hydrogen or argon which will substantially upset the system. This problem may be overcome by plotting the mixing curve

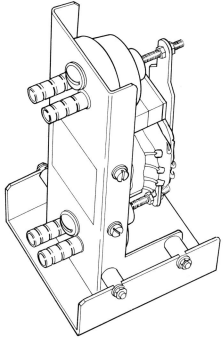

FIG. 3. Double diaphragm gas sampling pump.

during the test and extrapolation back to the axis to find the point of equilibration when mixing is complete. This is also a useful method to deal with small leaks in a gas analyser/spirometer apparatus, (see Fig. 4).

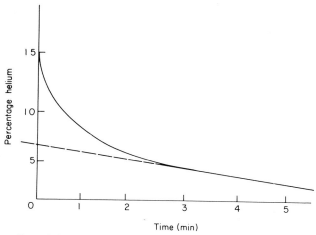

FIG. 4. Helium dilution curve in lung volume analysis.

The effect due to oxygen in the air/helium katharometer can only be ignored in lung volume determinations where the concentration of oxygen remains substantially the same throughout the test procedure. For the measurement of single breath diffusing capacity the subject inhales a mixture of 14.00% helium, 0.28% carbon monoxide, 17.80% oxygen with a balance of nitrogen. The inspired oxygen is recommended to be close to the normal alveolar oxygen level since diffusing capacity for carbon monoxide is inhibited by the mixed venous Po_2. After breath-holding, the subject exhales a mixture which may contain 14–15% oxygen. The drop in oxygen concentration will have a small effect on the helium katharometer and decrease the resulting measurement of alveolar volume.

When measurements of membrane diffusing capacity and pulmonary capillary blood volume are attempted a further measurement of single breath-diffusing capacity (transfer factor) is made with an inspired gas mixture containing 14.00% helium, 0.28% carbon monoxide with a balance of oxygen (85.72%). If the katharometer was set to zero with room air (20.8% O_2) the error at 85% O_2 would be approximately 1.8% He, which would have a serious effect on alveolar volume measurement. It is important, therefore, either to make graphical corrections for the error, or to use a katharometer with a correcting bridge potentiometer (Fig. 5).

The thermal conductivity effect on a filament bridge is not linear and

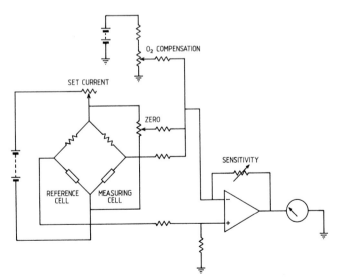

FIG. 5. Helium katharometer with oxygen compensation circuit.

it is necessary to calibrate direct reading galvanometers individually for each bridge. Alternatively, if a digital display meter is to be used then the output from the bridge to the meter should be linearized at input to the meter amplifier.

The principal disadvantages of the thermal conductivity analyser are non-specificity and slow response. It is possible to decrease the normal response time. If the sample gas is drawn into the analyser cell with a vacuum pump, and the flow into the unit restricted by a fixed orifice or a needle valve, measurements can be made at a total internal pressure of approximately 100 mmHg. This method dramatically improves the clearance time for the cell and response time of 90 ms for full scale deflection can be obtained.

When operating at low pressure, the molecular concentration of the sample gas is reduced and greater signal amplification must be used. Some instability and drift are inevitable but the analyser is able to follow breath by breath changes and measure the alveolar plateau concentration.

NON-DISPERSIVE INFRA-RED ANALYSERS
(Hill and Powell, 1965)

Radiation passing through gases and liquids is absorbed to an amount dependent on the wavelength of the energy and the characteristics of the substance. In optical gas analysers the range of radiation covers the UV and IR bandwidths.

While UV absorption is used for the analysis of some anaesthetic vapours the IR analyser is the instrument preferred for respiratory applications. All hetero-atomic gases absorb IR radiation and it is possible to prepare analysers to be quite specific for a particular gas.

Luft (1943) developed an instrument for the measurement of IR absorption in gases variations of which are widely used both in industry and medicine. From Fig. 6 it may be seen that while the absorption band for many gases is quite distinct, the overlap of CO and CO_2 is an unfortuante coincidence. The Luft principle, however, enabled this problem to be solved effectively.

The Luft detector consists of a sealed chamber fitted with quartz glass windows divided across the centre by a thin metal diaphragm. A fixed metal plate is mounted proximal to the diaphragm and electrically insulated from the body of the detector. The diaphragm and the plate thus form the two elements of a capacitor (Fig. 7). The chambers are filled at about half atmospheric pressure with the pure gas for which the analyser is to be calibrated.

E

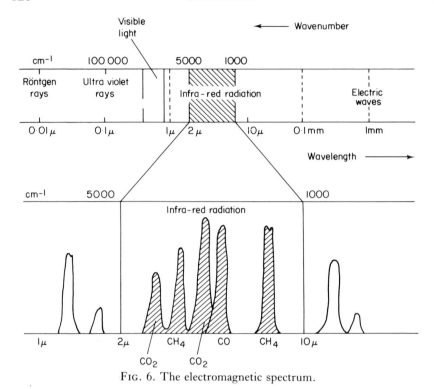

FIG. 6. The electromagnetic spectrum.

The design and manufacture of Luft detector cells is a very precise engineering science. Filling and testing requires great skill and special techniques; a well-constructed cell may be expected to remain leak-proof and sensitive for many years.

There is a wide variety of non-dispersive IR analysers in production. The most prevalent instrument found in medical laboratories employs the double beam selective detector system.

Infra-red Carbon Monoxide Meters

The carbon monoxide analyser is a good example of the use of a number of technical innovations to make the best use of this principle of measurement. Figure 8 shows how a double beam system is used to detect low concentrations of CO (0–0.3%) in the presence of water vapour, high concentrations of CO_2 (approx 5%) and oxygen.

Nitrogen and oxygen do not absorb IR radiation but water vapour and CO_2 are interfering gases and unless dealt with effectively upset the selectivity of the instrument. The IR emitter is a single element coil

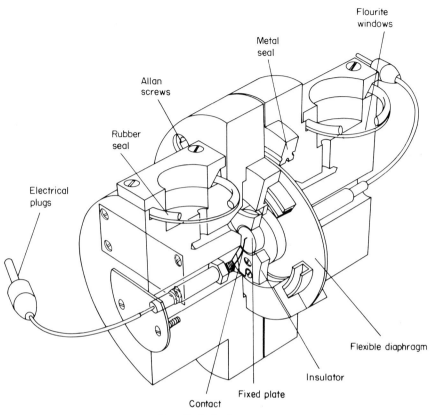

Flourite
windows

Metal
seal

Allan
screws

Rubber
seal

Electrical
plugs

Flexible diaphragm

Insulator

Fixed plate

Contact

FIG. 7. Luft detector.

fitted in a parabolic reflector sealed at the twin outlets with fluorite windows. All the cells and chambers are sealed with this material which has the property of transmitting IR radiation without substantially reducing the strength of the beam. The energy is passed alternatively through the reference chamber (usually filled with nitrogen) and the sample cells to be detected in the chamber. All the cells are highly polished on the inside and usually gold-plated to maintain maximum internal reflection and transmission. The emitter outlet windows are fitted with adjusting masks to equalize the energy falling on both valves of the detector chamber.

Since the detector chamber is filled with pure carbon monoxide the energy from the emitter is absorbed and the gas expands. The rise in pressure causes the diaphragm to distend in the direction of the cold side of the chamber thus altering the distance between the flexible

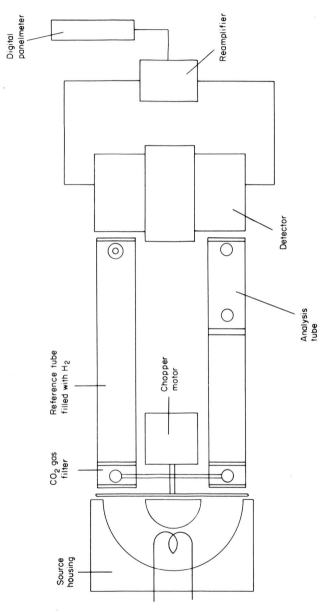

Fig. 8. Two range double beam carbon monoxide analyser designed for single breath diffusing capacity measurement.

diaphragm and the fixed plate causing a change in capacitance. A radio-frequency tuned bridge is unbalanced and an electrical signal emitted is proportional to the change.

The chopper blade running at 4–12 Hz causes the beam to be flashed alternately between the reference and the analysis tubes reversing the deflection with equal and opposite effect.

When a gas containing CO is introduced into either the short analysis cell or the longer cell, the energy on the analysis side will be absorbed prior to detection in the chamber and a one sided imbalance occurs causing a signal to appear on the meter. Optical absorption follows Beer's law which describes a hyperbola between 0 and 99% absorption. Analysers are devised to operate on the essentially linear portion of this curve between 10% and 30% absorption. The meter, therefore, may be calibrated to suit the range of the detection required, i.e. 0–0.3% CO.

To make maximum use of the meter scale for respiratory work two cells are constructed to be in the ratio 1:3 in length thus enabling the inspired mixture of the single breath test (usually 0.28% CO) to be measured in the short less-sensitive cell F and the expired mixture (usually around 0.09% CO) to be measured in the long cell E. A double changeover tap with double diaphragm sample pump is arranged to pass flushing room air through the cell not employed for measurement and the sample gas through the cell required. Range change is, therefore, effected by the changeover tap.

Because expired gas samples will contain less than 0.1% CO but also up to 5% CO_2 the slight overlap of the absorption spectrum will reduce accuracy of detection. Therefore, a gaseous filter cell in both reference and analysis beams has been fitted (C). The filter may be filled with pure CO_2 to absorb 99% of the energy in the wavelength responsible prior to arrival in the reference and analysis tubes. The analyser will then react only to CO and exclude the reaction to CO_2.

It is similarly possible to eliminate the effect of water vapour. The filter cell can be filled with a mixture of 50% carbon dioxide and 50% isobutane (which has similar absorption characteristics to water vapour). The instrument is then highly specific for very low concentrations of CO in a background of relatively high concentrations of interfering gases.

The use of the single element emitter and the parabolic reflector eliminate drift by "ageing" of the emitter. (Some instruments fitted with a pair of emitters suffered from this effect early in use, requiring frequent re-adjustment.)

Two weaknesses, however, appear in this otherwise highly successful design. The sample pump is arranged "downstream" from the analysis cells and it is, therefore, essential to calibrate and analyse at the same flow rate. The molecular concentration of the sample will be rarefied at higher velocities and result in a drop in sensitivity.

Because the effect of water vapour is eliminated from the analysis stream prior to the reference and analysing cell system it is essential to ensure that the gas is eliminated from the flushing gas distributed to the sample cell not in use. In humid atmospheres the effect can be considerable and a water vapour absorber (calcium chloride) should be fitted to the flushing gas inlet port. The interference from flushing gas water vapour is evident if a calibration gas of, say, 0.09% is set up on the sensitive range and then read on the 0–0.3% scale by switching the changeover tap. The 0.09% gas will read too high on the 0–0.3% scale due to the additional absorption of the humid air in the unutilized, but flushed, 0–0.1% analysis tube. The remedy is to ensure that the flushing gas is dry.

The response time of the IR analyser is determined by the volume of the sample cell and the modulating frequency of the chopper–detector cell combination. Medical CO analysers are involved with the measurement of concentrations of a low order and, therefore, the sample cells are generally large, having an optical length of 2–6 cms. The response time with a sample pump running at a flow rate of 500 ml min^{-1} will be around three seconds for full scale deflection. To some extent the rise time may be shortened by reduction of cell size and increase of amplification but ultimately loss of stability and the limitation of a low modulating frequency prevent further improvement.

CO$_2$ Analysers

The use of IR CO$_2$ analysers in physiology and anaesthesia has long been established and in this case the principle performs at its best. The higher concentration of the mixtures to be detected (0–10% CO$_2$) enable a different design of detector cell to be used which can be modulated by a higher chopper speed (12/20 Hz) and the volume of the sample cell can be reduced. A path length of sometimes less than 1 mm has been used with a lenticular cell shape to enhance rapid clearance. By these means the CO$_2$ analyser can be designed to achieve full scale deflection in less than 100 ms permitting the study of breath-by-breath expired air wave forms.

An electrical output to high speed recorders is always provided.

Because CO$_2$ analysers are most frequently used during anaesthesia special steps must be taken to avoid the interference due to the mixtures of gases involved. Gaseous optical filtration can be achieved by flushing the interstices of the emitter/cell detector unit with the anaesthetic mixture. A supply of flushing gas can be diverted from the anaesthesia machine and thus automatically correct as the anaesthetist adjusts his mixtures. Alternatively, high quality thin film optical filters with a narrow bandwidth in the IR range are now available and often these are used instead of gas filters for the exclusion of interference.

There remains, however, the effect of "pressure broadening" of the spectrum due to molecular interactivity in the mixtures. This has the effect of widening the spectral range over which a particular gas will absorb and, in a finely tuned instrument, reduces the gain. For accurate work this effect must be taken into account when setting up the instrument for calibration.

Luft detectors operate over the modulating frequency range 4–20 Hz which renders the system highly microphonic and precautions must be taken to reduce mechanical vibration to a minimum since this will cause the system to deflect. Excellent vibration-free mountings are available for analyser units and the problem can be effectively overcome. This feature does, however, preclude the mobile applications of interest to aviation and military medical investigations.

Solid state detectors for IR radiation have been available for many years but hitherto they have lacked the selectivity desirable for good specific performance. The improvement of thin film interference filters has enabled designers to produce satisfactory analysers with some distinct advantages over the Luft type instruments. The detectors are compact and rugged and can be modulated at much higher frequencies than the Luft chamber. They are insensitive to vibration but highly sensitive to temperature. This latter quality has been one of the inhibiting features in design and several commercially available solid state IR analysers exhibit unfortunate instabilities due to the lack of sufficient cooling applied to the cell.

There are already a number of good solid state instruments available for the measurement of CO_2 and CO gas but even these carefully designed units lack the freedom from interference from background gas changes exhibited by the Luft type analysers.

As use of the microprocessor controlling chip has advanced it is certain that the disadvantages referred to above will be overcome and that the solid state detector will be the device chosen by most gas analyser manufacturers because of the low cost, speed of response and simplicity of the electronic design requirement.

OXYGEN ANALYSERS

Paramagnetic Analysers

Oxygen is the only common gas which possesses the physical property of paramagnetism. Michael Faraday in 1851 demonstrated that a hollow glass sphere filled with oxygen and suspended on a silk thread could be attracted by a magnet. Faraday was interested in the magnetic suscepti-bility of all materials and examples of susceptibility or Faraday balances are still in existence today.

Before the second world war, German chemical engineers experimented with methods of using the paramagnetic properties of oxygen to create a physical analyser for production control methods. Senft Leben invented a magnetic wind oxygen analyser which used the change of paramagnetic effect with temperature. Paramagnetism decreases 0.8% per degree Centigrade rise in temperature.

In the United States in 1948 when high altitude flying problems stimulated an increased interest in oxygen analysis Linus Pauling used a quartz glass dumb-bell filled with nitrogen suspended in a magnetic field to measure the concentration of oxygen passing through the field.

The dumb-bell has a diamagnetic effect and will tend to be deflected out of the field (see Fig. 9). As the concentration of oxygen passing through the magnetic field increases the diamagnetic object is deflected with increasing force because the property of the gas has the effect of enhancing the magnetic field. Pauling added a quartz glass suspension for the dumb-bell and used electrostatic charges to restore the dumb-bell to its origin (Pauling et al., 1946). This apparatus worked well but

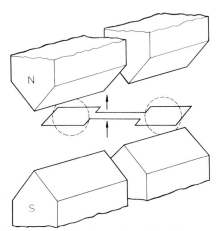

Fig. 9. Paramagnetic analyser. Dumb-bell in magnetic field.

was fragile and required 300V DC potential to create the electrostatic restoring field.

Charles Munday was the inventor of several improvements to the Pauling analyser which have led to the rugged and reliable analyser in use today. The quartz suspension was replaced by a flat platinum alloy strip and the dumb-bell was surrounded by a platinum electrical coil. This substitution created a rugged and practical instrument in which a mirror fixed to the suspension reflected a light onto a ground glass screen indicating the angle of deflection. This could be calibrated for oxygen concentration within the magnetic field.

Using the platinum coil fixed to the dumb-bell, however, it is possible to pass a current which tends to restore the deflection to the original position producing a null balance instrument controlled by a ten turn calibrated potentiometer. This analyser is very accurate (Nunn, 1964).

A more practical version of the analyser is provided by a meter readout display. This analyser still uses the null balance principle via twin photocells and a differential amplifier. The restoring current is measured by an indicating galvanometer (see Fig. 10). The relationship between feedback current and susceptibility is highly linear and, therefore, proportional attenuators allow a variety of ranges to be indicated on the one calibrated meter.

One version of this analyser is fitted with an off-set counter current to enable the scale to be set for a full deflection between 11% and 21% oxygen, the range of interest to respiratory physiologists.

Many variations on the same theme have been created for the wide range of interests in oxygen analysis but they all depend upon the use of the basic elements of permanent magnets, quartz dumb-bells and restoring coils. In practice, these elements are reduced to miniature size in the modern paramagnetic cell enhancing the rugged and reliable nature of the principle. There are a few interfering gases to consider. NO, NO_2 and ClO_2 all have magnetic susceptibility and would need to be considered if present in any mixtures under test.

The response time of the conventional design is rather prolonged and varies from 15 to 30 seconds for full scale deflection according to the flow rate of the sample through the cell. A bypass unit attached to the sample inlet system ensures that the flow through the cell is not high enough to do damage to the suspension. A recent instrument has a sample system which will permit up to 200 ml min^{-1} to pass through the measuring cell and a response time of between 3 and 6 s for full scale deflection is now possible.

Samples for analysis must be clean and dry. It is, therefore, necessary to fit a particular filter and a drying column to the sample inlet unit.

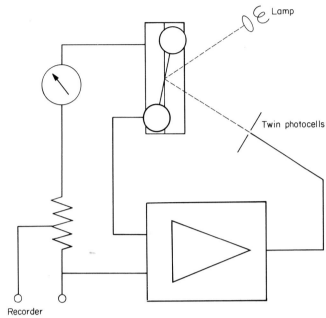

Fig. 10. Paramagnetic analyser. Modification employing twin photocells, lamp and mirror.

A sampling system has been devised for the paramagnetic oxygen analyser which ensures a rapid transit time through the cell by drawing the gas with a powerful vacuum pump through a needle valve restrictor. This produced an atmosphere of 150 mmHg in the cell. Gases entering the needle valve at atmospheric pressure are reduced to the low pressure and thus swept at high speed through the cell system. Response times of better than 200 ms were reported for this modification and the system was well capable of resolving alveolar plateau concentrations breath by breath.

Generally speaking there is much less need for high speed oxygen analysis in respiratory physiology. Breath by breath studies do not have the same importance as do measurements of CO_2 in respiration. The rapid oxygen analyser, has, therefore, not emerged as a standard tool for pulmonary physiologists, the respiratory mass spectrometer often being preferred for the simultaneous rapid analysis of several gases (Chapter 7).

Polarographic Analysers

An inexpensive and reliable analyser for use in oxygen tents and stable environmental measurements is available in several forms.

These analysers are slow in response (5–10 s for full scale deflection) and depend upon the use of the Clark electrode principle which is discussed in Chapter 5. Polarographic analyser cells are disposable and have a limited life varying from six months to as much as two years depending upon the electrolyte and the membrane used in construction.

Whilst the instrument is often less expensive than the paramagnetic unit the replacement electrodes are expensive. The units are very small and are battery operated, a useful point to remember when selecting analysers for use in hazardous conditions such as operating theatres and barometric chambers.

Zirconia Analyser

When the oxide zirconia is heated the material behaves rather like a pH electrode. An electrical potential difference developes across the zirconia membrane proportional to any partial pressure difference in oxygen concentration. The effect of hydrogen ion migration through the zirconia mass is very fast and oxygen analysers depending on this principle achieve response curves of better than 50 ms for full scale deflection.

Zirconia analysers will also resolve very low concentrations and the instruments can be calibrated to 0–10 parts per million full scale deflection.

The analysis cell can take the form of a tube of zirconia mounted in an electrical furnace coil where the sample gas flowing through the inside of the tube may be referred to atmospheric gas encompassing the exterior of the tube. A potential difference will develope across the wall of the tube when there is a difference between the oxygen concentration of room air and that of the sample under test.

To promote the flow of hydrogen ions it is necessary to heat the zirconia to approximately 800°C and maintain very close control on the heating current.

It is possible to arrange for the sample to be referred to a prepared reference gas thus creating a differential analyser. Recently, it has been shown that palladium oxide behaves rather like oxygen at high temperature and this material may be used instead of a gaseous reference.

Zirconia analysers are sensitive to water vapour which has the effect of offsetting the zero and reducing the gas. Care must be taken to avoid the induction of water from spirometers or any source available to the sample line. Cold water hitting the red hot zirconia cracks the oxide tube and destroys the analyser. The analyser is also sensitive to fluctuations of room temperature and the flow rate of the sample gas.

Factors Influencing Choice of Oxygen Analyser

Paramagnetic analysers are reliable and widely used, but have a low speed. Polarographic instruments are relatively inexpensive but have a restricted range. Zirconia analysers respond rapidly at low O_2 concentrations but are unstable and fragile.

EMISSION SPECTRAL ANALYSIS: NITROGEN METERS

The nitrogen meter was one of the first rapid continuous gas analysers to be introduced into respiratory physiology (Lilly, 1950). The analysis is spectrophotometric, depending on the emission of light in the blue range when a current is passed through nitrogen gas at a pressure of 15 mmHg (2 kPa) or less. Selective filters make the instrument almost specific for N_2.

Continuous analysis at 10 mmHg total pressure is achieved by a flow-through system, operated by a vacuum pump and controlled by a needle value, situated near the source of gas to be analysed. The sampling rate is 15 to 20 ml min^{-1} with a 99% response time of 100 ms.

The relationship between output and concentration is alinear. The response of the instrument is flat near 50% fractional concentration of N_2 and rises sharply above 90%, above which the instrument cannot function. A linearizing circuit is required to correct for this characteristic in the working range of the instrument.

Water vapour, which emits white light, causes a background error. If expired gases are to be analysed, the instrument can be set up using humidified room air. Alternatively, the meter and its tubing may be saturated with water vapour before calibration, by sampling expired gas for a few minutes. The instrument remains saturated during tidal breathing.

Formerly, a chopper blade was incorporated, rotating between the source and the detector, and yielding an AC output. As stable DC amplifiers are now available, this feature is no longer necessary.

References

Hill, D. W. and Powell, T. (1965). "Non-dispersive Infra-red Gas Analysers in Science, Medicine and Industry." Hilger and Watts, London.
Hill, D. W. and Dolan, A. M. (1976). "Intensive Care Instrumentation", Chapt. 8. Academic Press, London and New York.
Luft, K. V. Z. (1943). *Tech. Phys.* **24**, 97.
Lilly, J. C. (1950). *Amer. J. Physiol.* **161**, 342–344.
Nunn, J. F. (1964). *Bri. J. Anaesth.* **40**, 569–578.
Pauling, L., Wood, R. and Sturdevant, I. O. (1946). *Science NY* **103**, 336.

7. RESPIRATORY MASS SPECTROMETRY

Peter Scheid

University of Bochum, Bochum, F.R.G.

A respiratory mass spectrometer constitutes a device for continuous and simultaneous measurement of the partial pressures of several components in a gas mixture. Respiratory mass spectrometry developed in the early 1950s in co-operation between manufactures and scientists in biomedical laboratories (Kydd and Hitchcock, 1949; Miller *et al.*, 1950; Fowler and Hugh-Jones, 1957; Fowler, 1966; Goodwin, 1979; Reed and Hugh-Jones, 1979). Twenty-five years later, technical improvements and simplifications have led to manufacturing mass spectrometers that are not only more sensitive and stable, thereby allowing more reliable measurements in the research laboratory, but are also simpler in operation and maintenance and are thus applicable to the clinical routine (Guy *et al.*, 1976; Ayres, 1976).

The purpose of this brief review is to outline the principle of operation of respiratory mass spectrometry and to point at those specifications that are important for the user, with some examples of application of respiratory mass spectrometry to physiological and clinical measurements. I do not intend to contribute a comprehensive review of the technical state of the art of respiratory mass spectrometry, but will rather communicate some of our personal experiences with this method. The interested reader is referred to recent reviews (Milne, 1971; Buckingham and Denis, 1975; Dawson, 1976; Lundsgard *et al.*, 1976; Mastenbrook *et al.*, 1978; Watson, 1976; Smidt, 1980) and symposia reports (Symposium, 1967; Muysers and Smidt, 1971; Symposium 1975; Payne *et al.*, 1979). I will restrict the discussion to the analysis of the gas phase (see pp. 98–103).

PRINCIPLE OF OPERATION OF
RESPIRATORY MASS SPECTROMETERS

A typical respiratory mass spectrometer comprises three stages (Fig. 1).

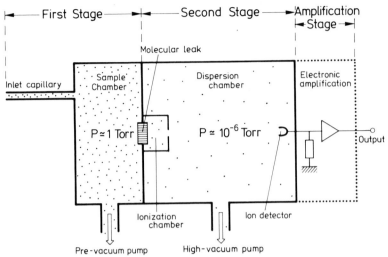

FIG. 1. Schema of a respiratory mass spectrometer with continuous sample inlet. For details, see text.

The *first stage* consists of the inlet capillary through which a continuous flow of gas is sucked, by means of a rotary pump, into a sample chamber. Only a small fraction of the gas entering the sample chamber reaches the *second stage*, through the molecular leak. In this stage, the molecules are ionized and separated according their mass-to-charge ratio, m/e, so that only ions of a given m/e ratio reach the ion detector and induce an ion current. This current is converted in the *third stage* by appropriate electronic circuits into a voltage signal that constitutes a quantitative measure of the partial pressure of the corresponding gas species in the sampled gas mixture.

First Stage: Sample Inlet

Inner diameter and length of the inlet capillary tube are the main determinants of the sample flow into the sample chamber.* The inner capillary diameter, typically around 250 μm, is adjusted to provide viscous flow down the capillary length which is important to keep the response time low (cf. Fowler, 1969) and to prevent separation of the gases on their way down the capillary according to their different molecular masses. Pumping speed and geometry of the pumping lines are adjusted to a pressure of around 1 mmHg in the sample chamber, as this is the lower limit for the viscous flow regime (Buckingham, 1979). The inlet capillary may be heated to prevent water condensation at its walls with ensuing delay to water soluble gases.

* The gas mixture to be analyzed as well as those parts of it that enter the mass spectrometer for analysis will be referred to as the (gas) sample.

Second Stage: Ionization and Mass Dispersion

The pressure in the second stage is sufficiently low ($\approx 10^{-6}$ mmHg) for molecular flow conditions to prevail. The undesirable gap between viscous flow condition in the first and molecular flow condition (flow independent of viscosity) in the second stage is bridged by a molecular leak in which molecular flow conditions prevail despite the relatively high pressure (cf. Buckingham, 1979). Molecular leaks are made of metal plates with thin holes (about 20 μm diameter) or by sintered porous leaks.

The molecules enter the ionizing chamber which is a part of the high vacuum system of the second stage. Molecules have to be ionized for separation, by electric or magnetic forces, in the dispersion tube. The conventional way of ionization is by electron impact. Electrons are emitted from a filament that is heated by electrical current (3–4 A), and are then attracted to an anode by a d.c. voltage of about 70 V. The focused electron beam crosses the molecular beam entering from the molecular leak. Energy is thereby transferred from the electrons onto the molecules, and positively charged molecular ions are produced. However, due to excess electron energy, some molecules are doubly or multiply charged or are fragmented. Therefore, electron impact ionization creates a characteristic fragmentation spectrum for each molecule species, typically comprising a major parent peak, at the m/e ratio of the singly-charged parent molecule, and several other peaks at smaller m/e ratios, resulting from fragmentation (smaller mass) or multiple ionization (larger charge).

Fragmentation may cause technical problems in mass spectrometry (see p. 154), and other, more gentle, ways of ionization have been applied as well (cf. Watson, 1976). In chemical ionization, for example, a reactant gas is introduced into the ion source at a much higher density than that of the sample. Electron impact ionizes the reactant gas molecules, which in turn react with the sample gas to exchange charge at a considerably lower energy. Hence, chemical ionization creates less fragmentation, and the resulting spectrum is cleaner. Other techniques of ionization involve negative ions, where electrons are attached to the sample molecule. A novel system has been developed by Hunt et al. (1976) by rapidly switching all electric potentials in a quadrupole mass spectrometer between positive and negative levels. Thereby, positive and negative ions are intermittently ejected from the ion source to enter the quadrupole which itself does not distinguish the ion charge (see below). Two electron multipliers detect the positive and negative ions. With this technique both electron impact and chemical ionization spectra can be recorded, and the detection threshold is extremely low (cf. Watkins, 1979).

High sensitivity and rapid response are achieved with a closed ionization chamber, attached directly to the molecular leak, the only exits being the source slits for extraction of ions and the holes for entry and exit of the ionizing electron beam. The advantages of the closed to an open ionization chamber are the higher density of gas molecules available for ionization and the fast response to a change of the composition of the gas sample (cf. Fowler, 1969).

After leaving the ionization chamber, the ions are separated in the dispersion tube of the second stage. The types of mass spectrometer differ basically in their methods of mass separation, and three types (magnetic, quadrupole, time-of-flight) will be briefly described below.

After separation, the ions of a given gas species reach an ion detector, and the amplitude of the induced current is proportional to the partial pressure of this species in the sample at the tip of the inlet capillary. Simultaneous measurement of several species in a sample mixture is possible either by an array of ion detectors, one for each gas component, or by successive measurement of all components by way of scanning procedures (see p. 138). The gas is eventually pumped off the high-vacuum chamber by a high-vacuum pump, and the turnover rate of this pumping determines largely the response time of the mass spectrometer (see p. 142).

Amplification Stage: Electronic Processing

In the amplification stage, the ion current signal is converted into a voltage signal which is then amplified and processed according to the specific needs of the mass spectrometer. Special electronic circuitry (multiplexing, sample-hold circuits) are needed when employing scanning (see p. 138).

TYPES OF RESPIRATORY MASS SPECTROMETER

This section will briefly introduce the three basic types of respiratory mass spectrometer, and discuss some of the advantages and disadvantages that result from their basic principle (cf. Watson, 1976).

Magnetic Sector Mass Spectrometer

A schematic diagram of this mass spectrometer is shown in Fig. 2. The assemblage of ions is extracted, by a high d.c. voltage, U, into a

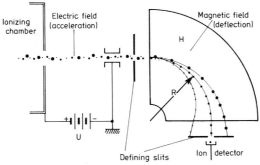

FIG. 2. Ion dispersion in a magnetic sector mass spectrometer. The magnetic field, H, of the 90° sector magnet is perpendicular to the plane of the figure. Three ion species of different m/e ratios are shown by different symbols. While the spectrometer is tuned to the ion of middle m/e (radius of curvature in magnetic field, R), the radius of the heavier ion (larger m/e) is too large, that of the lighter ion too small, to fall on to the ion detector through the defining slit.

homogeneous magnetic field, of strength H, which is perpendicular to the plane in Fig. 2. This magnetic field exerts a force on the ions which is perpendicular both to the magnetic field and to the direction in which the ions move. Thereby, the ions are forced onto circular trajectories while passing the magnetic field, and the radius of the ion trajectories is determined not only by U and H but, more importantly, by the mass-to-charge ratio, m/e, of the ion

$$R = \left(\frac{2U}{H^2} \cdot m/e \right)^{\frac{1}{2}} \tag{1}$$

Hence, given a radius of curvature, R, between the source and the ion detector, only those ions will reach the detector for which the m/e ratio satisfies eqn. (1).

An essential feature of respiratory mass spectrometers is their capability of measuring simultaneously several gas species. This can be achieved in the magnetic sector machine by attaching several ion detectors at different values of R that correspond to the desired m/e ratio of several gas species. The position of these ion detectors can be fixed by the manufacturer, thus predetermining the set of gases that can be analysed. More flexibility is obtained with adjustable detectors, as this allows selection of an assembly of gas species within an m/e range set by the specifications of the machine. Limits for the radius, R, are given by the geometry of the machine, and they define the range of m/e according to eqn. (1) when U and H are fixed. In addition, some mass spectrometers allow to change the high voltage, U, whereby the m/e range "window" may be moved across the m/e scale. From eqn. (1) it is evident that reducing U by a given factor results in increasing the m/e ratios of both the upper and the lower limits on the m/e scale by the same factor. Thus, as U is decreased, the window is moved towards higher masses and its width increases. Scanning the accelerating voltage provides a possibility to measure (quasi-) simultaneously many gas species in a sample using only one ion detector (see p. 138).

Quadrupole Mass Spectrometer

In this non-magnetic mass spectrometer separation of ions is achieved in a combined electric d.c. and r.f. (radio frequency) field. The ions are extracted from the ion source by a small voltage, of some 15 V, and enter the electric quadrupole field. This field is provided by an assembly of four metal rods, the diagonally opposite rods being electrically connected to a combined d.c. and r.f. generator (Fig. 3A). When the ions enter this quadrupole field with the axial momentum provided by the extraction voltage, they are subjected to attracting forces towards, and repelling forces from, the rods, and these forces are oscillating with the radio frequency. The ions thus follow complex trajectories, and only those ions pass the rods to be received by the ion collector that do not collide with the rods. Mosharrafa (1970) has described the quadrupole as a mass filter in which the rods with the positive d.c. potential act as high-pass mass filters, as they attract the light ions easily to collide with the positive rods, whereas the rods with negative d.c. potential act as low-pass mass filters, as they retain light ions. The whole quadrupole assembly can then be compared with a band-pass in which only ions of a narrow m/e range can pass without collision with the rods.

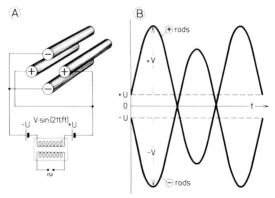

FIG. 3. Rods of a quadrupole mass spectrometer (A) and rod voltages (B). For details, see text.

The mass resolution (width of the pass-band) of the quadrupole is given by the ratio of the r.f. amplitude to the d.c. voltage, V/U. If $V \leqslant U$, the bandwidth is zero, i.e. no ions pass the rods. A typical value to obtain acceptable mass resolution is $V/U = 6$.

While the voltage ratio determines the resolution, the absolute values of V and U (at constant V/U ratio) determine the m/e ratio of the ion that passes the rods as

$$m/e = k \ V/f^2 = k' \ U/f^2 \tag{2}$$

where f is the radio frequency and the values of the constants k and k' involve geometry of the quadrupole rods. Appropriate adjustment of U and V, while maintaining their ratio unaltered, will thus allow measurement of ions with m/e ratios over a wide range. Scanning facilities are needed to obtain a (quasi-) simultaneous output for a number of gases (see p. 138).

Time-of-Flight Mass Spectrometer

This mass spectrometer involves measurement of the time necessary for an ion to travel from the ion source to the ion detector. A discrete bunch of ions is extracted from the ion source during a short time interval and subjected to an accelerating voltage, U. All ions receive thus the same kinetic energy, eU, but the speed they attain (v) depends on their mass as

$$eU = mv^2/2 \tag{3}$$

Thus the flight time, T, from the accelerating grid to the ion detector a distance L away, is

$$T = L \left(\frac{1}{2U} \cdot m/e \right)^{\frac{1}{2}} \tag{4}$$

and depends on the m/e ratio of the ion. In typical instruments, L is 100–200 cm and U is 3000 V (cf. Watson, 1976). Hence, at the upper limit of the m/e range of interest in respiratory mass spectrometry, 150 amu (for units of m/e, see p. 140), the time of flight would be around 20 μsec. After this time all ions of interest have (successively, in order of their m/e ratio) reached the ion detector, and a new bunch of ions can be extracted from the ion source and accelerated. At the ion detector a spectrum will be recorded in synchrony with the pulsed acceleration of each ion bunch. Multiplexing and sample-hold electronics are needed to enable (quasi-) simultaneous and (quasi-) continuous records of a multicomponent mixture.

The rather long flight path needed for appropriate resolution results in a rather bulky set-up, which does not appear appropriate for clinical application. However, time-of-flight mass spectrometers have successfully been used in the respiratory research laboratory and appear to have distinct advantages over magnetic sector or quadrupole machines (Lacoste, 1967).

Signal Processing in Scanning Mass Spectrometers

A requirement set for respiratory mass spectrometry is the simultaneous and continuous analysis of a number of gases in a gas mixture. Of the instruments described, only the sector magnet with several ion collectors strictly fulfils this requirement. However, special electronic circuitry enables in particular the quadrupole mass spectrometer to operate in a quasi-continuous and quasi-simultaneous mode.

Figure 4A is a schematic diagram of a spectrum in the range between 10 and 50 amu, obtained e.g. in a quadrupole mass spectrometer in the scanning mode. The d.c. and r.f. voltages, U and V, are made to increase as a linear ramp. The diagram at the top of Fig. 4A constitutes a schema of a spectrum recorded in expired air, showing N_2 at m/e (in amu) 28, O_2 at 32, Ar at 40 and CO_2 at 44. Aside from these peaks there

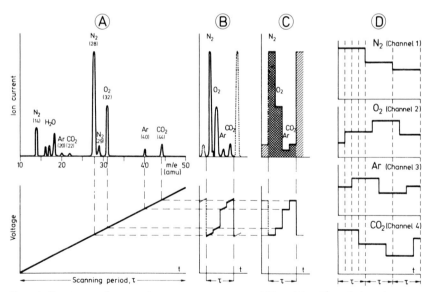

FIG. 4. Spectrum of a scanning mass spectrometer (A) and its abbreviations by ramp segments (B) and by segments of constant voltage (C). (D) shows the simultaneous recording of 4 masses. For details, see text.

are peaks of naturally abundant isotopes (e.g. N_2^{29}), of fragmentation or double charged ions (N_2 at 14, Ar at 20, CO_2 at 22), and of H_2O (16, 17, and 18), which are not important for the analysis. Also, there is a considerable fraction of time during which the voltage sweeps through "empty" mass regions.

An abbreviated spectrum, that contains only peaks of interest, can be produced by replacing the ramp by a series of short, discontinuous ramps (Fig. 4B), whereby the total scanning period can be considerably reduced. If the ramp series is replaced by discrete voltage steps, the magnitude of each corresponding to the highest level of the respective peak in the spectrum, the histogram of Fig. 4C is obtained.

The output from the ion detector can now be gated into different amplifier channels, one for each voltage step and its corresponding m/e. This gating is synchronized with the voltage step so that each amplifier receives a signal only when "its" ion falls on the ion detector. Since each channel is fed with a signal from the ion detector only during a fraction of the scan duration, electronic sample-hold circuits have to maintain the signal for the remaining period, until the channel is updated (for electronic details, see Mable, 1979).

A schema of the output signals of the four channels corresponding to the four masses of Fig. 4C is depicted in Fig. 4D. Three scan cycles are displayed and it can be seen that N_2 is updated during the first quarter of the scan cycle, O_2 during the second and so on. This results in steps for each mass with phase shifts between them. It is thus evident that scanning allows only for quasi-simultaneous and quasi-continuous measurement. However, the scan period, τ, can be made short enough (<100 ms) that for most problems the signals appear as truly simultaneous and continuous.

Scanning can also be applied to sector magnets equipped with only one ion detector. Both the electric and the magnetic fields can be scanned, but only electric scanning is practicable in respiratory mass spectrometry as magnetic scanning is too slow (Watson, 1976).

SPECIFICATIONS AND REQUIREMENTS FOR RESPIRATORY MASS SPECTROMETERS

The specifications required for a respiratory mass spectrometer (cf. Fowler, 1969; Mosharrafa, 1970) depend largely on the application. The following section attempts to define the limits for some important parameters and some basic requirements of respiratory mass spectrometers for use in the clinical routine. Although this list will not be comprehensive and will reflect the personal view of the author, it may be useful for the reader to select the proper mass spectrometer from the commercially available machines.

Mass Range

The important variable for mass separation in the mass spectrometer is the m/e ratio of an ion. Usually m is expressed as relative atomic mass (relative to the molecular mass of carbon, which is set at 12.000) and e as multiples of the electron charge. Thus the m/e ratio of a singly-charged ion corresponds to its (relative) molecular mass, the unit being atomic mass units, amu. For multiply-charged ions, the m/e ratio is expressed as the amu of the corresponding singly-charged ion of same m/e. Thus, the m/e ratios of the following ions are (in amu): O_2^-, 32; O_2^{--}, 16; O^-, 16. The generally used notion that O_2 can be recorded on "mass 16" refers to the m/e ratio of the doubly-charged ion which creates a peak at the same location as a singly-charged ion of mass 16. This is the basis for using mass units on a scale which strictly pertains to m/e units.

TABLE I

Some gases used in respiratory mass spectrometry

	Gas species	Atomic mass
Respiratory gases:	N_2	28
	O_2	32
	CO_2	44
Inert gases: low solubility	H_2	2
	He	4
	Ne	20
	CO	28
	Ar	40
	SF_6	146
medium solubility	C_2H_2	26
	Cyclopropane	42
	N_2O	44
	Freon 22	86
high solubility	Acetone	58
	Diethyl ether	74
	Halothane	197
Stable istotopes:	$^{13}C^{16}O$	29
	$^{12}C^{18}O$	30
	$^{13}C^{18}O$	31
	$^{15}N_2$	30
	$^{18}O_2$	36
	$^{13}C^{16}O_2$	45

The atomic masses of some molecules that have been used in respiratory mass spectrometry are compiled in Table I. With an m/e range between 2 and 200 amu all these gases can be measured as singly-charged, non-fragmented ions. However, for practical purposes this requirement may be too restrictive. In fact, with electron impact ionization peaks of significant amplitude will be produced at m/e ratios below that for the parent peak. For example, in the schema for Fig. 4, both N_2 and Ar produced peaks at half their main m/e ratios, due at least for Ar, to double-ionization. Fragmentation peaks occur mainly for complex compounds of higher molecular mass (e.g. Freon 22, Chloroform, Diethyl ether, Cyclopropane in Table I), and their amplitudes can in fact be larger than that of the parent peak. By resorting to measurement of fragmentation peaks, the upper end of the mass range necessary in respiratory mass spectrometers can readily be lowered to 80. The higher mass range may be desirable for some research applications, but for most problems it constitutes no essential requirement, as suggested by Mosharrafa (1970).

Mass Resolution

The resolving power of a mass spectrometer can best be visualized when scanning the spectrum. Ideally all ions, derived from a given gas species and bearing a given m/e ratio, should be imaged at the same location in the spectrum thus producing an infinitely sharp line. However, realistic inhomogeneities in the dispersing electric and magnetic fields, as well as finite width of the collimating slits result in more or less broad peaks for a given mass, and the peak width determines mainly the mass resolution. Two masses are defined as properly separated when the valley between their peaks (of equal height) does not exceed 10% of the peak height (cf. Goodwin, 1979). When under these conditions m constitutes the (mean) mass underlying the two peaks, and Δm their mass difference, $m/\Delta m$ is defined as the mass resolution. (Strictly, m/e and $\Delta(m/e)$ should be used in this definition; see p. 140).

In quadrupole mass spectrometers, m/e is a linear function of the rod voltages (cf. eqn. (2)). Hence, the spectrum produced by linear voltage ramps is linear in m/e and the separation of ions is identical in the high and the low mass range. This constitutes a distinct advantage of the quadrupole compared with the magnetic sector in which the radii for ions of unit mass difference converge towards higher masses. Hence, the separation for higher masses is less than for lower masses.

For respiratory mass spectrometers unit mass resolution ($\Delta m = 1$) for higher masses (e.g. $m = 50$) is quite sufficient, and hence a resolution of $m/\Delta m = 50$ is desirable. This resolution is not sufficient for separating isotopes of almost identical molecular masses. For example the molecular mass of $^{14}N_2$ is 28.006 and that of $^{12}C^{16}O$, 27.995; the difference is $\Delta m = 0.011$ amu. Separation of both gases in a mass spectrometer would thus require a resolution of about $28/0.011 \approx 2500$ which would necessitate special techniques (cf. Leck, 1979) that are expensive and impracticable for respiratory mass spectrometry in medical application. Use of stable isotopes constitutes an interesting alternative for measuring gases that can normally not be separated (see p. 158).

Unit mass resolution cannot prevent contamination by fragmentation peaks. For example, the gas of interest, x, may produce its main peak at the same m/e ratio as a fragment of gas y. The contamination by y can be corrected by using appropriate electronic circuits (see p. 154).

In the magnetic sector with various adjustable ion collectors, the minimum mass difference between two recorded masses is usually set by the geometry of the ion detector rather than by the mass resolution in the spectrum. However, special ion collectors can be built that enable unit mass resolution even with multi-detector magnetic sector machines (see p. 158).

Delay Time and Response Time

When the gas mixture at the tip of the inlet capillary is suddenly altered from one to another constant composition, it usually takes a finite time for the mass spectrometer output to respond to this input step, and this response is typically gradual rather than instantaneous. Two variables are generally used to quantify this response (Fig. 5), the delay time and the response time. Generally, the delay time is referred to as the time

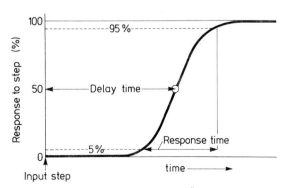

FIG. 5. Definition of delay and response time in a mass spectrometer.

from the step change until a change is seen in the mass spectrometer output, and the response time as the period from this onset of change to its 95% completion. We prefer to define the delay time as the duration between the input step and 50% of the response, and the respone time as the period between 5% and 95% of the response. This definition is practical as the "onset of response" is difficult to measure with the usually gradual response.

For viscous inlet systems, delay and response time are largely independent variables. The delay time reflects the finite transit time of the gas front between the tip of the inlet capillary and the analyser. The response time is mainly determined by the pumping time constant in the ionization chamber (cf. Fowler, 1969). Length of the inlet capillary and sample flow rate into it are the major variables that determine delay time, but dispersion along the capillary length does not add significantly to the finite response time (Goodwin, 1979). Therefore, long inlet probes can be used with acceptably short response time, and this is of practical importance for patient monitoring (Davies and Denison, 1979). With the advancement in electronic development, time constants in the electronic circuits should not limit the response time (see, however, below for scanning mode), and this can be checked by recording the signal directly from the ion detector with appropriately fast responding devices.

Delay and response times can easily be measured in the following way. Connect the inlet capillary to a constant gas mixture in which the concentrations of the relevant gases differ from those in air. Provide two electric wires which, when disconnected, produce a signal on the recorder. Hold both wires and the inlet capillary so that when pulling the capillary off the gas mixture reservoir, the electric wires are disconnected. Measure the time on the record as in Fig. 5 relative to the electric signal produced by disconnecting the wires. Depending on the length of the inlet capillary and on its sampling rate, the delay time typically varies between 0.1 and 1 s, there being not much difference between different masses recorded simultaneously. When the delay time appears to be prolonged, the most likely reason is plugging of the inlet capillary, e.g. with mucus when recording near the mouth. Compensation of the delay time is only necessary when the phase between the mass spectrometer output and other signals is important (e.g. plot of expired concentration against expired volume). With modern electronic aids, this compensation usually imposes no major problem provided the delay time is known.

More critical is the response time as it affects the fidelity of the recorded signal. It is evident that any change in the input signal (gas to be analysed) occurring over a shorter time period than the response time, is distorted in the mass spectrometer output. Hence, the mass spectrometer acts as a low-pass filter whose bandwidth is directly related to the response time. For normal purposes in respiratory physiology, a response time of 0.1 s is sufficient. It should, however, be realized that the finite response time may become limiting, e.g. in the analysis of the shape of Phase II in expirograms. In this case, expiration must either be slowed or attempts must be made to account mathematically for the response time.

In mass spectrometers that employ scanning and sample-hold electronics, particular problems arise when recording rapidly changing signals. If it is accepted that five points are sufficient to identify the response curve of Fig. 5, the scan period should not exceed one fifth of the response time of the mass spectrometer, e.g. 20 ms when the response time is 100 ms. The scanning frequency should thus be at least 50 Hz.

Linearity

The output of the mass spectrometer for a given gas species is directly related to its partial pressure in the sample mixture (see p. 150). This relationship should be linear for each gas over the significant range of concentration. For some applications it may even be required that there exist proportionality (zero output for zero gas partial pressure; cf. p. 150). This requires that a constant background (either from rest ions in the vacuum system or from electronic offset voltages) can be zeroed electrically. This back-off facility which most mass spectrometers provide as an option only, is very helpful if not necessary.

Sensitivity: Detection and Discrimination Thresholds

These factors deserve an exact definition since much confusion exists in the specification provided by manufacturers of respiratory mass spectrometers.

Signal-to-noise-ratio

Consider measurement of a gas species in a gas mixture of constant composition using a sector magnet or a quadrupole mass spectrometer. Assume that the machine is tuned to the mass in question (no scanning mode). The output of the mass spectrometer amplifier will yield a signal that ideally is constant in time, but in reality displays some variation

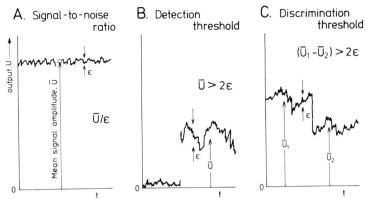

FIG. 6. Definition of signal-to-noise ratio (A) and of the derived estimates for the sensitivity in a mass spectrometer, detection threshold (B) and discrimination threshold (C).

about the mean (Fig. 6A). Generally, the random variation occurring on a short time scale is called noise, and the variations that occur over longer periods, drift. Noise or drift may derive from several factors including variations in ionizing current or ionization efficiency; variation in pumping rate; or may reflect unsteadiness in the electronic components. Correspondingly these variations may be random or systematic.

The essential factor to determine the sensitivity of a mass spectrometer is the ratio of the signal amplitude to the noise (or drift) amplitude, the signal-to-noise ratio. An unequivocal measure of noise, ε, is its root-mean-square average, defined as the standard deviation of the signal, U, from its mean, $\bar{U}$:

$$\varepsilon = \left[\sum_{i=1}^{N} (U_i - \bar{U})^2/N \right]^{\frac{1}{2}} \tag{5}$$

where N is the discrete sample size. Its determination is easily possible with computer aids, but an estimate can be obtained by one quarter of the noise band that appears on a slow record of the signal on a strip chart recorder.

The noise level, and thus the signal-to-noise ratio, depends on the recording conditions, which therefore must be stated when quoting a signal-to-noise ratio. The bandwidth of recording is important as the noise amplitude diminishes when the cut-off frequency of the low-pass filter is reduced. The bandwidth of the electronics and the recording devices should be higher than that of the mass spectrometer, which is determined by its response time (see above). For a response time of 0.1 s, a bandwidth of 30–50 Hz is desirable and sufficient.

Secondly, the signal-to-noise ratio depends on the level of the signal. The noise level generally grows with the signal, but less than proportional to it. Hence, the signal-to-noise ratio increases with increasing signal, and a plot of the signal-to-noise ratio against the signal amplitude would be desirable to characterize the mass spectrometer (see p. 156).

Using the signal-to-noise ratio, two different thresholds can be defined to characterize the sensitivity of a mass spectrometer, the detection threshold and the discrimination threshold.

Detection Threshold

The sensitivity may be defined as the capability of the mass spectrometer to detect a gas species present in the sample in trace amounts. If one accepts a signal-to-noise ratio of 2–3 as sufficient to identify a signal against the background noise, the detection threshold can be defined as the smallest signal amplitude that exceeds the noise level by a factor of 2–3 (Fig. 6B). Since the noise amplitude of mass spectrometers diminishes with the signal (see above), the detection threshold is usually very low, the detection sensitivity hence very high, reaching in most respiratory mass spectrometers the ppm level. (The fractional concentration corresponding to 1 ppm (part per million) is 10^{-6}.)

This favourably high detection sensitivity is generally quoted by manufacturers. While this specification is important for analysis of trace amounts of compounds, it bears only limited significance in respiratory mass spectrometry.

Discrimination Threshold

In respiratory physiology, the relevant gas concentrations often vary within a range set by finite upper and lower limits. For example, the O_2 fraction in respired air normally stays between 0.21 and 0.15, and this range may be substantially narrowed when ventilation is increased without increased metabolic rate (e.g. inspired CO_2 sensitivity test). In these cases, the noise level must be small enough to allow discrimination between the two finite signals (Fig. 6C). The discrimination threshold can thus be defined as the smallest signal difference that can be detected against the noise with a signal-to-noise ratio of at least 2–3. As the noise level increases with the signal level (see above), the discrimination threshold is generally larger (discrimination sensitivity lower) at higher than at lower signal levels, and much larger than the detection threshold.

The discrimination threshold required depends mainly on the application. The user must specify the upper and lower concentration limit within which the gas in question varies in his application. If this range is displayed full scale on a recorder, a noise level of below 1% full scale is very good, of 2% is acceptable, and of 5% is liminal. These noise levels define the discrimination threshold.

If, for example, respired O_2 and CO_2 levels are to be monitored in air-breathing normal subjects, the recording sensitivity should be between 0.21 and 0.15 for O_2, and between 0 and 0.06 for CO_2. For acceptable discrimination, the noise levels must not exceed 2% of the respective differences, or 0.0012 for both gases. Hence, the signal-to-noise requirement for O_2 is $0.21/0.0012 = 175$ at an O_2 fraction of 0.21, and for CO_2, $0.06/0.0012 = 50$ at a CO_2 fraction of 0.06. If, however, the inspired–expired differences recorded narrow in the experiment in question, so that O_2 varies between 0.21 and 0.20, the required signal-to-noise ratio increases to over 1000. Examples will be given on p. 156.

Noise Level and Scanning

It has been assumed in the above discussion that the recorded signal was continuously available to the ion detector as is the case in the magnetic sector with multiple ion collectors. In quadrupole (and in scanning magnetic) mass spectrometers, however, the signal is available to the ion collector during a fraction of the scan time only. Typically, when N masses are to be recorded, the signal can at best be gated during a fraction $1/N$ of the scan time to one channel. Usually the time during which the signal can be processed is even smaller (cf. Mable, 1979), and $1/(3N)$ is a more realistic fraction. With 8 masses recorded, only $1/24$ ($\sim 4\%$) of the total ions are available for measurement due to the scanning and multiplexing. Thereby the scanning mode severely reduces the signal-to-noise ratio. This must be kept in mind when testing a scanning mass spectrometer.

This reduction in the available signal constitutes a severe disadvantage of the quadrupole as compared with the multiple-detector magnetic mass spectrometer. It also imposes an upper limit on the number of masses that can be recorded with sufficient sensitivity. It constitutes a helpful feature of some scanning machines that the number of masses measured in the peak select mode is adjustable. Hence, if only O_2, CO_2, and N_2 are to be measured, it is not necessary to waste the remainder of the scan time to scan across masses without interest. Another important feature in some machines is that the relative dwell time assigned to each mass may be adjusted. This is helpful since the signal-to-noise requirements are usually different for the different gases measured simultaneously.

Signal-to-noise-requirements

It is evident from the above discussion that a unique value cannot be given to specify the sensitivity of a respiratory mass spectrometer and that the requirements needed depend largely on the application. It would be desirable that the manufacturer provides plots of the signal-to-noise ratio against the level of the signal (cf. Fig. 10), individually for the most interesting gases (e.g. O_2, CO_2, N_2, Ar, He, C_2H_2 etc.); these plots should contain statements about how the measurements were performed (e.g. bandwidth of recording, scan parameters etc.). The user, on the other hand, should estimate the signal-to-noise requirements for his analytical problem. Examples for a high-performance magnetic sector mass spectrometer will be given on p. 155.

Analog vs Digital Electronics

Advancement of digital electronics and the desire to adapt the mass spectrometer output directly to digital data processing units have led some manufacturers to adopt digital techniques in their mass spectrometers. This is particularly attractive in scanning machines where multiplexing and demultiplexing is much more reliably achieved by digital technique (Marlowe, 1979). However, this approach imparts problems that result from the discussion in the preceding section.

With an AD (analog-to-digital) converter of 12 bit resolution, each bit corresponds to $(1/2)^{12} \approx 0.025\%$ of the signal. This is obviously satisfactory when the signal is displayed between zero and its maximum level. When, however, the significant variation occurs only within a narrow range around a finite value (e.g. O_2 fraction changing between 0.21 and 0.20), the bits pertaining to this range are reduced as most bits are assigned to an unused part of the signal. Similarly, when recording "wash-out" curves, the signal diminishes with time, and after reaching, say, 5% of the original value one may want to increase the amplifier gain to display the tail of the curve in more detail. Increasing the gain at the recorder 100-fold reduces the number of resolving bits to $(2)^{12}/100 \approx 40$, and the recording sensitivity hence to 2.5%. Thereby one reaches the range where the entire inspired–expired difference in the signal is one bit or less apart.

Appropriate hybrid techniques can solve these problems. It may in particular be useful to employ zero offset before AD conversion, e.g. in the first amplifier, whereby the full resolving power of the AD conversion is available to the window in which the significant signal variation occurs. Similarly, gain control of the first amplifier is a useful requirement.

Stability

The quantitative relationship between gas partial pressure and the corresponding mass spectrometer readout should be stable over sufficient periods of time in order to avoid the necessity of frequent recalibration. Drift (instability) and noise are the same phenomena in that they create (random or directed) sensitivity variations, but they occur on different time scales, e.g. fractions of seconds vs multiples of seconds. Typical causes of drift are variations in sample inlet rate; in ionizing electron current; in suction rate of pumps; or in amplifier gain. Drift (and noise) affecting all recorded ions proportionately (equivalent to a change in overall sensitivity) can electronically be compensated for (see p. 150).

The requirement for stability depends on the application. For use in a clinical routine laboratory or for patient monitoring, drift should be less than 5% of the recorded signal (e.g. the recorded partial pressure difference, see above) over a period of 2 h. For more exact measurement in the research laboratory, calibration should be checked before and after each crucial measurement.

Multi-Component Analysis

Simultaneous analysis of more than one gas in a mixture is a prerequisite for respiratory mass spectrometry. The preceding discussion shows, however, that the number of gas species to be measured by a respiratory mass spectrometer must carefully be chosen, particularly when using the scanning mode, where increasing the number of channels inevitably reduces the signal-to-noise ratio (see p. 147). It appears that facilities for recording five gases at adjustable m/e ratios suffice for most purposes, and that a number of eight is rarely needed in research projects.

Sample Inlet Rate

The amount of gas sampled by the mass spectrometer for analysis should be a small fraction of the gas mixture available. Hence, when sampling in flowing gas (e.g. in respired gas), the sampling rate should be small compared with the flow rate at the measuring site (see p. 161); when measuring in a closed gas volume, the amount sampled until a stable reading is obtained (usually 5–10 s) should be small compared to the volume of the supply (see p. 163). Typically, the sampling rates of respiratory mass spectrometers are 10–50 ml min^{-1}, and this may at times be too large. A possibility to reduce this figure is to introduce a wire into the inlet capillary. If properly chosen, the sampling rate can be largely reduced, thereby prolonging the delay time, but without changing the response time (see p. 163). The sensitivity of the mass spectrometer can be maintained despite the lowered sampling rate when the pressure in the first stage is readjusted (see p. 156).

Other Requirements

Other requirements include ease of operation and of service, mobility, reliability, short pump-down time, low cost, quiet operation (see Mosharrafa, 1970). Although respiratory mass spectrometers have been considerably simplified, they still require some servicing that usually has to be done by representatives of the manufacturer. Reliability of these service representatives is a requirement that is worth checking before deciding on the mass spectrometer to be purchased.

ELECTRONIC DEVICES FOR IMPROVING SIGNAL OUTPUT

The following electronic circuits have specially been designed to improve the signal-to-noise ratio, the stability and versatility of respiratory mass spectrometers. Some manufacturers have built them into their machines, but for most part they can easily be added on later.

Water Vapour Compensation and Automatic Stability Control

Water Vapour Compensation

In the respiratory mass spectrometers described above the output signal is a linear function of the partial pressure of the gas under study in the analysed gas mixture. The partial pressure, Px, of a gas species in a gas mixture depends on its fractional concentration, Fx (i.e. the ratio of the amount of X to the amount of all dry gas components in the mixture), on the total pressure, P_B, and the water vapour pressure, P_{H_2O}

$$Px = Fx \cdot (P_B - P_{H_2O}) \qquad (6)$$

P_{H_2O}, in turn, depends on both temperature and water vapour saturation in the sample mixture at the tip of the inlet capillary (see Fig. 7).

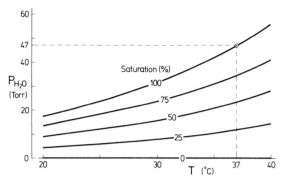

FIG. 7. Water vapour partial pressure (P_{H_2O}) at various temperatures (T) and various water vapour saturation levels.

Consider the case that alveolar partial pressure of O_2 is to be determined mass spectrometrically from a deep expiration. The P_{H_2O} at the measuring site (e.g. mouth piece) is usually lower than that in the alveoli (full water vapour saturation at 37°C; $P_{H_2O} \approx 47$ mmHg). When the P_{H_2O} at the measuring site is known, eqn. (6) can be used to first calculate F_{O_2}, and then to calculate P_{O_2} for alveolar conditions ($P_{H_2O} = 47$ mmHg). This calculation is, however, generally not possible, as neither temperature nor water vapour saturation at the measuring site are known, and the P_{H_2O} at the measuring site remains thus unknown.

Scheid *et al.*, (1971; cf. Slama and Scheid, 1975) have proposed a simple method by which the output signal of a mass spectrometer becomes independent of water vapour pressure, whereby it measures gas fraction rather than partial pressure. This conversion makes use of the fact that the fractions of all dry gas components in a mixture add up to 1.0, independent of P_{H_2O}. Figure 8 shows a schema of the feedback circuits used for the water vapour compensation. The mass spectrometer is calibrated with a dry gas mixture (Fig. 8A), and the output of each channel is adjusted by its gain to the respective fraction $F_X = P_X/P_B$ (e.g. 1 V for fraction of 0.1). In a summing amplifier, S, all F signals are added and compared with a signal of 1.0. During calibration the output of the summing amplifier is therefore zero. The effect of the water vapour, generally present in analysed samples, is to dilute each dry gas component of a mixture and hence to attenuate the mass spectrometer output. Compared with the measurement in the dry mixture, the attenuation factor of the humid mixture of same dry gas composition is $(P_B - P_{H_2O})/P_B$. With unity gain, the summing amplifier would hence

F

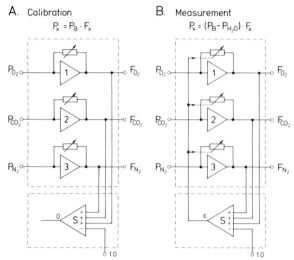

Fig. 8. Diagram of the water vapour compensator and automatic stability control circuit for 3 gas components during calibration with dry gases (A) and measurement in humid gas (B). Outputs of channel amplifiers (1, 2, 3) are summed in the summing amplifier (S) and compared with constant reference signal (1.0). An error signal, ε, during measurement in humid gas is used to adjust all channel gains by the same factor. For details, see text.

give a signal

$$\varepsilon = 1 - \frac{P_B - P_{H_2O}}{P_B} \tag{7}$$

which may be used in a negative feedback circuit to increase the gain of each channel amplifier by the same factor, $P_B/(P_B - P_{H_2O})$, until the output of S is minimized. Hence, with this feedback control the output from each channel becomes proportional to Fx and independent of water vapour. Px for alveolar conditions can then easily be calculated using eqn. (6) with the alveolar P_{H_2O} of 47 mm Hg.

It is important for proper functioning of the feedback that the output of the mass spectrometer is zero for zero partial pressure of each component gas. Back-off facilities must therefore be provided with the mass spectrometer that allow to compensate for background.

Automatic Stability Control

The essence of the feedback circuit described above is that it compensates for any change in the mass spectrometer reading that affects the partial pressures of all dry gas components by the same factor. Aside from changes in water vapour partial pressure, variations in total pressure, P_B, constitute such a mechanism, and the feedback circuit can eliminate the effects of total pressure variations on the output signals. This is particularly useful when measuring gases at fluctuating total pressure (e.g. during rebreathing).

Other factors may cause variations in the over-all mass spectrometer sensitivity, e.g. partial blockade of the inlet capillary; variations in ionization current or in pumping rates. As these variations tend to attenuate all mass spectrometer output signals by the same factor, the feedback control circuit compensates for them. It may hence be addressed as an *automatic stability control*. The time constant of compensation depends on the time constant of the feedback system, which should be shorter than the response time of the mass spectrometer.

There are several ways in which the feedback control circuit can be realized (see Scheid *et al.*, 1971; Slama and Scheid, 1975). Its use generally results in a significant increase in the signal-to-noise ratio and in long-term stability of the mass spectrometer, and in many cases it is necessary for a correct interpretation of the mass spectrometer signals. There are, on the other hand, applications when Px is needed rather than Fx, and a modern mass spectrometer should provide the alternative option of reading the output as partial pressure (no feedback circuit) or as fraction (with feedback circuit).

Automatic Peak Control

A requirement for optimum measurement is that the mass spectrometer is tuned, and remains tuned, to the peak of the mass under study. Several factors may cause the peak to fall off the ion detector and this results in changing sensitivity which appears as drift. We have developed a feedback circuit for automatic peak control of one selected mass in respiratory mass spectrometry (H. Slama and P. Scheid, unpublished).

Figure 9 is a diagram to explain the operation of this control circuit. It shows a segment of the spectrum, displaying the mass spectrometer output for a range of the voltage U_B (e.g. accelerating voltage in magnetic sector; d.c. or r.f. voltage in quadrupole). The peak is represented by the voltage U_P. If U_B is now modulated at a frequency, f, with an amplitude, U_M, of about 1/4 of the peak half-width, the output signal, $I(t)$, will be modulated with an amplitude and a phase that depends on the position of U_B relative to U_P. If there is perfect tuning, i.e. $U_B = U_P$ (Fig. 9A), $I(t)$ will oscillate with a frequency $2f$, while for $U_B \neq U_P$, this oscillation, with frequency f, is of higher amplitude.

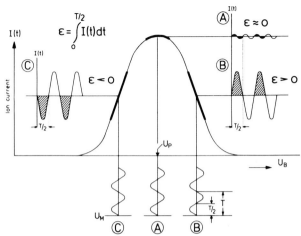

FIG. 9. Schema of operation of the automatic peak control circuit. See text for details.

Relative to the phase of U_M the phase angles are 180° different when $U_B > U_P$ (Fig. 9B) compared with $U_B < U_P$ (Fig. 9C). Hence, phase-related integration of the output over the first half of the modulating cycle will result in a positive signal, $\varepsilon > 0$, in Fig. 9B, in a negative signal, $\varepsilon < 0$, in Fig. 9C, and in a zero signal, $\varepsilon \sim 0$, in Fig. 9A. This signal ε may thus be used in a feedback circuit to adjust the d.c. level of U_B until ε is minimized and $U_B \sim U_P$.

This automatic peak control circuit reduces the drift in respiratory mass spectrometers as most factors affecting peak tuning modify the peaks of all gases simultaneously. It is, however, also very useful for tuning the mass spectrometer to a given peak while reading the respective ε on a meter.

Cross-Talk Correction

The spectrum of a given compound produced by electron impact ionization usually comprises several peaks at different m/e ratios (see p. 133). This fragmentation spectrum becomes increasingly complex with increasing number of atoms in a given compound. Cross-talk may thus result with complex fragmentation spectra of a gas mixture.

Assume gas x and y are measured on their main peaks, $(m/e)_x$ and $(m/e)_y$ [$\neq (m/e)_x$]. Assume further, that a fragmentation peak of gas y occurs at $(m/e)_x$. The output on $(m/e)_x$ will thus depend on the concentrations in the sample of both gases x and y. This cross-talk of gas y on the output of x can be corrected for by subtracting from the output of x an appropriate fraction of the output of y. This fraction is determined by zeroing the output of x when only y, but not x, is present in the sample.

With electron impact ionization CO_2 produces a peak at 28 amu with an intensity of about 10% of the main peak at 44 amu (Muysers and Smidt, 1969). This peak, which interferes with that of N_2, is due to formation of CO^-. Without cross-talk compensation, the error can be avoided by measuring N_2 on 14 amu with a relative sensitivity of about 10% of the main peak; to this peak, CO_2 contributes insignificantly (about 0.02% of the main peak). Cross-talk correction, however, allows measurement at the stronger main peak of 28 amu. For more complex compounds of higher molecular mass the fragmentation spectrum in the available mass range may be so complex that no two contamination-free peaks may be found. In this case, cross-talk correction is mandatory.

The cross-talk correction can be built into the amplification stage of the mass spectrometer. It is, however, necessary to provide facilities for adjusting the cross-talk fraction, even in mass spectrometers set at fixed masses, since the cross-talk fraction may vary. For the use of the automatic sensitivity control (see p. 152), cross-talk correction is mandatory.

APPLICATION OF RESPIRATORY MASS SPECTROMETRY

This section will demonstrate some applications of respiratory mass spectrometry to problems in the respiratory laboratory. In the examples described below a redesigned magnetic sector mass spectrometer has been employed, and the discussion will start with a short outline of the modifications applied.

Redesign of a High Performance Mass Spectrometer

We have redesigned the magnetic sector mass spectrometer Varian M3 (MAT, Bremen, Germany) which was on the market until a few years ago. The set-up and performance of this machine has been described in detail by Muysers and Smidt (1969). Briefly, it has 4 adjustable ion collectors that yield a mass range of 4 to 80 with a resolution of $m/\Delta m = 50$. Vacuum system and electronics had been designed according to the technical standard of the 1960s.

Technical Realization

The changes that have mainly contributed to the improvement of the performance include the following.

Vacuum system. The oil diffusion pump is replaced by a turbo-molecular pump (TPH 200 or 270, Pfeiffer, Wetzlar, Germany). These pumps yield a constant high vacuum in the second stage of about 10^{-6} mmHg. They do not need a cold trap in the vacuum system and can be cooled with a small external cooling unit. A major advantage is their high pumping efficiency for gases of high molecular mass so that there is no back-diffusion of oil vapour from the rotary pump back through the turbomolecular pump into the high vacuum. This results in a very clean spectrum.

An adjustable valve is introduced between the sample chamber and the pre-vacuum pump of the first stage by which the pressure in the sample chamber can be maintained at 1 mmHg even when changing the sampling rate. This pressure assures optimum conditions in the inlet capillary (see p. 132).

First-stage amplification. High-impedance FET-input IC electrometer amplifiers (AD 515 L, Analog Devices, Nordwood, Mass.) are used in conjunction with low-noise high-impedance resistors ($10^9 - 10^{11}\Omega$; type RX-1, Victoreen, Cleveland, Ohio) as impedance converters at the ion detector.

Automatic stability control. The feedback control circuit of Scheid *et al.* (1971) in the technical version of Slama and Scheid (1975; see p. 150) is incorporated into the second amplifiers. This allows for choosing between partial pressure or fraction as output signals.

Automatic peak stability. This feedback circuit (see p. 153) is added and can be used for tuning each ion collector to its peak maximum and for controlling proper peak tuning for any selected mass.

Temperature stabilization. The temperature of the analyser (first and second stage) is stabilized by an analogue feed-back which eliminates drift in the sensitivity for the masses due to temperature fluctuations.

Number of channels. A fifth ion collector is added. Although this collector, unlike the initial four, is fixed, it can be adjusted to the desired m/e by adjusting the accelerating high voltage. The remaining masses can then be set by adjusting the position of the collectors relative to this fixed collector.

Sensitivity of the Redesigned Mass Spectrometer

The sensitivity was measured by the signal-to-noise ratio for O_2 and

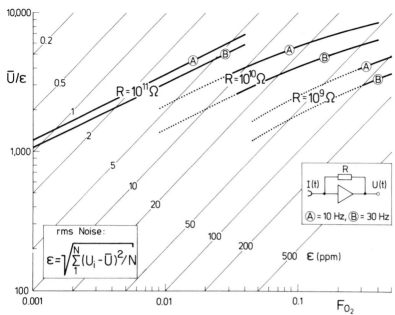

FIG. 10. Signal-to-noise ratio, $\bar{U}/\varepsilon$, against O_2 fraction, F_{O_2}, in the redesigned magnetic sector mass spectrometer. For details, see text. In the range of the dotted lines, which are based on measurements, use of the higher resistance is recommended (larger $\bar{U}/\varepsilon$ ratio).

CO_2 at various fractions of these gases. For determination of noise, the signal, after appropriate back-off and amplification, was fed into a minicomputer (MINC 1103) using a 12 bit AD converter at a sampling rate of 115 Hz. (115 Hz was used to avoid synchronization with line a.c. frequency, 50 Hz.) A total of $N = 4000$ points, U_i, were thus collected during about 40 s and the signal-to-noise ratio, $\bar{U}/\varepsilon$, was determined using eqn. (5).

Figure 10 shows the results of measurements for O_2 with 3 different high-ohm resistors in the head amplifier, each at two different low-pass frequencies (filter frequency corresponds to the 3 dB point of an active 3-pole filter). At any given O_2 fraction, F_{O_2}, $\bar{U}/\varepsilon$ is larger, hence the noise smaller, the higher the resistor. The upper F_{O_2} limit for a given resistor is, however, set by the overload limit of the head amplifier (10 V in this case). This is reached for $R = 10^{11}\Omega$ at $F_{O_2} = 0.04$, and for $R = 10^{10}\Omega$ at 0.4. It is thus advisable to choose R so that the head amplifier will yield 10 V for the largest concentration expected in the sample.

The signal-to-noise ratio for any given resistance, R, increases with the signal. For constant noise level, this increase would occur along lines parallel to the constant-noise lines in Fig. 10. If, on the other hand, the noise increased in proportion to the signal, $\overline{U}/\varepsilon$ would remain constant. The increase in $\overline{U}/\varepsilon$ occurs approximately in proportion to the square root of the signal (slope equal to 0.5 in the double-logarithmic plot of Fig. 10).

The noise increases with the bandwidth, however, less than in proportion to the square-root of the bandwidth. This is probably because the mass spectrometer itself acts as a low-pass, cutting out significantly between 10 and 30 Hz. With $10^{11}\Omega$ this bandwidth is sufficiently small to yield no major differences between 10 and 30 Hz filtering at the output.

In the range of respiratory variation in F_{O_2}, the signal-to-noise ratio is about 4000 at 30 Hz ($R = 10^{10}\Omega$), resulting in a discrimination threshold of less than 0.00005 ($= 50$ ppm) (see Fig. 10). At trace levels, $F_{O_2} < 0.001$, the signal-to-noise level is still above 1000 yielding a discrimination threshold of 1 ppm or less. Measurements for other gases yielded comparable results.

Application of the Redesigned Mass Spectrometer

Rebreathing: Use of Stable Isotopes at Trace Concentrations

Rebreathing has been used by many investigators as a non-invasive method for measuring pulmonary capillary blood flow ($\approx$cardiac output, $\dot{Q}$) in normal subjects and in patients (cf. Piiper and Scheid, 1980). In this method, the subject breathes in a closed system, and the disappearance rate of a moderately soluble inert gas (e.g. C_2H_2) is continuously monitored for calculating $\dot{Q}$. The method has later been applied to the measurement of lung diffusing capacity, D_L, using O_2 as the measured gas (Adaro *et al.*, 1973; cf. Piiper and Scheid, 1980).

Two major problems arise, however, during the measurement of $D_L O_2$ by this method: (1) as D_L is obtained from the rate of approach of alveolar ($=$ end-expired) to mixed venous P_{O_2} ($P_{\bar{v}}O_2$), $P_{\bar{v}}O_2$ must be measured with high precision. (2) The analysis requires knowledge, and assumes constancy, of the slope of the blood O_2 dissociation curve. It can be shown that the use of a rare (stable) isotopic O_2, e.g. $O^{18} - O^{18}$, circumvents these problems, and the only requirement is that the level of the rare isotope is much smaller than the $P_{\bar{v}}O_2$ of the abundant isotope.

Use of rare isotopes provides yet another advantage. CO cannot simply be measured by mass spectrometry as it cannot easily be sepa-

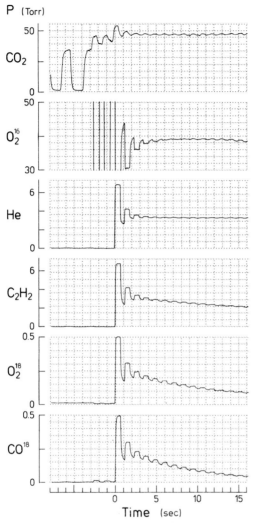

FIG. 11. Typical recording of various gases during rebreathing. All gases except CO_2 were simultaneously recorded with a magnetic spectrometer. Noise levels are undetectable.

rated from N_2 (see p. 142). However, the stable isotopes $C^{12}O^{18}$ and $C^{13}O^{18}$ can easily be analyzed in the presence of respired gases.

Recently, Meyer *et al.* (1981) have simultaneously measured D_LO_2 and D_LCO in healthy subjects at rest and at exercise using stable isotopes. Figure 11 shows a recording in a typical rebreathing manoeuvre. The mass spectrometer was adjusted to record O_2^{16}, He (lung volume determination), C_2H_2 (cardiac output), O_2^{18} (D_LO_2), and $C^{12}O^{18}$ (D_LCO) (CO_2 in the upper trace was recorded by other techniques). The recording shows virtually undetectable noise levels which are less than 1% of the full-scale recording. Hence, the noise level (in mmHg) are: O_2^{16} : < 0.2; He and C_2H_2 : < 0.06; O_2^{18} and CO^{18} : < 0.005. The corresponding signal-to-noise ratios were thus: $O_2^{16} > 200$ at 40 mmHg; He and C_2H_2 : > 100 at 3 mmHg; O_2^{18} and $CO^{18} > 100$ at 0.25 mmHg. Figure 10 shows in fact that the signal-to-noise ratio of the mass spectrometer used was still appreciably higher at these signal levels.

In another study, both CO isotopes, $C^{12}O^{18}$ and $C^{13}O^{18}$, were used to measure D_L simultaneously at two different levels of CO (Meyer et al., 1981). This study involved construction of a double ion detector to utilize the mass resolution capability of the machine in distinguishing m/e of 30 and 31. The noise levels were similarly undetectable in the records. Piiper et al. (1980) have recently used the stable isotope $C^{13}O_2^{16}$ to measure the rate of CO_2 equilibration in the human lung by rebreathing mass spectrometry.

Pattern of Respired Gases during Hyperventilation:
Discrimination sensitivity

When ventilation is stimulated without elevating metabolism, e.g. by inspired CO_2 administration, the tidal variations of partial pressures of respired gases diminish. Scheid et al. (1979) have measured gas-blood CO_2 equilibration in dogs during hypercapnia. Figure 12 shows a recording where the dog inspired about 10% CO_2 in air ($F_1O_2 = 0.19$). The high level of CO_2 had stimulated ventilation to about tenfold the resting level without appreciable changes in metabolic rates, thereby reducing the inspired–expired differences of both F_{CO_2} and F_{O_2} to about 0.01. In order to measure the pattern of respired gases, and in particular to determine end-expired levels, the sensitivity of recording had to be increased compared with the air-breathing control. The noise level,

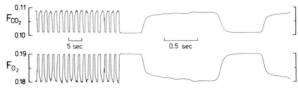

FIG. 12. Typical recording of F_{CO_2} and F_{O_2} at the mouth of a dog during spontaneous breathing of a hypercapnic mixture. Note, enhanced recording sensitivity. Different time scales to the left and to the right.

however, remained undetectable, thus below 0.0001 (100 ppm) at the recording level. The signal-to-noise ratio required in this case is 0.1/ 0.0001 = 1000, and Fig. 10 shows that the actual value at this level is even higher, but not much. In fact, similar recordings in our laboratory with a commercially available quadrupole respiratory mass spectrometer yielded serious impairment of the recording by appreciable noise.

Regional Sampling in the Lung: Mass Spectrometry during Bronchoscopy

Hugh-Jones and West (1960) were the first to use a respiratory mass spectrometer for regional sampling from single bronchi during bronchoscopy in patients. Denison and his colleagues at the Brompton hospital in London have adopted and extended this technique during fibreoptic bronchoscopic diagnosis in patients (cf. Williams *et al.*, 1979). They have mainly used Argon and Freon 22 to measure accessible lung volume and pulmonary capillary blood flow to lung regions distal to the sampling probe.

Recently this method has been extended to include measurement of pulmonary CO diffusing capacity during a single exhalation (Denison, Davies, Meyer, Pierce and Scheid, 1980). The subject inhaled one breath of a mixture containing 1% He, 1% C_2H_2 and 0.07% $C^{12}O^{18}$ in air while the tip of the mass spectrometer inlet tube, advanced through a fibre-optic bronchoscope, sampled from a given lobar bronchus. The three gases were monitored during the following exhalation, which was performed at a constant flow rate. Figure 13 is a typical recording, where the three signals are plotted on top of each other. Most of the irregularity in the signals derives from small variations in the expired flow rate. The noise level, however, is undetectably low in this record. For CO, for example, the inspired peak level is 0.07% (see above), and hence the noise level below 0.0007% (7 ppm).

A necessary requirement for these measurements is that the sampling rate is low compared with the flow rate at the sampling site. Total expired flow rate was 200 ml s^{-1} in these experiments, hence on the average 35 ml s^{-1} for each of the 6 lobar bronchi studied. The sampling rate was only 0.04 ml s^{-1} (cf. Denison *et al.*, 1980).

Application to Small Animals: Measurement at Reduced Sampling Rate

The small sampling rate of the mass spectrometer inlet becomes particularly important when working with small animals. Recently, Powell

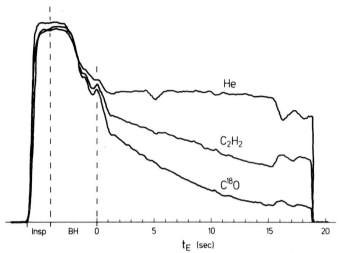

FIG. 13. Tracings of recordings of three gases during single exhalation in healthy man. The inlet probe samples through a fibre-optic bronchoscope from a lobar bronchus. Test gas was inspired during the period labelled Insp. Expiration, at constant rate, started after a period, of breath-holding, BH.

et al. (1981) have measured the respiratory gas profiles while sampling with a mass spectrometer at various sites in the bronchial system of birds. The avian lung is structurally and functionally much different from the mammalian alveolar lung (cf. Scheid, 1979), and these measurements yielded information on the pattern of airflow in the respiratory system.

Figure 14 shows two patterns of respiratory variations of F_{CO_2} and F_{O_2} both recorded at the same site in the main bronchus. The sampling

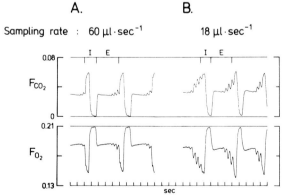

FIG. 14. Measurement of O_2 and CO_2 respiratory profiles in the duck lung at two sampling rates. I and E refer to inspiratory and expiratory phases. See text for details.

rate of 60 μl s^{-1} (=3.6 ml min^{-1}) in A was reduced in B to 18 μl s^{-1} (=1.1 ml min^{-1}) by inserting a length of wire into the inlet capillary. Rapid changes in the signal toward the end of the expiratory phase (E), due to the mechanical action of the heart, are particularly prominent at the low sampling rate (B) and are virtually completely damped out at the higher sampling rate (A).

When reducing the sampling rate it is important to check the response time of the mass spectrometer. In the above experiments, the response time was slightly larger than 100 ms, which probably did not compromise the amplitude of the cardiogenic oscillations in Fig. 14B which had a period of about 500 ms.

Measurement of Gas Solubility: Sampling from Closed Volume

Meyer and Scheid (1980) have measured solubility of C_2H_2 in liquids using mass spectrometry. In this method a liquid (e.g. blood) sample is equilibrated in a tonometer and transferred into a gas-tight vessel for re-equilibration of the gas in study between the blood phase ($\approx$2 ml) and the gas phase ($\approx$150 ml). Measurement of the partial pressure in the gas phase of the vessel allows easy calculation of the solubility coefficient of the gas in the liquid. Hlastala et al. (1980) have applied this method to low-solubility gases (He, Ar, SF_6), where the gas partial pressure becomes extremely low. For He, the signal to be analysed was 160 ppm, and for SF_6 even lower at 50 ppm. However, these signals could be measured with a signal-to-noise ratio exceeding 100 for He and 10 for SF_6.

The signal can be increased in this method by using a smaller vessel so that the given amount of gas gives rise to a larger partial pressure. There is, however, a lower limit to vessel volume set by the sampling rate and by the time required for recording a stable signal. Typically, recording for 10 s was enough in these experiments to obtain a reasonably well averaged signal, and with the sampling rate of 3.7 ml min^{-1}, the amount of gas collected from the closed system, 0.6 ml, was small compared with the total gas volume (150 ml), and decreases in total and partial pressures in the closed vessel were thus avoided.

Bridges and Scheid (1982) have modified this technique to measure CO_2 dissociation curve and buffer capacity of tissue homogenates.

CONCLUSIONS AND PERSPECTIVES

The above discussion intends to give an impression of the multitude of fields in which respiratory mass spectrometry can be applied. Of particular interest may be the use of stable isotopes as radioactive isotopes become increasingly banished from routine application. Theoretical and economic reasons demand use of trace levels of stable isotopes and this, in turn, puts considerable constraints onto the requirements of the mass spectrometer, notably on its signal-to-noise ratio and stability.

Respiratory mass spectrometers have been successful in entering the clinical routine, both for patient monitoring and for use in the diagnostic laboratory. This is due to the development of compact, movable machines that are easy to operate. These features constitute key advantages of the quadrupole compared with the magnetic sector mass spectrometer. However, the need for scanning entails a serious loss in signal-to-noise ratio of the quadrupole mass spectrometer, and we know of no commercially available quadrupole machine with sensitivity specifications as high as those of our redesigned magnetic sector. It is thus doubtful if refined lung function tests, e.g. rebreathing, stable isotopes, bronchoscopic sampling, can be performed with the quadrupole mass spectrometers that are currently on the market. It will be necessary for manufacturers and users to cooperate to design mass spectrometers with improved specifications that meet the requirements for these clinical applications.

References

Adaro, F., Scheid, P., Teichmann, J. and Piiper, J. (1973). *Resp. Physiol.* **18**, 43–63.
Ayres, S. M. (1976). *Critical Care Medicine* **4**, 219–222.
Bridges, C. R. and Scheid, P. (1982). *Resp. Physiol.* **48**, 183–197.
Buckingham, J. D. and Denis, N. T. H. (1975). *Vacuum* **25**, 489–492.
Buckingham, J. D. (1979). *In* "The Medical and Biological Application of Mass Spectrometry" (Eds J. P. Payne, J. A. Bushman and D. W. Hill), pp. 35–43. Academic Press, London and New York.
Davies, N. J. H. and Denison, D. M. (1979). *Resp. Physiol.* **37**, 335–346.
Dawson, P. H. (1976). "Quadrupole Mass Spectrometry and Its Application". Elsevier, Amsterdam, Oxford, New York.
Denison, D. M., Davies, N. J. H., Meyer, M., Pierce, R. J. and Scheid, P. (1980). *Resp. Physiol.* **42**, 87–99.
Fowler, K. T. and Hugh-Jones, P. (1957). *Br. Med. J.* **1**, 1205–1211.
Fowler, K. T. (1966). *Scand. J. resp. Dis. Suppl.* **62**, 73–82.
Fowler, K. T. (1969). *Physics Med. Biol.* **14**, 185–199.
Goodwin, B. (1979). *In* "The Medical and Biological Application of Mass Spectrometry". (Eds J. P. Payne, J. A. Bushman and D. W. Hill), pp. 49–64. Academic Press, London and New York.
Guy, H. J., Gaines, R. A., Hill, P. M., Wagner, P. D. and West, J. B. (1976). *Am. Rev. resp. Dis.* **113**, 737–744.
Hlastala, M. P., Meyer, M., Riepl, G. and Scheid, P. (1980). *Undersea Biomed. Res.* **7**, 297–304.
Hugh-Jones, P. and West, J. B. (1960). *Thorax* **15**, 154–164.

Hunt, D. F., Stafford, G. C., Crow, F. W. and Russel, J. W. (1976). *Annal. Chem.* **48**, 2098–2105.

Kydd, G. H. and Hitchcock, F. A. (1949). *Fedn Proc. Fedn Am. Socs exp. Biol.* **8**, 89–90.

Lacoste, J. (1967). *Bull. Physio-Path. Resp.* **3**, 491–502.

Leck, J. H. (1979). *In* "The Medical and Biological Application of Mass Spectrometry". (Eds J. P. Payne, J. A. Bushman and D. W. Hill), pp. 1–10. Academic Press, London and New York.

Lundsgaard, J. S., Petersen, L. C. and Degn, H. (1976). *In* "Measurement of Oxygen". (Eds H. Degn, I. Balslev and R. Brook), pp. 168–183. Elsevier, Amsterdam, Oxford, New York.

Lundsgaard, J. S., Groenlund, J. and Einer-Jensen, N. (1978). *J. appl. Physiol.* **44**, 124–128.

Mable, S. E. R. (1979). *In* "The Medical and Biological Application of Mass Spectrometry". (Eds J. P. Payne, J. A. Bushman and D. W. Hill), pp. 11–33. Academic Press, London and New York.

Marlowe, S. (1979). *In* "The Medical and Biological Application of Mass Spectrometry" (Eds J. P. Payne, J. A. Bushman and D. W. Hill), pp. 21–33. Academic Press, London and New York.

Mastenbrook, S. M., Massaro, T. A. and Dempsey, J. A. (1978). *J. appl. Physiol.* **44**, 634–639.

Meyer, M. and Scheid, P. (1980). *J. appl. Physiol.* **48**, 1035–1037.

Meyer, M., Scheid, P., Riepl, G., Wagner, H.-J. and Piiper, J. (1981). *J. appl. Physiol.* **51**, 1643–1650.

Miller, F. A., Hemmingway, A., Nier, A. O., Knight, R. T., Brown, E. B. and Varco, R. L. (1950). *J. thorac. Surg.* **20**, 714–728.

Milne, G. W. A. (1971). "Mass Spectrometry: Techniques and Applications". Wiley-Interscience, New York.

Mosharrafa, M. (1970). *Res. Develop.* **21**, 24–28.

Muysers, K. and Smidt, U. (1969). "Respirations-Massenspektrometrie". Schattauer, Stuttgart and New York.

Muysers, K. and Smidt, U. (1971). "Kolloquium über Respirations-massenspektrometrie". Schattauer, Stuttgart and New York.

Payne, J. P., Bushman, J. A. and Hill, D. W. (1979). "The Medical and Biological Application of Mass Spectrometry". Academic Press, London and New York.

Piiper, J., Meyer, M., Marconi, C. and Scheid, P. (1980). *Resp. Physiol.* **42**, 29–41.

Piiper, J. and Scheid, P. (1980). *In* "Pulmonary Gas Exchange, Vol. 1". (Ed. J. B. West), pp. 131–171. Academic Press, London and New York.

Powell, F. L., Geiser, J., Gratz, R. K. and Scheid, P. (1981). *Resp. Physiol.* **44**, 195–213.

Reed, J. W. and Hugh-Jones, P. (1979). *In* "The Medical and Biological Applications of Mass Spectrometry". (Eds, J. P. Payne, J. A. Bushman and D. W. Hill), pp. 109–116. Academic Press, London and New York.

Scheid, P., Slama, H. and Piiper, J. (1971). *J. appl. Physiol.* **30**, 258–260.

Scheid, P. (1979). *Rev. Physiol. Biochem. Pharmacol.* **86**, 138–186.

Scheid, P., Meyer, M. and Piiper, J. (1979). *J. appl. Physiol.* **47**, 1074–1078.

Slama, H. and Scheid, P. (1975). *Pneumonologie* **151**, 247–249.

Smidt, U. (1980). *In* "Biochemical Applications of Mass Spectrometry, First Supplementary Volume". (Eds G. R. Waller and O. C. Dermer), pp. 703–711. Wiley, New York and Chichester.

Symposium (1967). "Mass Spectrometer Applied to Lung Physiology". *Bull. Physio-Path. Resp.* **3**, 377–538.

Symposium (1975). *Pneumonologie* **151**, 241–295.

Watkins, P. (1979). *In* "The Medical and Biological Application of Mass Spectrometry". (Eds J. P. Payne, J. A. Bushman and D. W. Hill), pp. 85–92. Academic Press, London and New York.

Watson, J. T. (1976). "Introduction to Mass Spectrometry". Raven Press, New York.

Williams, S. J., Pierce, R. J., Davies, N. J. H. and Denison, D. M. (1979). *Br. J. Dis. Chest* **73**, 97–112.

8. TREADMILLS AND CYCLE ERGOMETERS

James W. Kane

*McMaster University, Medical Centre,
Hamilton, Ontario, Canada*

The treadmill and cycle ergometer are commonly used in the laboratory for the examination of the physiological response of subjects to exercise. Their relative use varies in different parts of the world (Atterhög *et al.*, 1979; Stuart and Ellestad, 1980), and the choice between them will rest upon a review of the intended applications and the preference of the buyer.

The cycle ergometer has the advantage that the workload presented to the exercising subject is measured accurately, and since the power output of the subject to a standard load is similar for all subjects, the oxygen consumption can be more easily predicted than with other forms of exercise. Because the energy output of subjects to a given submaximal load on the ergometer is nearly independent of their age and weight, exercise performance may be compared over a number of years.

The power output on a treadmill is determined by the speed and grade of the treadmill, and by the body weight of the subject. At a standard treadmill setting subjects of different weight have different total oxygen uptakes but a similar oxygen uptake per kilogram of body weight. This is different from cycle ergometer exercise where most of the body weight is supported and at a given load setting the total oxygen uptake is predictable.

The upper body of the subject is stable during exercise on the cycle ergometer and recording of blood pressure, the electrocardiogram and ventilation is more easily made than during treadmill exercise. Indwelling catheters for venous or arterial blood sampling are also more easily maintained because of the stability of the arms when the subject exercises on the ergometer. For exercise during cardiac catheterization, some cycle ergometers can be adapted for use by the supine subject. For subjects unable to cycle with their legs, the cycle ergometer may be used for arm exercise by mounting the ergometer before the subject at an appropriate height. It is sometimes argued that treadmill walking requires less skill and, therefore, requires less learning, than a cycling form of exercise. However, in practice this is not an important consideration and, indeed, some subjects find treadmill walking difficult at first. Because of the difficulty in fitting an adult ergometer to a young child (less than about eight years old) and because of the difficulty of some elderly subjects in maintaining cycling rhythm, the treadmill may be the best apparatus for exercise in these individuals. It is also sometimes easier for the very obese subject to walk on a treadmill than to mount and operate a cycle ergometer.

Differences of about 7% in the maximum oxygen uptake are found between the cycle ergometer and treadmill forms of exercise, the treadmill producing the higher value (Shephard, 1971). This difference can be explained by the greater muscle mass employed in treadmill running than during cycle ergometer exercise.

CYCLE ERGOMETERS

The two broad categories of cycle ergometer in general use are those which are braked by friction and those in which a braking effect is produced electromagnetically.

Friction Braked Ergometers

The mechanical, friction braked ergometers are characterized by their relative cheapness, mechanical ruggedness and ease of calibration. These features make them well suited for transporting between laboratories and to field studies since no electrical power supply is needed for their operation. During exercise on these ergometers the work done by the subject is calculated from the braking force applied to a wheel rotated by the subject multiplied by the circumference of the wheel and the number of times it is moved against the force (force × distance). When the time required to perform this physical work is considered the external work done per unit time by the subject is expressed as the power output (force × distance/unit of time). The production of power is expressed in watts, W, (joules per second, $J s^{-1}$) according to the System Internationale and formerly as kilopond metres per minute ($kpm min^{-1}$). The simplest form of laboratory ergometer is shown in Fig. 1. A strap brake is fitted to the smooth circumference of a wheel and the two ends of the strap are attached to spring balances.

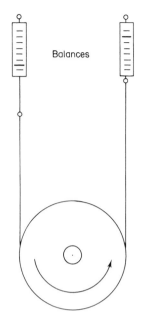

Balances

FIG. 1. A simple ergometer.

The pull on the strap can be adjusted and the frictional braking effect against the wheel during its rotation is read as the difference in tension between the two balances.

The difference multiplied by the wheel circumference and number of wheel roations is the work done in rotating the wheel. A disadvantage of this ergometer is the reliance placed on the accuracy of the spring balances and the inconvenience of adjusting the difference between the balance readings for each load. This simple form of ergometer was modified (von Döbeln, 1954) by the use of a weighing device called the sinus balance, Fig. 2. This balance which replaces the spring balances of the simple ergometer works on the following principle. If a tension T_1 is applied to a strap attached to the circumference of the balance wheel the pendulum arm will be deflected to a position which is dependent upon the force acting on the strap, the radius of the wheel, and the length and weight of the pendulum. The deflection resulting from the applied force will vary with the sine of the angle between the pendulum and the vertical starting line. If a second strap is attached to the circumference of the wheel and an opposing tension T_2 is applied, the balance will indicate the difference in the forces acting on the wheel. Thus this balance can be used to measure the braking force of a strap

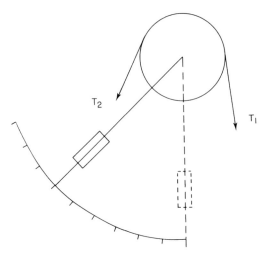

FIG. 2. Sinus balance.

applied to the circumference of the ergometer flywheel, Fig. 3. Tension in the strap is adjusted by a rack and pinion and maintained by a spring which is interposed in the strap. Work on the wheel can be measured accurately with this system, but frictional losses in the transmission from the pedals are not taken into account, and may account for an additional 5–10% in load.

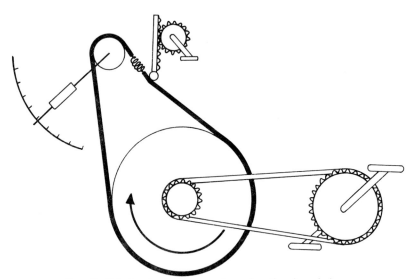

FIG. 3. Friction braked ergometer using the sinus balance.

A different approach to the use of a flywheel and belt brake was taken by Fleisch (1950), Fig. 4. The mechanism is more complex than that described by von Döbeln, does not use a balance, and provides automatic compensation for changes in friction which may occur during use from heat at the contact surface of the belt and flywheel. In the Fleisch ergometer one end of the braking strap of the flywheel is attached to a constant weight, the other end attached to an arm fixed to a wheel. The reaction to the friction of the belt against the moving flywheel will cause the arm and wheel to rotate. If a variable weight is attached to the wheel it will produce a force tending to rotate it and the belt in a direction opposite to that of the flywheel. Therefore the heavier the variable weight, the larger the surface area of belt applied to the flywheel and the larger the force needed to turn it. To suppress the tendency for the belt and weight arrangement to oscillate during use a cylinder surrounding the fixed weight acts as an air-damping device. A visual indicator is used as an aid to maintaining a constant preselected pedalling rate and total

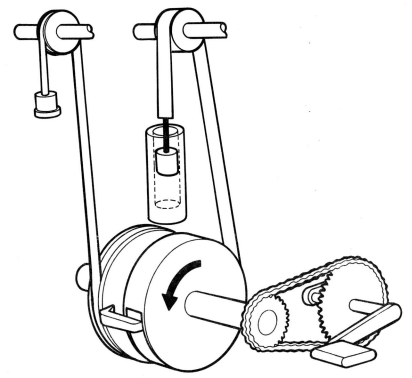

FIG. 4. The Fleisch ergometer.

pedal rotations are accumulated during exercise on a counter. The potential losses in the chain and crank transmission, which might result in a higher power output than indicated, are compensated in this ergometer by small adjustments in the variable weight related to the speed.

Another form of friction braked ergometer uses a brake pad against a wheel and a spring balance; this is not sufficiently accurate or consistent to be used in laboratory exercise testing but is of value in exercise training. Other forms of braking to produce a reproducable load which are less often seen use an oil pump and adjustable flow resistances (Dahlström, 1949); and a bicycle wheel with paddles which are moved against the resistance of air during rotation (Telford *et al.*, 1980). The former has a more expensive mechanism than the belt friction brake and the latter is simple but has a logarthmic relationship of pedalling rate and power output which makes the power output very sensitive to pedalling rate. Doubling the pedalling frequency in the belt friction braked ergometer requires a doubling of power output; in the air braked system, doubling the rate results in nearly an eightfold change in power output.

Electromagnetically Braked Ergometers

In all of the above forms of ergometer the power output (work/unit of time) is dependent on the applied braking force and the pedalling rate, which must be kept constant. This disadvantage has been overcome in a number of electromagnetically braked ergometers in which the braking force varies in an inverse ratio to the pedalling rate, within limits, through the following principle. The braking force on a copper disc spun in the field of an electromagnet is proportional to the speed of the disc and the area over which the magnet and disc interact. If the speed of the disc is increased above a certain level then the braking force of the magnet begins to decrease hyperbolically (Lanooy and Bonjer, 1956). The gear ratio of a cycle ergometer can be arranged so that a copper disc forming part of a flywheel will exceed this critical speed of rotation at the lowest usable choice of pedal revolutions and, under these conditions, the product of pedalling rate and braking force will remain constant over a range of speeds. The load is changed by changing the current through the electromagnet.

A different design which uses electromagnetic braking to maintain a preset load within the pedalling rates of 45–75 revolutions per minute uses a generator and a regulator circuit to control the current to the generator field coil and so the braking effect (Holmgren and Mattsson,

1954). The armature is driven by pedals and chain transmission and delivers its output to a loading resistor. The circuit compares the voltage drop across the resistor with a reference voltage and regulates the current to the field coil of the generator, to maintain this difference at zero, Fig. 5. A change in field coil current alters the braking effect on the armature so that the product of pedalling rate and load remains constant. Changes in load are made by changing the loading resistance and thus the voltage drop across it.

A small generator added to the circuit can provide a speed-dependent correction for potential frictional losses in the ergometer.

A more precise regulation of the current to the field coil of a generator is obtained by using the reaction torque of the stator to drive a control circuit (Atkins and Nicholson, 1963). In this device the magnetic coupling that exists between the armature and the field coil, and which tends to rotate the field coil in the direction of pedalling, is mechanically coupled to a potentiometer or strain gauge. The voltage output of the potentiometer is proportional to the reaction torque. When linked to the output from a tachometer, which is proportional to the pedalling speed, a combined voltage proportional to power is obtained. This voltage is compared with a reference voltage and a controller regulates the current to the field coil to maintain a constant load. Changes in load are made by changing the reference voltage. An advantage of this mechanism is that the deflection of the stator, which in this modified generator is permitted limited rotation, can be calibrated statically by suspending known weights at known distances from its axis and measuring the output of

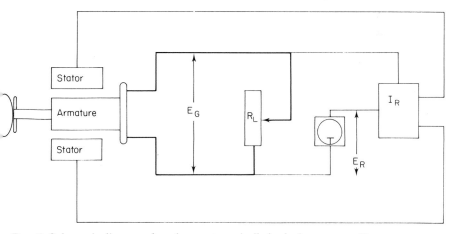

FIG. 5. Schematic diagram of an electromagnetically braked ergometer. E_G: generator voltage; E_R: Reference voltage; R_L: Loading resistor; I_R: Current regulator.

the potentiometer. None of the ergometers described above measure the frictional losses of the chain drive or the energy required to accelerate the flywheel. The actual power input to the pedals has been determined by measuring the applied torque on the pedal shaft using strain gauges (Atkins and Nicholson, 1963; Hoes *et al.*, 1968). However, to date, this approach to the determination of power output has not been adopted in commercially-available ergometers.

In both the mechanically and electromagnetically braked ergometers the mass of the flywheel when rotating reduces the irregularity of the pedalling movements by storing sufficient energy to maintain a constant velocity. The mechanical advantage during pedalling, is at a maximum when the pedals are horizontal and at a minimum in the vertical position. An ergometer with a rotating flywheel with an energy storage capacity of greater than about 110 J at 60 r min^{-1} is comfortable to pedal and smooths the cyclic variations in applied force. Toe-clips help subjects who are unfamiliar with cycling to maintain their feet on the pedals. A fixed wheel transmission maintains a constant cycling tempo after the flywheel is in rotation, but may become a danger in no load or low load cycling if the subject stops exercise abruptly or the feet slip off the pedals because of the continued rotation due to the momentum of the flywheel.

The initial high torque which is required to accelerate the flywheel can be overcome if exercise is started with no tension on the friction belt and the observer turns the pedals by hand until the required speed is achieved. The electromagnetically braked ergometer should be designed so that there is a delay in applying the load until the subject has reached the correct pedalling rate. Alternatively, a motor may be used to provide energy to spin the flywheel until the working speed is reached.

Both mechanically and electrically braked ergometers may be obtained with continuous or with discrete increments of loading. Provided that the discrete load increments are small enough to meet the needs of the exercise procedure, usually a minimum of 8 W (50 kpm) for children or the elderly and 16 W (100 kpm) for adults, the method has the advantage of speed and reproducibility.

Some electromagnetically braked machines can be programmed to increment load at predetermined times or to continuously increase load at a predetermined rate. Ergometers are available in which the heart rate of the exercising subject is continuously monitored and used in a feed-back circuit to regulate automatically the braking of the ergometer. In this way the heart rate can be brought to a predetermined rate and maintained during a period of exercise. This may be of value during exercise training or for such studies when the blood pressure, for example, is compared in subjects at a standard heart rate.

It is an advantage if the control circuit of the electromagnetically braked ergometer is not an integral part of the ergometer but a unit which can be located for the convenience of the observer. A control unit which does not clearly indicate that the electrical power supply has been switched on may result in tests that are performed without a load ever being applied. All ergometers require an indicator of the pedalling rate displayed so that it is clearly visible to both the subject and the observer. In cycle ergometers where the power output of the subject is proportional to pedalling rate an acoustic indicator of the required rate may be used. On these ergometers an accumulating revolution counter allows calculation of total external work performed by subjects who have been unable to maintain the required predetermined pedalling rate, (work = circumference of flywheel × revolutions × applied torque).

Since oxygen uptake is not strictly determined by the load alone but varies with pedalling frequency, the rate should be recorded even on ergometers which regulate the load with changes in rate. The most efficient pedalling rate, that is the rate which produces the lowest oxygen uptake at a standard load, is between 50 and 70 r min^{-1}, the subject feeling better able to maintain pedalling if the rate is higher near maximal loads. A change in pedalling rate from 40 to 80 r min^{-1} increases the oxygen uptake of an average subject pedalling an ergometer with no added load by about 25% (Gaesser and Brooks, 1975). As maximum levels of exercise are approached it becomes increasingly difficult to maintain a fixed pedalling frequency and the subject may stop abruptly; an important measurement may be salvaged if the subject slows the pedalling rate of the rate dependent ergometer, or if the observer decreases the ergometer load. A further advantage of decreasing the required power output when the subject's maximum is reached is that venous pooling in the legs and the chance of fainting is reduced. Both the comfort and performance of the subject will be affected by the position taken on the ergometer. A seat height which is about 5–10 cm more than the inside leg measurement is optimum.

Increasing the saddle height to 112% of the leg length will increase the oxygen uptake by about 6%, (Shennun and de Vries, 1976). The seat height is measured from the top of the saddle, through the pedal axis, to the top of the pedal when it is at a point farthest from the saddle. Using this height, the knee is just flexed when the ball of the foot is on the pedal and the pedal is at its most distant point from the saddle.

The radius of the crank arm is usually about 17 cm on ergometers intended for adult use, providing a comfortable leg excursion and good mechanical advantage. Children may require a shorter crank length to keep the upper leg below the horizontal when the pedal is at its shortest distance from the saddle. It is an advantage to use an ergometer with an adjustable crank length rather than cranks of different lengths if tests are to be performed on both adults and children. Interchangeable seats for adults and children are needed, and most subjects are appreciative of seats which are more generously proportioned than those used in conventional cycling.

The constraints imposed by the equipment used for measuring ventilation usually prevent the subject from adopting the cycling positions which might be used in heavy bicycling, when dropped handlebars are an advantage. However, an attempt should be made to ensure that the subject is in a position which permits comfortable stabilization of the upper body during exercise: handlebars at approximately the waist height of the seated subject and a saddle to handlebar distance which brings the subjects trunk forward of vertical with the elbows slightly flexed. The saddle height and other adjustments of the ergometer position are recorded with the subject information so that they may be reproduced for the subject at subsequent tests. A handlebar and saddle stem calibrated in centimeters is an aid to making these adjustments.

Ergometers which are adapted to arm cranking exercise use a longer crank arm radius than is used in leg cycling. This is usually between 21 cm and 30 cm with the crankshaft height at about the waist level of the subject (Atzler and Herbst, 1927). The optimum speed for arm cranking is lower, 40–50 r min^{-1} than in cycling. The physiological responses to arm cranking are different from those of cycling (Bobbert, 1960) and the oxygen cost of cranking with both hands on the same handle and one hand on alternate handles, is different. Some ergometers advertised as being suitable for both cycling and arm cranking make the transition from one form to the other only with considerable effort on the part of the laboratory staff. If an ergometer is intended for both uses, at frequent intervals, the ease of conversion should be examined before purchase.

Safety

The electrical safety of the electromagnetically braked ergometer must meet local medical standards and be tested regularly for electrical leakage, keeping in mind the risk of electrically conductive paths to other equipment from skin electrodes or intra-arterial and venous catheters. The protective covers now found on many ergometer cranks, chains and wind paddles protect against serious lacerations, and even lost digits in children. No ergometer should be in general use without such protection.

Calibration

Friction belt ergometers using a balance may be statically calibrated by hanging a known weight from the balance at the point of belt attachment after checking the zero.

Errors in the balance are unusual, once accurately set, unless the mechanism has been damaged. The balance on von Döbeln type ergometers can be made to read accurately by adjusting the centre of gravity of the balance arm. This procedure, of course, only calibrates the measuring device of the ergometer as does the static calibration of the stator in some electromagnetically braked ergometers.

Dynamic calibration of cycle ergometers is the method of choice and calibrates the complete system including the frictional resistance of the transmission from the pedal shaft (Cumming and Alexander, 1968). In the dynamic calibrator, or torque balance, a direct current motor and step-down gear box drives the ergometer from the pedal shaft. The housing of the motor is mounted on bearings so that it can turn freely and an arm is attached to the housing. In use, the motor is driven at a known rate at each of the ergometer load settings. The electromagnetic coupling between the housing and drive shaft of the motor tends to rotate the housing but is restrained by the attached arm which rests on a balance. The housing arm and balance indicate the torsional force exerted at the pedal shaft and the power output, p, can be calculated:

$$p = f \times l \times 2\pi \times n$$

where f = balance reading; l = length of lever; n = revolution of pedal shaft per unit time.

Conversion to watts can be made by multiplying kpm min^{-1} by 0.1635. Calibration may be different at different pedal rates and change as the ergometer heats up during use. Dynamic calibration in a number of laboratories has shown that large errors are not uncommonly present in electromagnetically braked ergometers (Jones and Kane, 1979).

In the absence of a continuously available calibrating device large changes in ergometer calibration can be detected by regularly exercising one or two laboratory subjects and comparing their measured physiological variables with previous values.

Maintenance

Ergometer maintenance is straightforward but essential; a poorly maintained friction belt ergometer can have a frictional load in the transmission which is more than twice that found in one which is well maintained. Transmission maintenance is similar to that for a bicycle; the chain should be lubricated with light machine oil as required and the tension adjusted so that the chain moves vertically about half an inch. The ball bearings of the pedal axle and balance are checked for damage and greased once or twice yearly. Ergometers with totally enclosed transmissions require oil changes in accordance with the manufactures recommendations, at least every second year of use.

Accumulated grease and dust on the friction belt and flywheel of the ergometer will cause an erratic balance reading which is cured by cleaning the wheel surface with alcohol and reversing or changing the belt.

TREADMILLS

The treadmill is a continuous belt which is moved across a platform by an electric motor. The belt speed and angle (grade) can be changed. The most obvious difference between treadmills is one of size, (the smaller treadmills being only suited to training and rehabilitation). Treadmills having a motor with a rating of greater than one horsepower are generally suited to the commonly used exercise testing protocols.

For medical applications a treadmill speed which is variable to 11 km h^{-1} (7 mph) and an elevation to 11 degrees (20% gradient) is adequate. Research applications may require the higher speed and elevation in large and more expensive treadmills. The belt is driven from the main motor through a continuously variable transmission which is controlled by a subsidiary motor from the control box when a change in belt speed is desired. More recently, electronically controlled d.c. drive motors have been used in this application. Elevation is achieved using a hydraulic system or, more frequently, with a fractional horsepower electric motor. A consideration, other than the maximum speed and elevation, is the response time to a command from the control box; a long transition time from one speed or elevation to another could create inaccuracies in the application of a chosen test protocol. The change in speed with a heavy subject walking on the belt should be insignificant. Treadmills using a belt material and platform which need lubrication will slow from increased friction if this service is neglected.

Polyester and nylon belts have generally replaced belt materials such as wood filled phenolic compounds and are more durable than rubber, although the latter runs more quietly and presents a more comfortable walking surface. A belt tread surface area of 46 cm × 150 cm is adequate for the stride of most subjects, except athletes, during walking and running exercise. A braking system is important in an emergency and should stop the treadmill in 2–3 s from 11 km h^{-1}. The braking mechanism is usually electromagnetic and operation should be possible from the treadmill and control panel.

Before purchasing a treadmill it will be necessary to consider the space it will occupy and the electrical power needed. A large treadmill may be too wide to pass through a doorway and a tall subject at maximum elevation might not have head room to run. A small room is unsuitable for the use of a large treadmill because of the space requirements for other equipment associated with the exercise procedure, for safety if the subject loses balance or collapses, and for acoustic reasons. A 3-phase drive motor is preferable to a single phase motor, if the necessary power can be provided, because it is quieter in operation. A great advantage in the clinical setting is a treadmill on which a subject can stand while the operator slowly increases the speed from zero until the desired speed is reached. For research purposes a few treadmills are available which may be elevated at either end, making them suitable for studies involving negative work. The control panel, which should be mounted separately from the treadmill, indicates belt speed and elevation and changes may be made using continuous manual adjustment, or manual step adjustments according to a particular protocol. As with cycle ergometer control systems automatic programme circuits and heart rate controlled circuits are also available. A revolution counter on the control panel will show the distance the subject has travelled during a study.

The power output of a subject on the treadmill is governed by the subject's weight, and the treadmill speed and grade. The oxygen uptake may be predicted using one of a number of formulae van der Walt and Wyndham, 1973; Givoni and Goldman, 1971). The oxygen uptake is higher in running than walking at the same speed and holding the handrails during exercise can reduce the oxygen uptake by about 17%. The inexperienced subject will often feel apprehensive on first approaching the treadmill which is more noisy and imposing than the cycle ergometer; every attempt should be made to give the subject a feeling of security. The subject should be shown how to get on and off the moving belt by grasping the handrails on either side of the platform, putting the weight on one foot, taking a good step forward with the other, and immediately following with the first foot so that the subject is then walking on the treadmill. The subject should be instructed to walk upright and not look down at the belt or feet. When walking confidently, the subject should, if possible, remove his hands from the handrails which, in any case, should not be gripped hard. It is easier to get off the treadmill if it is first brought down to the minimum tread speed and then stopped, or alternatively, the subject moves backwards and steps off the belt with one foot which is quickly followed by the other. The subject should be allowed to walk on the treadmill before being connected to a mask or mouthpiece. The potential danger in an emergency of rigidly fixing a valve holder to the subject's head should be considered before this technique is used.

Safety

A handrail is essential and preferably will extend along the side of the treadmill. An emergency stop switch should be available on the treadmill for the subject to operate if needed, and an automatic switch, actuated by a bar behind the subject, will stop the treadmill in the event of the subject falling. In children and the elderly, the risk of losing a footing on the treadmill is great and, for these subjects and others at risk, there should always be an observer standing behind the treadmill to help the subject in an emergency. In one treadmill system the subject wears a harness attached to an overhead gantry and is free to walk and run. Should the subject stumble or fall, the harness not only provides support but actuates a treadmill stop switch. On all except the smallest treadmills, side platforms are needed which elevate with the treadmill. This facilitates close contact with the subject for physiological monitoring and safety purposes. The treadmill may also be hazardous to laboratory staff and these hazards can be reduced by guards fitted to the ends and underside of the treadmill where the moving belt could contact the operator's feet or clothes (see also Chapter 14).

It if is possible to turn the treadmill on at a high speed an indicator on the control panel should give a clear warning that the treadmill is in this condition so that the speed may be reduced before the subject steps on to the belt.

The importance of electrical safety has been mentioned previously.

Calibration

It is reasonable to demand that the speed and elevation of a treadmill to be accurate to within 5% of the indicated setting. Speed indication is derived from a tachometer generator and the elevation from a multiturn potentiometer driven by the elevation pinion gear.

Tread Speed

The tread speed can be determined by marking a line across the belt and measuring the length of the belt, setting the control to the desired speed and, together with a stopwatch, counting the number of belt revolutions per minute. The tread speed is then:

$$\text{speed (km h}^{-1}) = \frac{\text{r min}^{-1} \times 60 \times \text{belt length}}{1000}(\text{m})$$

This calibration should be made at several tread speed settings and the indicator adjusted or a calibration graph constructed showing the correct speed values. The treadmill speed should also be measured with a subject on the belt at near maximum elevation. The belt may run faster unless the treadmill has been equipped with a regenerative braking mechanism to overcome this error.

Elevation

The accuracy of the elevation meter is checked after levelling the treadmill platform using a carpenter's level and shims under the treadmill feet as required. The zero position of the indicator is read and, if necessary adjusted by changing the position of the multiturn potentiometer on the treadmill, and then elevated to a setting near maximum incline. The angle of the platform from the horizontal can be read using a large protector or inclinometer, or by measuring off a fixed distance on the floor and measuring the difference in height over this distance. The gradient is calculated by simple trigonometry, Fig. 6. Other elevation settings can be checked in the same way and the indicating meter control reset if necessary.

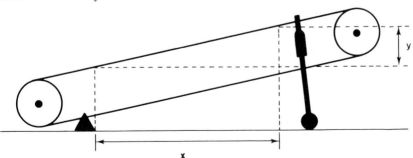

FIG. 6. Calibration of treadmill elevation. % grade = $y/x \times 100$; angle of elevation = tan y/x.

Maintenance

Treadmills with belts which need regular lubrication are waxed with dance floor wax or lubricant supplied by the manufacturer. This is applied, approximately weekly if the treadmill is used daily, on the inner surface of the belt so that it lubricates the walking platform. This wax may become a slipping hazard to the laboratory personnel, if scattered on the floor around the treadmill. Inadequate lubrication will result in excessive belt wear and drive motor overloading.

The belt tension and alignment may require adjustment after considerable use and will wander across the platform when this is necessary. Realignment is carried out with an unloaded treadmill by making small changes to the adjustable roller position to bring the belt to the centre of the rollers and platform. The treadmill is run at about $10\,\mathrm{km\,h^{-1}}$ for about one minute to allow the belt to find its new position between adjustments. If the adjustment is made at the front of the treadmill the belt will move away from the side of the roller which is being adjusted towards the front of the machine. To prevent slipping low friction nylon and polyester belts are run at a higher tension than rubber or phenolic material belts, but this imposes a greater demand on the bearings of the drive and take-up rollers of the treadmill. Care should be taken to follow the manufacturers lubrication instructions for these bearings.

The final drive chain requires lubricating at approximately monthly intervals or it may become noisy and wear rapidly. A loose or worn drive chain will cause the treadmill belt to hesitate momentarily with each foot-fall.

Lubrication of the other components should follow the manufacturers recommendations and will greatly extend the trouble-free life of the treadmill. A thorough service should be performed after approximately every 1000 hours of use.

References

Atkins, A. R. and Nicholson, J. D. (1963). *J. appl. Physiol.* **18**, 205.
Atterhög, J. H., Jonsson, B. and Samuelsson, R. (1979). *Scand. J. Clin. Lab. Invest.* **30**, 87.
Atzler, E. and Herbst, R. (1927). *Pflüger's Arch. ges. Physiol.* **215**, 291.
Bobbert, A. C. (1960). *J. appl. Physiol.* **15**, 1007.
Cumming, G. R. and Alexander, W. D. (1968). *Can. J. Physiol. Pharm.* **46**, 917.
Dahlström, H. (1949). *Svenska Läk-sällsk. for handl.* **46**, 944.
Fleisch, A. (1950). *Helv. med. Acta Ser. A.* **17**, 47.
Gaesser, G. A. and Brooks, G. A. (1975). *J. appl. Physiol.* **38**, 1132.
Givoni, B. and Goldman, R. F. (1971). *J. appl. Physiol.* **30**, 429.

Hermansen, L. and Saltin, B. (1969). *J. appl. Physiol.* **26**, 31.

Hoes, M. J. A. J. M., Binkhorst, R. A., Smeekes-Kuyl, A. E. M. C. and Vissers, A. C. A. (1968). *Int. Z. angew. Physiol. einschl. Arbeitsphysiol.* **26**, 33.

Holmgren, A. and Mattsson, K. H. (1954). *Scand. J. Clin. Lab. Invest.* **6**, 137.

Jones, N. L. and Kane, J. W. (1979). *Medicine and Science in Sports* **11**, 368.

Lanooy, C. and Bonjer, F. H. (1956). *J. appl. Physiol.* **9**, 499.

Repco Health System Company, P.O. Box 349, Victoria, 3175 Australia.

Shennum, P. L. and de Vries, H. A. (1976). *Medicine and Science in Sports* **8**, 119.

Shephard, R. J. (1971). *In* "Frontiers of Fitness", (Ed. R. J. Shephard). Charles C. Thomas, Springfield, Illinois.

Stuart, R. J. and Ellestad, M. H. (1980). *Chest* **77**, 94.

Telford, R. D., Hooper, L. A. and Chennells, M. H. D. (1980). *Aust. J. Sports Med.* **12**, 40.

van der Walt, W. H. and Wyndham, C. H. (1973). *J. appl. Physiol.* **34**, 559.

von Döbeln, W. (1954). *J. appl. Physiol.* **7**, 222.

9. MEASUREMENT OF THE MECHANICAL PROPERTIES OF THE THORAX, LUNGS AND AIRWAYS

G. J. Gibson

Freeman Hospital, Newcastle upon Tyne, U.K.

To move air into the lungs the respiratory muscles must overcome forces of three different types, elastic, resistive and inertial, which are related respectively to changes in volume, flow and acceleration of gas and tissue. The magnitude of each is determined by the compliance (or elasticity), resistance and inertia of the chest wall, lungs, airways and thoracic gas. Except when breathing with a very rapid frequency, the contribution of inertial forces is small (Mead, 1961) and usually ignored. The major site of resistive forces is in the airways; flow resistance of lung tissue has been the subject of many studies but the current view is that it is very low and much of what was previously described as "tissue resistance" is more correctly a reflection of the elastic properties of the lungs (Bachofen and Scherrer, 1970). The major compliant structures are the alveolar ducts, alveoli and the chest wall; the conducting airways are also elastic but the volume of gas they contain is small relative to the gas-exchanging part of the lung.

The mechanical properties of the respiratory system are therefore largely determined by the resistance of the airways and the distensibility of the lungs and chest wall. Elegant techniques have been developed for the measurement of these variables and will be described. Their theoretical background is straightforward but the practical difficulties of direct determination of resistance and compliance are such that neither measurement is routine in most lung function laboratories. Instead, the elastic properties of the respiratory system are usually inferred from the simpler measurements of static lung volumes and resistive properties assessed by tests of forced expiration. The latter are less demanding of equipment and expertise and may even in certain situations give information which is clinically more useful than the "purer" index of resistance, but the theoretical background of the forced expiratory manoeuvre is more complex.

The basic items of equipment necessary for assessment of the mechanical properties of the respiratory system have been described in earlier chapters, i.e. devices for measuring pressure, flow and volume. One further piece of equipment which is frequently used in measurements of lung mechanics is the whole body plethysmograph and its principles will be described before more detailed accounts of the individual measurements.

BODY PLETHYSOMOGRAPHS

When an individual inspires, the volume of gas in his lungs changes for two reasons. First, the transfer of gas from the surrounding air into the lungs, and second, the rarefaction of gas in the lungs (both resident and inspired) accompanying the associated fall in intrathoracic pressure (Boyle's law). Converse effects occur on expiration when intrathoracic pressure is above atmospheric. During normal breathing, the effect of transfer of gas into and out of the lung is quantitatively much more important but the whole body plethysmograph (or box) utilizes this additional "Boyle's Law effect" to measure the volume of gas in the lungs.

Body plethysmographs are of two main types: constant volume (DuBois *et al.*, 1956a) and variable volume (Mead, 1960). The essential difference in design is that in the constant volume instrument (Fig. 1(a)) the subject is seated in an enclosed box and breaths air from within the box itself, while in the variable volume box the subject breathes directly from the room and the plethysmograph measures the resulting changes in thoracic volume by displacement either into a spirometer (Fig. 1(b)) or through a flow measuring device whose output is electrically integrated to give volume (Fig. 1(c)).

The constant volume box is the most commonly used in routine lung function laboratories and is more suitable for measurements of airways resistance and absolute thoracic gas volume. With a subject breathing inside a constant volume box there is, if we ignore any changes due to temperature and humidity differences, no nett change in volume of the total system (box + subject) but the alternating rarefaction and compression of intrathoracic gas will be reflected in reciprocal changes in the pressure of gas in the box. This phenomenon is used in two different ways so that box pressure, with appropriate calibration signals, can be

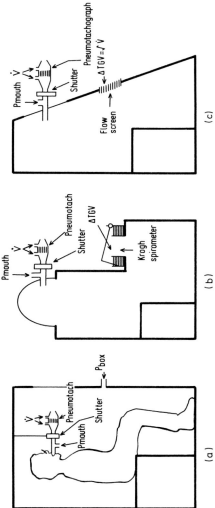

FIG. 1. Three types of whole body plethysmograph. (a) Constant volume plethysmograph—the subject is seated completely within the box and breathes in and out from the box. The mouth pressure and box pressure are measured by separate transducers and the mouthpiece is attached to a shutter assembly and pneumotachograph across which flow is measured by a third transducer. (b) Variable volume box with Krogh spirometer: the mouthpiece is connected to the exterior and attached to a shutter and pneumotachograph assembly as in (a). Changes in TGV are recorded directly with a low impedance spirometer. (c) Variable volume box with flow screen: similar to (b) except that change in TGV is obtained by integration of flow across a flow screen with linear resistance in the wall of the box.

used to measure either change in thoracic gas volume (during volume measurements) or in alveolar pressure (during measurements of airways resistance); the details are described below. The constant volume box therefore needs to be sensitive to small pressure changes and is used during fairly rapid manoeuvres which require a good frequency response. It should be as rigid and leak-free as possible but these requirements are not absolute.

In the variable volume box (Fig. 1(b) and (c)) the volume displaced is due to both mass transfer of gas and Boyle's Law effects. Such instruments are sometimes incorrectly described as "constant pressure" which they cannot be, since a pressure has to develop in the box before a volume change is produced; this immediately presents a problem in that a square wave volume change in the box will not be precisely reproduced by the pressure measuring device (Fig. 2). Attempts have been made to overcome this by "compensating" the volume signal by the addition of a signal related to pressure in the box, (van de Woestijne and Bouhuys, 1969; Leith and Mead, 1974). This can be done whether volume is measured by an external spirometer (Fig. 1(b)) or by integration of air flow through the wall of the box (Fig. 1(c)). In practice it is usually simpler with the latter: flow is measured by a sensitive transducer which is as nearly linear as possible. The volume displaced is then the integral of flow with respect to time ($\int d\dot{V}_{box}$) and with a linear resistance (where flow is directly proportional to pressure drop) this

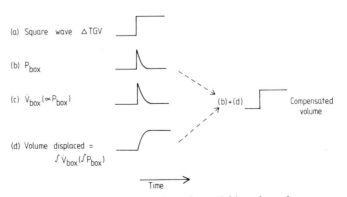

FIG. 2. Principle of pressure compensation of a variable volume box: a square wave change in volume (a) produces a transient rise in box pressure (b). If the flow screen has a linear resistance the resulting flow through the box wall ($\dot{V}_{box}$) is directly proportional to P_{box} (c) and on electrical integration gives volume displaced (d) which has a blunted profile and lags slightly behind (a). Addition of signals (b) and (d) with appropriate amplification reconstitutes (a).

equals $\int k dP_{box}$ (where k is a constant). To this signal is added electrically a signal proportional to box pressure itself with the aim of reconstituting a square wave change in the volume recorded (Fig. 2). A variable volume plethysmograph "compensated" in this way for pressure changes is sometimes known as a pressure–volume plethysmograph. Further details of setting up such an instrument are given by Leith and Mead (1974). Although this type of box can be used for direct measurements of thoracic gas volume (TGV) it is in practice less convenient for measurements of airways resistance. The variable volume box is also used for manoeuvres where knowledge of changes in TGV is required, e.g. during the measurement of flow–volume and pressure–volume curves (see below). Because it may be used for measurements over several minutes, it is necessary to keep the air in the plethysmograph at constant temperature. This is usually achieved by a refrigeration circuit.

ASSESSMENT OF ELASTIC PROPERTIES OF LUNGS AND CHEST WALL
(See also Gibson and Pride (1976))

Theoretical Aspects

The lungs and chest wall may be regarded as two elastic structures arranged mechanically in series so that they share the same volume change and the pressure distending the total respiratory system (P_{RS}) is given by the algebraic sum of the pressures distending the lungs and chest wall individually (Fig. 3). The pressure distending each structure

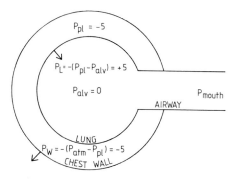

FIG. 3. Balance of static pressures acting on lungs and chest wall. Each component develops a recoil pressure equal and opposite to the distending pressure. During relaxation at FRC, $P_{alv} = 0$ (glottis open) and then $P_L = -P_{pl}$, $P_W = P_{pl}$ and $P_L = -P_W$.

is opposed by an equal and opposite elastic recoil pressure, whose value is used to characterize the distensibility of each. In the case of the lungs the distending static transpulmonary pressure is given by the difference between the pleural surface pressure (P_{pl}) and the pressure within the alveoli (P_{alv}) and this is equal and opposite to the elastic recoil pressure of the lungs (P_L)

$$\text{i.e. } P_L = - (P_{pl} - P_{alv}) = P_{alv} - P_{pl} \qquad (1)$$

With the chest wall the distending pressure is given by the difference between the nett pressure resulting from contraction of the respiratory muscles (P_{mus}) and the pleural surface pressure and this is opposed by the recoil pressure of the chest wall (P_W)

$$\text{i.e. } P_W = - (P_{mus} - P_{pl}) = P_{pl} - P_{mus} \qquad (2)$$

For the intact respiratory system the total recoil pressure (P_{RS}) is given by the sum of eqns (1) and (2) and is equal and opposite to the difference between P_{mus} and alveolar pressure

$$\text{i.e. } P_{RS} = P_L + P_W \qquad (3)$$

$$P_{RS} = - (P_{mus} - P_{alv}) = P_{alv} - P_{mus} \qquad (4)$$

In the particular situation of complete muscular relaxation ($P_{mus} = 0$) eqns (2) and (4) simplify respectively to:

$$P_W = P_{pl} \qquad (5)$$

$$P_{RS} = P_{alv} \qquad (6)$$

Since the chest wall is partly composed of muscles, its elastic behaviour may be dependent on their degree of tone. Measurements of chest wall recoil pressure or compliance during complete muscular relaxation (e.g. under anaesthesia or after use of neuromuscular blocking drugs) may therefore differ from those made during "voluntary" relaxation.

The compliance ($\Delta V/\Delta P$) of normal lungs is dependent on their size, so that, for example, the left and right lungs contribute in relation to their respective volumes. Although the bulk of the volume change occurs in alveoli, the alveolar ducts and even the conducting airways also contribute to the overall compliance of the lungs. The shape of the pressure–volume (PV) curve of the lungs above resting lung volume (FRC) resembles a monoexponential curve with a gradually diminishing compliance as volume increases (Fig. 4). Below FRC the measured curve often deviates from a simple monoexponential. Opinions differ on the cause of the apparently lower compliance below FRC—in

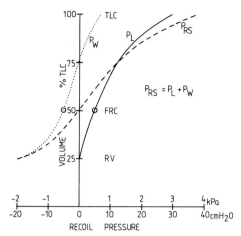

FIG. 4. Pressure volume curves of lung (solid line), chest wall (dotted line) and total respiratory system (broken line). At FRC (open circles) P_{RS} equals zero and P_L equals $-P_W$; below approximately 75% TLC chest wall recoil is outwards (negative) and above this volume both the lungs and chest wall have an inward (positive) recoil.

some circumstances it may be due to oesophageal artefacts (see below) but there is also evidence indicating progressive closure of airways during deflation, with the result that lung units below their closing volume no longer contribute to volume change and thus the total compliance falls below FRC (Glaister et al., 1973; Ingram et al., 1974). The static pressure–volume curve of the lungs also depends on the previous volume history and measurements during interrupted inspiration show higher recoil pressure and lower values of compliance than during expiration (Fig. 5). This difference results partly from hysteresis of lung tissue but quantitatively more important is the difference in numbers of lung units contributing to the volume change on inspiration and expiration, i.e. at a given lung volume on inspiration it is likely that fewer units are contributing but each individual unit is more distended than at the same overall volume on expiration.

Because the pressure–volume curve of the lungs is curvilinear it is difficult to characterize the elastic properties simply. A single value of compliance (C_L) remains the most frequently used index but, because of difficulty in measuring a tangent to the curve, the relationship is usually approximated to a straight line over the tidal breathing range, e.g. FRC + 0.5 l; alternatively, values of lung recoil pressure at standard lung volumes may be used but preferable is examination of the whole curve either visually or mathematically by fitting an exponential function (Salazar and Knowles, 1963; Gibson et al., 1979). The spe-

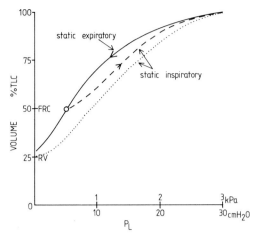

FIG. 5. Pressure volume curves of the lung determined during interrupted expiration (solid line) and during interrupted inspiration from both FRC (broken line) and RV (dotted line). The expiratory curve below FRC often shows a reduction in compliance (slope of the line). Curves obtained during interrupted inspiration are displaced to higher values of recoil pressure and show lower compliance in the tidal breathing range.

cific compliance (C_L/V) is sometimes used to compare individuals of different sizes but note that (unlike specific airways conductance) this cannot be used to compare measurements at different lung volumes *within* a subject as compliance and volume above FRC have an inverse relation.

Changes in the pressure–volume curve of the lungs may result from alterations in shape, in slope or in position (Fig. 6). With normal aging the slope increases a little but the major change is a reduction in recoil pressures at all lung volumes. In patients with emphysema there is more marked loss of lung recoil and much greater increase in the compliance in the tidal range together with a pronounced increase in the total lung capacity (TLC). In asthma the TLC also increases and the PV curve again shows some loss of recoil but there is little change in compliance in the tidal range. The situation in chronic airways obstruction without significant emphysema is probably similar to asthma, while with the typical restrictive defect of pulmonary fibrosis the compliance is greatly reduced as is the total lung capacity (Gibson and Pride, 1977).

Measurements are sometimes made of the so called "dynamic compliance" of the lungs when, during tidal breathing, pressure and volume are measured at points of zero air flow at the mouth. Such measurements are often not a true reflection of the static elastic properties of the lungs because events at the mouth may be out of phase with events in

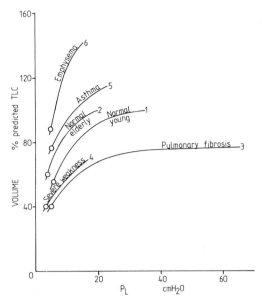

Fɪɢ. 6. Pressure volume curves of the lung in various physiological and pathological states. For each curve the open circle represents the position of FRC and the upper end of the curve the position of TLC. Compared to the curve for a healthy young subject (1), that for an older normal subject (2) shows slightly increased compliance, but predominantly a displacement to lower recoil pressures. With a reduced TLC due to pulmonary fibrosis (3) very high recoil pressures at TLC are generated whereas with severe respiratory muscle weakness (4) recoil pressure at TLC is less than normal. In asthma (5) the curve is displaced to lower values of recoil pressure but the compliance is close to normal, while in emphysema (6) the recoil pressures are much lower and both the compliance and TLC are greatly increased.

the lungs; the difference between "dynamic" and static compliance is however sometimes used as a relatively sensitive index of increased resistance in the peripheral airways.

The normal static pressure–volume curve of the chest wall (Fig. 4) is less well established because reproducible measurements are more difficult and need to be made during relaxation—either "voluntary" or under anaesthesia. At volumes below FRC the chest wall is much less compliant, probably due to passive stretching of the diaphragm as it is displaced further up into the chest rather than to inability to compress the rib cage (Agostoni, 1970). In infancy, the chest wall is very compliant and with age it becomes relatively stiffer compared to the lungs, with an increasing outward recoil at low volumes (Agostoni and Mead, 1964). Disease of the chest wall is much less common than disease of the lungs: severe curvature of the spine (scoliosis) may cause a reduction in chest wall compliance but in younger patients this measurement may remain normal even with fairly severe deformity (Caro and DuBois, 1960).

Techniques
(see also Macklem (1974))

Measurement of the pressure–volume curve of the lungs requires apparatus for recording changes in lung volume and in transpulmonary pressure. The volume change may be determined by either a spirometer or a variable volume plethysmograph. The advantage of the latter is that measurements can be made during interrupted inspiration or expiration with the subject relaxing against a closed mouthpiece and the associated changes in thoracic volume due to gas compression are immediately evident on the volume record. With a spirometer, unless a correction is applied, the subject has to maintain an open glottis and cannot relax during breath holding. Oesophageal pressure is usually measured with a thin walled latex balloon in the mid or lower oesophagus (Milic Emili et al., 1964). Various artefacts are well recognized, for example too much air in the balloon may distend the oesophagus itself and produce a pressure reflecting the elasticity of the oesophagus rather than the lungs. In general the smallest volume compatible with negligible recoil of the balloon itself is chosen (Milic Emili et al., 1964) and this is usually between 0.2 and 0.5 ml. This in turn demands a catheter and transducer system with a very small volume. Further artefacts may arise from the mediastinum and measurements of pleural pressure in the supine posture may therefore be unreliable. Cardiac oscillations are seen on the record and for greater accuracy measurements at a fixed time in the cardiac cycle may be used (Trop et al., 1970).

The balloon is usually introduced after local anaesthesia of the nostril to the lower third of the oesophagus and its depth adjusted until pressure at end expiration is most negative and the cardiac artefact least. With a 10 cm long balloon this is usually 38–42 cm from the nostril, depending on the subject's height. Alternatively, the balloon may be introduced to a standard depth of ($\frac{height}{5}$ + 9) cm (Zapletal et al., 1976).

Measurement of the pressure–volume curve is usually made during interrupted expiration after at least three full inspirations. The subject is asked to maintain an inspiratory effort at TLC until a reasonably steady pressure is recorded, the airway is then occluded, he is allowed to relax and subsequently to breathe out in convenient volume decrements with repeated interruption for periods of 1–2 s (Fig. 7). Stress relaxation is usually seen at TLC, especially when recoil pressures are high and presents particular problems of measurement—most authors record a peak transpulmonary pressure and in addition a "static" value at TLC obtained after a full inspiratory effort has been sustained for 4–5 s. At lower volumes during stepwise expiration stress recovery may be seen and 1–2 s at each volume may be necessary to achieve a plateau of pressure. The readings of transpulmonary pressure and change in volume are then plotted against each other and a direct determination of lung volume (see p. 198) allows reference to an absolute volume scale. Some investigators prefer to record a complete PV curve during a single slow expiration; such a quasi-static PV curve is convenient for direct recording on an oscilloscope or XY recorder but the static transpulmonary pressure may be slightly overestimated. Similar measurements may be made during interrupted or very slow inspiration from either FRC or RV: this measurement is usually preceded by one full inspiration but the conventions are less well established.

If dynamic compliance is being measured, especially at rapid breathing frequencies, the frequency response characteristics of the system are much more critical and a pneumotachograph is necessary at the mouth to measure points of zero air flow. The subject is asked to take a full inspiration followed by an expiration to FRC and then to breathe, usually with a predetermined tidal volume and constant end

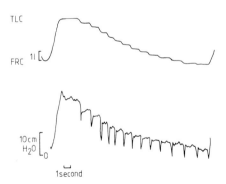

FIG. 7. Record of volume expired (upper tracing) and transpulmonary pressure ($P_{mouth} - P_{pl}$) during interrupted expiration. During breath holding $(P_{mouth} - P_{pl}) = (P_{alv} - P_{pl}) = P_L$ (eqn (1)). From the plateau values of volume and pressure the static expiratory PV curve can thus be constructed. During the brief expirations between breath holding P_{pl} becomes less negative and therefore $(P_{mouth} - P_{pl})$ falls. Oscillations on the pressure record represent cardiac artefacts. Note that the peak pressure at TLC is greater than the sustained pressure.

expiratory volume which are displayed to him on an oscilloscope. The dynamic compliance is calculated for each breath by dividing tidal volume by the change in transpulmonary pressure between the points at zero flow and the mean of at least 10 breaths is usually taken. To investigate the frequency dependence of dynamic compliance the procedure is repeated at selected breathing frequencies.

The pressure–volume curve of the chest wall is usually obtained by determining the curve for the total respiratory system and subtracting the lung curve (Fig. 4). The relevant pressure here is transthoracic i.e. the difference between alveolar pressure and body surface during muscular relaxation (eqn (6)) and volume is measured as for lung PV curves. Some trained subjects can produce consistent results during "voluntary" relaxation of the respiratory muscles but most patients cannot. An alternative is to use the method of Heaf and Prime (1956) in which positive and negative pressures are applied at the mouth.

STATIC LUNG VOLUMES

Theoretical Aspects

In practice, the distensibility of the lungs can usually be assessed by measuring lung volumes. The simplest measurement is the vital capacity (VC). This may be reduced not only when the lungs are small ("restrictive" ventilatory defect) but also in patients with diffuse airways obstruction whose lungs cannot be emptied normally. These may be distinguished by measuring TLC (which is usually increased in airways obstruction and decreased when there is reduced distensibility). A restrictive defect (i.e. reduced VC and TLC) may result from either intrapulmonary disease (e.g. fibrosis of the lungs) or from extrapulmonary factors such as muscle weakness or pleural disease. Theoretically, measurements of compliance should distinguish between these conditions but in practice the compliance is reduced not only in patients with intrapulmonary disease but also in many with respiratory muscle weakness (Gibson et al., 1977) (Fig. 6). The distinction may be made by measurement of maximum respiratory pressures (p. 212).

The two main techniques for the measurement of absolute lung volume are described below; either helium dilution or plethysmography is usually used to estimate FRC whence TLC and RV are easily calculated by addition of the inspiratory capacity or subtraction of the expiratory reserve volume respectively. In normal subjects both methods give similar results but large differences are seen in patients with airways obstruction. The first technique uses helium as a marker gas which is breathed in a closed circuit so that it is diluted with resident gas in the lungs and when a stable concentration is reached it is assumed full equilibration has taken place with intrathoracic gas. Using a dilution equation, the volume of thoracic gas with which the helium has been mixed is then easily calculated. In patients with significant airways obstruction equilibration is much slower and a stable end point may not be reached in a convenient time if the lungs contain areas which are very slowly ventilated. An extreme example occurs with large air-containing cysts or bullae which are effectively unventilated and therefore their volume will not be measured. Such areas will however be exposed to pressure changes and therefore measured by the plethysmographic technique which in general estimates all intrathoracic gas. Abdominal gas also contributes to the plethysmographic estimate to the extent that it shares similar pressure changes; this will depend on which muscles are used during the respiratory efforts (Fig. 8). If the subject makes inspiratory efforts predominantly with the inspiratory intercostal and accessory muscles, changes in abdominal pressure are in the same direction as the changes in alveolar pressure and TGV will be slightly overestimated; the effect of diaphragmatic contraction, however, is to reduce the intrathoracic pressure but to increase the abdominal pressure so that if efforts are made with the diaphragm alone TGV is underestimated. In practice most subjects during this measurement pant in the former way but since the volume of abdominal gas is small, the overestimation of TGV is unlikely to be more than 200 to 300 ml (Habib and Engel, 1978).

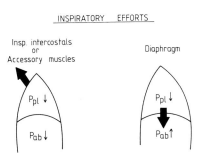

Fig. 8. Inspiratory efforts performed in two different ways: use of the inspiratory intercostals or accessory muscles (left hand diagram) produces a fall in pleural pressure which, if the diaphragm is relaxed is transmitted to the abdomen so that abdominal pressure also falls and abdominal gas is therefore subject to similar pressure changes as thoracic gas. If the diaphragm alone is used it also lowers pleural pressure but increases abdominal pressure so that abdominal gas is compressed as thoracic gas is rarefied.

Techniques

Helium Dilution Technique

The technique evolved from earlier versions which used oxygen or hydrogen. The advent of the katharometer (Chapter 4) rapidly established helium as the gas of choice as it is both inert and safe (Meneeley and Kaltreider, 1949). The subject rebreathes in a closed circuit from a spirometer; the circuit also includes a soda-lime canister for absorbing CO_2, a fan to mix the gases and a supply of oxygen which is continuously added to compensate for the oxygen consumed by the subject and to maintain the total volume of the system (apparatus + subject) constant. For greatest accuracy the total volume of the apparatus should be approximately equal to the volume being measured (i.e. the FRC of the subject). The patient is connected to the closed system at end expiration and the flow of oxygen is adjusted as necessary to keep the end-expiratory level in the spirometer constant. The patient breathes from the circuit until the helium reading stabilizes; the recommended tolerance is a range of not more than 0.02% over a 30 s interval (Ferris, 1978). Although the apparatus is simple, it is essential that it be airtight and the procedure is time-consuming if repeated measurements are to be made. In patients with severe airways obstruction equilibration may require more than 15 min and an arbitrary end point may have to be taken. Prolonged rebreathing exaggerates any errors due to leaks or to the swallowing of gas from the circuit.

Plethysmographic Technique

Although the constant volume plethysmograph is more commonly used, the principle is more easily appreciated with the variable volume box and the method using the latter will be described first. To make a measurement a shutter in the mouthpiece is closed and the subject is asked to make inspiratory and expiratory efforts. Since the airway is closed there is no movement of air into or out of the lungs but during inspiratory efforts the negative alveolar pressure produces some rarefaction of alveolar gas. The accompanying expansion of the thorax displaces a small volume of gas out of the plethysmograph into the spirometer or through the flow screen. From Boyle's Law the original thoracic gas volume (V) is related to the change in TGV (ΔV) and change in alveolar pressure (ΔP) by the relationship:

$$V = P\Delta V/\Delta P \qquad (7)$$

(where P is barometric pressure—water vapour pressure). During panting against a shutter the change in alveolar pressure is normally equal to pressure at the mouth where it can easily be measured with a suitable transducer and ΔV is measured directly as the displaced volume. In practice mouth pressure (i.e. alveolar pressure) is displayed against ΔV on an oscilloscope or XY recorder and the slope of the resulting line is measured and substituted in eqn (7). Mouth pressure is generally a reliable index of alveolar pressure provided the subject does not close his glottis and supports his cheeks with his hands while panting against the closed shutter. As soon as the shutter opens the subject is asked to take a full inspiration and the inspiratory capacity is directly recorded and added to the measured thoracic gas volume to give TLC.

With a constant volume plethysmograph the principle is identical, the only practical difference being that ΔV is not directly measured but is reflected in changes in box pressure, i.e. with an inspiratory effort against the shutter the increased TGV within a closed box produces a proportional rise in box pressure. The latter is calibrated in terms of volume by use of a pump with a stroke of 50–100 ml, usually with the subject seated in the box holding his breath. The inspiratory capacity is conveniently measured by integrating flow across a pneumotachograph at the mouth after opening the shutter.

The initial cost of the equipment is greater than for the helium dilution technique and greater technical expertise is required. Most patients can perform the manoeuvres satisfactorily with a little training and several determinations can be made rapidly.

AIRWAYS RESISTANCE

Theoretical Aspects
(see also Pride, 1971)

The calibre of an individual airway depends on both the intrinsic properties of its wall, including the degree of smooth muscle tone, and on the transbronchial pressure which is largely determined by the degree of lung inflation and retractive force. In normal subjects, the bronchial tree branches in such a way that, although the diameters of individual airways become progressively smaller towards the alveoli, the total cross-section of all airways of the same generation increases considerably from the trachea to the terminal bronchioles. In consequence, in normal subjects the major site of resistance during quiet

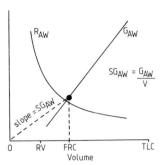

FIG. 9. Relation of airways resistance and conductance to lung volume. The slope of the G_{AW}–volume relationship would only equal SG_{AW} if the line passed through the origin, otherwise SG_{AW} varies slightly depending on the volume at which it is measured.

breathing is the central airways, in particular the larynx or, if breathing through the nose, the nasal passages. The resistance therefore tends to be dominated by the calibre of the central airways. Measurements of airways resistance are aimed at an assessment of resting airway dimensions, i.e. minimizing any dynamic effects and for this reason they are usually performed with low pressures and flows (tidal breathing or panting).

The relationship of overall airways resistance (R_{AW}) to lung volume is illustrated in Fig. 9 and is approximately hyperbolic; for this reason the reciprocal of resistance, that is airways conductance (G_{AW}) is often used since its relationship to volume is approximately linear. The important effect of lung volume can be largely removed by dividing

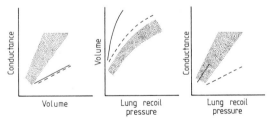

FIG. 10. Effect of loss of lung recoil on airways conductance: schematic diagram showing results in two patients with airways obstruction, one (solid line) with severe emphysema the other (broken line) with bronchial disease alone. Both show abnormally low conductance in relation to the lung volume (left). The patient with emphysema has a grossly abnormal lung pressure volume curve but that for the patient with bronchial disease is only mildly abnormal so that if conductance is related to static transpulmonary pressure (i.e. lung recoil pressure—right), the value of conductance in the patient with emphysema is within the lower end of the normal range whereas that for the patient with bronchial disease remains abnormal.

conductance by the volume at which it is measured to give the index specific airways conductance (SG_{AW}). The extrapolated plot of conductance against volume does not pass through the origin so there may be slight variation of specific conductance at different volumes but for most purposes this may be ignored. Airways conductance may also be related to lung recoil pressure (Fig. 10) which allows the distinction between intrinsic airways disease (in which conductance is low in relation to distending pressure) and loss of lung elasticity, as in emphysema, where conductance is reduced in relation to lung volume but conductance is normal in relation to lung recoil pressure. Measurements of airways resistance and conductance are usually abnormal in patients with symptomatic chronic airflow obstruction but are not sensitive to early changes which result from narrowing of the peripheral airways.

Techniques

Airways resistance is defined as flow divided by the difference between alveolar and mouth pressure. The methods of measurement of airways resistance differ mainly in the technique of estimating alveolar pressure.

Subtraction Method (Mead and Whittenberger, 1953)

This method involves use of an oesophageal balloon to estimate pleural pressure; airflow at the mouth is displayed on an oscilloscope against pleural pressure during tidal breathing. Part of the pleural pressure is required to overcome elastic forces and part to produce flow; the former is subtracted by impressing on the pressure axis a voltage proportional to lung volume and adjusting the gain until the loop of flow against pressures closes. The slope of the resulting line is then an estimate of airways conductance and the gain of the volume signal applied is inversely related to the dynamic compliance. The technique is time consuming and inconvenient and now largely obsolete.

Interruptor Method

Alveolar pressure is estimated by making measurements of mouth pressure during transient interruption of airflow. Clements *et al.* (1959) devised a rotating valve which obstructs airflow 10 times a second. The determination depends on the assumptions that mouth pressure rises to equal alveolar pressure when flow stops and that there is no significant change in alveolar pressure during the interruption. Neither of these is strictly true, especially in disease. The technique tends to give results in normal subjects which are rather higher than the oesophageal balloon method but has the advantage of simplicity.

Plethysmographic Technique (constant volume instrument)

Plethysmograph pressure (P_{box}) is used to estimate alveolar pressure. The measurement is made in two stages—firstly, the subject breathes with open airway through a pneumotachograph and the relationship between flow and P_{box} is obtained on a suitable oscilloscope or XY recorder; the shutter at the mouth is then closed, the subject continues to make breathing efforts against it and the relationship between mouth pressure (now approximating alveolar pressure) and box pressure is established. By multiplication of $\dfrac{P_{mouth} \text{ (i.e. } P_{alv})}{P_{box}} \times \dfrac{P_{box}}{\dot{V}}$, P_{box} cancels out and the result is a measure of airways resistance. It is important to emphasize that the measurements are made during airflow and the closure of the airway is simply used as a calibrating technique to express box pressure in terms of alveolar pressure. P_{box} with the airway open is only a function of alveolar pressure if there are no changes due to temperature or humidity of the gas inspired and expired. This can be achieved in one of two ways—if the pneumotachograph is heated to 37°C and the subject pants very gently the front of gas moving in and out of the mouth can be limited to the pneumotachograph mesh avoiding any significant mixing with gas at ambient temperature in the box. Panting also has the advantage of minimizing the laryngeal contribution to airways resistance because it causes abduction of the vocal cords. This technique is favoured in Britain and North America. Alternatively, the subject can inspire warmed humidified gas from a separate rebreathing bag which allows measurements to be made with larger tidal volumes, e.g. during normal tidal breathing—this technique is favoured by some centres in continental Europe. The plethysmographic method has the extra advantage that TGV is measured during the same manoeuvre when the shutter is closed (see p. 198) and is therefore immediately available for expression of the results as specific conductance.

The relationship between flow and P_{box} should approximate a straight line and looping should be minimal. Formation of loops can result from various factors including temperature differences between inspired and expired gas, unequal time constants in parallel compartments of the lung or phase differences in the different amplifiers used for recording—the various factors are analysed by Jaeger and Bouhuys (1969).

Forced Oscillation Method

With this technique alveolar pressure is not measured but airflow is induced by the application of fluctuating pressure at the mouth. This is generated by attaching to a mouthpiece an oscillator and loudspeaker whose output superimposes a flow signal, measured by a pneumotacho-graph, on the subject's normal tidal breathing. The imposed oscilla-tions of pressure are sinusoidal and, as originally proposed, are applied at a frequency which minimizes the summed impedance due to elastic and inertial properties. At low frequencies elastic impedance domin-ates, while at very high frequencies inertial impedance dominates. Since they are 180° out of phase with each other it is possible to choose a frequency (the resonant frequency) at which elastic and inertial forces cancel out so that pressure is in phase with airflow and the values of pressure and flow can be used directly to calculate the resistance of the respiratory system. The resonant frequency of the normal respiratory system is approximately 5 Hz, but in patients with airways obstruction it may be considerably higher. Goldman *et al.* (1970) modified the technique to allow estimation of respiratory resistance by forced oscilla-tion at frequencies lower than the resonant values by utilizing points in the induced cycle where the components of applied pressure due to elastic and inertial properties are both equal to zero.

The volume amplitude of the sinusoidal oscillations used in adults is approximately 40 ml and is smaller for children. The pressure applied is measured together with airflow at the mouth and flow can also be integrated so that immediately after the measurement a full inspiration can be performed to calculate the volume at which the resistance was measured. The technique is usually simple to perform, rapid and suitable for use even in fairly small children, although some subjects require several minutes of acclimatization. Attempts to resist forced oscillations result in narrowing of the upper airway but this can be recognized by the appearance of large variations in amplitude of the signals. The cheeks should be supported during measurement.

FORCED EXPIRATION
(see also Pride, 1971)

Tests based on forced expiration are the most commonly performed measurements of lung function in clinical practice. The measurements are deceptively simple to make but the underlying physiology is complex. Because the airways are elastic they are susceptible to distending and compressing forces and during a forceful expiration the intrathoracic airways are exposed to the surrounding positive pleural pressure. When a subject makes a forceful expiration he may develop an alveolar pressure of the order of 100 cm H_2O which is dissipated between the alveoli and the mouth. Since from eqn (1) the alveolar pressure is equal to the sum of lung recoil pressure and pleural pressure, a value of P_{alv} of 100 cm H_2O at a volume in the middle of the vital capacity ($P_L \simeq 10$ cm H_2O) corresponds to a pleural pressure of approximately 90 cm H_2O and clearly therefore part of the intrathoracic airway is potentially exposed to a nett compressing force (Fig. 11). Equal pressure points (EPP) arise where intra- and extra-airway pressures are equal (Mead *et al.*, 1967) and downstream from the EPP (i.e. on the mouth side) the intrathoracic airways will tend to narrow. The location of the EPP during a forced expiration depends on the instantaneous lung volume and at low lung volumes (and therefore low recoil pressure) the EPP migrate further upstream towards the alveoli. Mead *et al.* pointed out that the total airway could therefore be considered as two segments defined by the position of the EPP; they went on to analyse events in the segment "upstream" from the EPP i.e. between the alveoli and EPP: the pressure drop along this segment is equal to P_{alv} minus the pressure at EPP; the latter is however by definition P_{pl} and therefore the driving pressure for airflow along the "upstream" segment equals $P_{alv} - P_{pl}$. But this also equals P_L (eqn (1)) and hence lung recoil pressure is a major determinant of maximum expiratory flow. This analysis immediately demonstrates how in patients with emphysema where P_L is reduced, maximum expiratory flow will be low, without necessarily any alteration in the airways themselves.

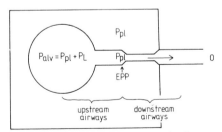

FIG. 11. Schematic diagram of events during forced expiration: at some point along the airway (EPP), the pressure inside becomes equal to the surrounding pleural pressure. Downstream from these EPP there is a tendency for dynamic compression as extrabronchial pressure is now greater than intrabronchial pressure. The pressure driving flow along the airway upstream from EPP equals $P_{alv} - P_{pl}$ i.e. lung recoil pressure.

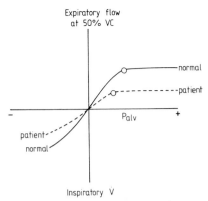

Fig. 12. Isovolume pressure flow (IVPF) curve for normal subject (solid line) and patient with airways obstruction (broken line) both recorded at 50% of the individual's vital capacity. The expiratory curve shows a plateau of flow and beyond the effective maximum pressure (open circles) increasing driving pressure does not increase expiratory flow. In the patient maximum flow is markedly reduced and the maximum effective pressure is less. With inspiratory efforts no flow plateau is achieved. The slope of the relationship close to the origin represents airways conductance at that particular volume.

The major determinant of P_L is lung volume and Fig. 12 shows the relationship of expiratory and inspiratory flow at a constant lung volume to the effort applied—this is the isovolume pressure flow (IVPF) curve, introduced by Fry and Hyatt (1960) which proved a major step forward in analysis of the factors influencing airflow during voluntary manoeuvres. Expiratory flow is obviously dependent upon effort to some extent but with applied pressures well short of the maximum which the expiratory muscles can generate, a plateau of flow is produced which represents the maximum possible at that volume. Beyond this "maximum effective pressure" greater efforts do not produce increased flow because, in simple terms, more forceful contraction of the expiratory muscles increases both alveolar pressure and pleural pressure further compressing the intrathoracic airways. At other volumes different flow maxima are achieved (Fig. 13) and in general the smaller the lung volume the less the maximum effective pressure necessary to achieve maximum flow. Tests of forced expiration are therefore often described as "effort independent" and this is largely true, provided that at least 10–20% of the maximum available effort is applied. At large lung volumes a true plateau is not achieved and the peak expiratory flow (which is measured close to TLC) is completely effort dependent. Nevertheless, it is very useful in practice as a simple guide to airway narrowing because it is usually quite reproducible after

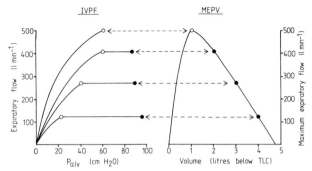

FIG. 13. Relation of IVPF to maximum expiratory flow volume (MEFV) curve in a normal subject. Each IVPF curve is recorded at a single volume and curves for four different volumes are shown, 1, 2, 3 and 4 litres below TLC respectively. Note that at the highest volume no plateau of flow is achieved whereas at lower volumes plateaux are seen; the maximum effective pressure (○) is less at low volumes and the maximum flow achieved falls with lung volume. The relationship of maximum flow to lung volume during a single forced expiratory manoeuvre is shown on the right and the closed circles represent corresponding points of flow, volume and pressure.

a few practice attempts. In patients with airways obstruction these tests become even less dependent upon effort because the more rapid dissipation of pressure along the narrower airways produces flow limitation due to dynamic compression at higher lung volumes and with smaller maximum effective pressures.

Figure 12 also illustrates an IVPF curve during forceful inspiration with different voluntary efforts. Although the relationship of flow to applied pressure is curvilinear, no plateau is achieved and the greater the effort the higher the airflow. During forceful inspiration the airway is always exposed to a nett distending force and therefore no flow limiting mechanism due to dynamic compression operates. Maximum inspiratory flow is, however, dependent on lung volume since this determines the static dimensions of the intrathoracic airways and it is also determined by the strength and rate of contraction of the inspiratory muscles.

It is useful to compare the information obtained by, on the one hand, tests of airways resistance and, on the other, tests of maximum flow. Although both usually tend to move in the same direction in disease there is no reason to expect a proportional change in the different indices. Although the IVPF curve is never constructed simply to measure airways resistance, the latter is directly represented on the curve (Fig. 12), since the slope of the line passing through the origin represents airways conductance and clearly there is no *a priori* reason why this sould bear a direct relationship to the plateau value of maximum expiratory flow. For reasons explained above SG_{AW} is sometimes regarded as an index of "large" airway calibre since in normal subjects it is mainly determined by the more central airways and early changes in peripheral airways are more readily detected by examining flow at small lung volumes (see below). In established generalized airways obstruction, however, this distinction becomes blurred. In practice, the IVPF curve is used as a tool for research and teaching rather than clinical investigation and all indices based on forced expiration (and inspiration) are derived from two related curves, the flow–volume curve and volume–time curve, which will now be described.

Flow–Volume Curve

The IVPF curve examines events at a single lung volume and clearly there is an infinite number of such curves over the vital capacity. If the flow maxima from each volume are taken and related to the volume expired the resulting maximum flow volume curve, also introduced by Fry and Hyatt (1960), has a characteristic, and in an individual highly reproducible, shape (Fig. 13). At the start of a forceful expiration maximum flow rises rapidly to a peak (approximately equivalent to the value recorded by a peak flow meter) and then in a young normal subject declines in an approximately linear relation to lung volume. With age (Fig. 14) the curve tends to become more convex towards the volume axis, i.e. there is a disproportionately greater reduction in maximum flows at lower volumes. Maximum inspiratory flow volume curves are

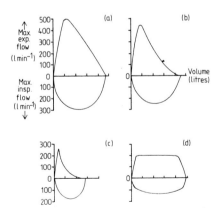

FIG. 14. Examples of maximum flow curves in (a) normal young and (b) elderly subjects, (c) in severe intrathoracic airways obstruction (e.g. asthma) and (d) upper airway obstruction (e.g. tracheal stenosis).

much more symmetrical with peak inspiratory flow close to the middle of the vital capacity. Various indices have been derived from the curve, such as maximum flow rates at standard lung volumes (e.g. 50% VC), but in routine testing the overall shape of the curve may be the most useful feature and certain characteristic patterns are immediately recognizable (Fig. 14). With generalized intrathoracic airways obstruction, such as in asthma and emphysema, all flows are reduced; this is most evident at low volumes and the appearance of the flow–volume curve is an exaggeration of the normal change with age. In early airways obstruction there is some evidence that examination of maximum flow rates at low lung volumes detects changes before they are apparent with simple indices such as the FEV_1. Another characteristic pattern appears in patients with obstruction of the upper (extrathoracic) airway (Miller and Hyatt, 1973). Here a further resistance is in effect added in series with the normal resistance of the dynamically compressed intrathoracic airways. The effects are similar to those of an incomplete effort, i.e. a reduction of maximum flow rates at high lung volumes but not at low, and a reduction of maximum inspiratory flow rates at all volumes (Fig. 14(d)). Maximum expiratory flows at low lung volumes remain unchanged because flow is here less effort dependent and pressure can be dissipated across the narrowed upper airway without any effect on the flow, which is determined by dynamic compression of the intrathoracic airways. At higher volumes, however, flow limitation by this mechanism is less complete and the result of the addition of a series resistance is apparent. Similar appearances result from inability to apply the necessary force, e.g. in patients with weakness of the respiratory muscles.

Flow is usually measured at the mouth either with a pneumotachograph or by electrical differentiation of the expired volume signal. Volume may be recorded by integration of flow or by having the subject expire into a spirometer with an electrical output so that flow can be displayed against volume on a suitable recorder. An oscilloscope is preferable because the frequency response of XY plotters is not usually sufficient to cope with the more rapid events at higher volumes. An alternative means of recording volume which has some advantages is by use of a variable volume plethysmograph; the volume recorded by a spirometer reflects only bulk transfer of gas from the lungs into the spirometer and the inevitable compression of thoracic gas by the positive alveolar pressure is not seen. If any detailed assessment of lung mechanics is being performed it may be desirable to relate expiratory flow directly to thoracic volume and in particular to lung recoil pressure of which thoracic volume and not expired volume is the relevant

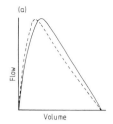 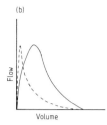

FIG. 15. Maximum expiratory flow volume curves obtained by measurement of flow at the mouth and either Δ TGV (solid line) or volume expired (broken line) in (a) a normal subject and (b) a patient with severe airways obstruction. There is little difference in the normal but a marked difference in the patient and the difference in volume at a given flow represents the effects of gas compression which is only seen in a plethysmograph.

determinant. Two different curves may therefore be recorded—flow against expired volume and flow against change in TGV (Ingram and Schilder, 1966); the differences in normal subjects are not large but they may be considerable in patients with significant airways obstruction who have a large residual volume (Fig. 15). In such a patient, a 10% reduction in thoracic volume resulting from the application of an alveolar pressure of 100 cm H_2O (1/10th of an atmosphere) may represent a large proportion of the limited vital capacity.

In an individual subject differences in repeat measurements of flow volume curves most commonly result from slight inconsistencies in the preceding maximum inspiration. At least three manoeuvres should be performed and the vital capacity during the manoeuvre should not vary by more than ±5% or ±0.1 l, whichever is greater (American Thoracic Society, 1979). The flow indices recorded are usually the best achieved during at least three attempts. Various methods of reading flow–volume curves have been analysed in detail by Peslin et al. (1979).

Volume–Time Curve

It is clear from examination of the maximum expiratory flow–volume curve that during a forced expiration the initial rate of lung emptying is rapid and becomes progressively slower as more of the vital capacity is expelled. In normal subjects the volume expired within the first second represents the majority of the vital capacity (the FEV_1/VC ratio in healthy young subjects exceeds 75% and in older subjects exceeds 70%). Other intervals have been used for measurement of forced expiratory volume ($FEV_{0.5}$, $FEV_{0.75}$ etc.) but they convey little additional information. The FEV_1 may be expressed as a ratio of either the vital capacity or the forced vital capacity (FVC)—the latter is performed during the same manoeuvre and the former is the maximum volume expired during either a forced or relaxed manoeuvre. Use of the VC has the advantage that this is also the measurement used for the calculation of the other subdivisions of lung volume and therefore it avoids an extra measurement on a lung function test report. In normal subjects there is little difference between VC and FVC but in patients with significant airways obstruction the FVC usually underestimates the VC and when testing responses to bronchodilator drugs the relaxed measurement often gives more useful information. The FEV_1/VC (or FEV_1/FVC) ratio is the simplest and in practice most useful guide to the presence of significant airways obstruction and, although normal in the early stages, it will inevitably be reduced in symptomatic patients; however, quantitative changes in its value should be interpreted with caution—a larger improvement in VC or FVC than in FEV_1 is often seen, resulting in a fall in the ratio with undoubted improvement of the patient's airways obstruction.

A further derivative of the volume–time curve which has been widely applied especially in North America is the maximum mid-expiratory flow (MMEF also known as $FEF_{25-75\%}$) which is the mean expiratory flow rate measured between 25 and 75% of the vital capacity (Leuallen and Fowler, 1963). In general it gives similar information to the FEV_1/VC ratio.

A more recent development has been the application of mean transit time (MTT) analysis to the forced expiratory spirogram (Tockman *et al.*, 1976). The principle is derived from the estimation of the mean transit time of an indicator injected into the circulation and represents

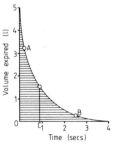

FIG. 16. Record of expired volume against time during a forced vital capacity manoeuvre: gas molecules expired early have a short transit time from alveoli to the mouth, (e.g. 0.2 s at point A) while later in the breath the transit time is longer (e.g. 2.5 seconds for gas molecules arriving at the mouth at point B). The mean transit time (c) is given by the integrated area under the curve divided by the FVC.

the average time for gas molecules to travel from alveoli to the atmosphere during a forced expiration. The MTT is calculated by integration of the area under the volume time curve and then dividing the area by the forced vital capacity (Fig. 16); the measurement is particularly sensitive to the presence of slowly emptying alveoli with very long transit times and may therefore be useful in detecting early changes in peripheral airways. In this respect it is comparable with measurement of maximum flow at low lung volumes on the flow volume curve but its value remains to be fully assessed.

Measurements during forced inspiration (e.g. FIV_1) are of value in the recognition of patients with upper airways obstruction, especially if the facility is not available for measuring flow–volume curves.

RESPIRATORY MUSCLE POWER

Theoretical Aspects

Muscle power is conventionally described by the force–length relationship. Ideally the power of the respiratory muscles would be assessed by measuring the force generated either during voluntary efforts or after application of standard stimuli. In practice force cannot be directly measured and respiratory muscle function is usually inferred from measurements of the pressure generated statically (usually at the mouth) during maximum voluntary inspiratory and expiratory efforts. A pressure volume relationship rather than a force–length relationship can be established. The relationship between force and pressure is determined by the geometry of the thorax and in the case of the diaphragm, its radius of curvature determines the pressure developed across the diaphragm for a given linear tension. As originally pointed out by Rohrer (1916), the pressure recorded at the mouth during a static effort is not the same as the pressure generated by the muscles (P_{mus}) since the recoil pressure of the respiratory system has to be taken into account. By rearrangement of eqn (4), $P_{mus} = P_{alv} - P_{RS}$ (or under static conditions $P_{mus} = P_{mouth} - P_{RS}$). Rohrer demonstrated that by measurement of mouth pressure during relaxation (which allowed calculation of P_{RS}) and during static voluntary efforts the relationship of P_{mus} to lung volume could be derived (Fig. 17). Expiratory pressures tend to be greatest close to full inflation and inspiratory pressures greatest (i.e. most negative) at FRC or below. In practice, measurements of expiratory pressure initiated at TLC and of inspiratory pressure initiated at FRC or RV are sufficient to detect moderate or severe respiratory muscle weakness. The volume dependence of the

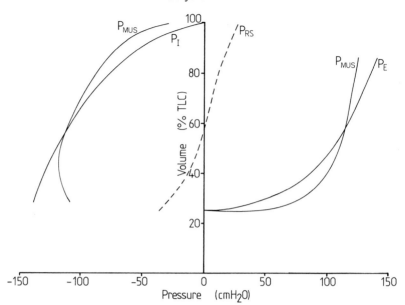

FIG. 17. Pressure volume relationships during maximum efforts (redrawn from Rohrer (1916)). The lines labelled P_I and P_E represent values of mouth pressure (equal to P_{alv}) recorded during a series of maximum inspiratory and expiratory efforts against a closed airway. P_{RS} (broken line) is the recoil of the total respiratory system, obtained by measurements of mouth pressure at various lung volumes during relaxation (closed airway). The nett pressure generated during maximum efforts by the inspiratory and expiratory muscles respectively (P_{mus}) is then equal to P_I (or P_E) $- P_{RS}$ (c.f. eqn (4)).

pressures recorded in normal subjects would suggest that in hyperinflated patients (with severe airways obstruction, e.g. emphysema) less negative inspiratory pressures might result and this is usually the case though some adaptation of inspiratory muscle function seems to occur. Considerable interest has been shown in recent years in the possible role of fatigue of the respiratory muscles (Macklem and Roussos, 1977) and elegant electromyographic methods have been developed to detect evidence of fatigue. This is an expanding area of research but so far the techniques have not been widely applied and the exact role of "failure" of the respiratory muscles (perhaps akin to failure of cardiac muscle) is not clearly defined.

Techniques

Measurements of maximum respiratory pressures vary considerably depending on the technique used and they are entirely dependent on the co-operation of the subject. It is therefore particularly important to

compare the values obtained with normal data recorded with identical
techniques rather than to rely on data from the literature. The mouthpiece arrangement may considerably influence the results and greater
pressures are recorded with specially designed mouthpieces (Cook *et
al.*, 1964). Use of a tight fitting face mask may produce greater pressures in very weak patients if they have associated weakness of the facial
muscles. Artefactually high pressures may sometimes be produced by
the cheek muscles if the glottis is closed and can be avoided by introducing a small leak in the mouthpiece (Ringqvist, 1966). In practice such
artefacts can usually be identified by a sudden increase in the pressure as
the subject tries to maintain his effort. Some authors record transient
pressures but most prefer the pressure sustained for one or two seconds.
Since the pressures recorded are usually static the requirements for
frequency response of the equipment are not stringent and a simple
pressure transducer will suffice.

A further refinement which is being increasingly applied in clinical
assessment is direct measurement of transdiaphragmatic pressure. This

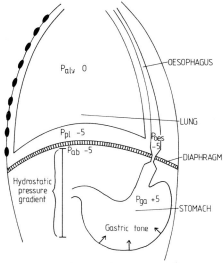

Fig. 18. Estimation of transdiaphragmatic pressure. Pressures are measured in the
oesophagus (P_{oes}) and in the stomach (P_{ga}) by two balloons. P_{oes} is assumed to equal P_{pl}
and P_{ga} is used as a guide to subdiaphragmatic pressure (P_{ab}). During relaxation at FRC
as illustrated the diaphragm is assumed to be relaxed and therefore $P_{pl} = P_{ab}$, in a
normal subject approximately −5 cm H_2O. P_{ga} is more positive that P_{ab} due to the
hydrostatic pressure gradient in the abdomen and the effects of gastric tone. It is
assumed that the difference between P_{ga} and P_{ab} remains approximately constant and
the standing pressure ($P_{ga} - P_{oes}$) at FRC is therefore subtracted from subsequent
measurements of P_{ga} to give P_{ab} from which P_{di} is calculated.

is achieved by the use of two balloon and catheter systems, one in the oesophagus and the other in the stomach (Agostoni and Rahn, 1960). The requirements for the oesophageal balloon are as described above in the measurement of lung recoil pressure but the performance of the gastric balloon is less critical; usually a short balloon containing 2–4 ml air is used. Theoretical considerations suggest that the pressure recorded in the stomach is more positive than the pressure immediately below the diaphragm because of both hydrostatic gradient and gastric tone (Fig. 18). In practice it is usually assumed that during relaxation at end expiration the pressures immediately above and below the diaphragm are identical and the standing pressure between the two balloons is subtracted from all subsequent gastric pressure measurements to estimate abdominal pressure (P_{ab}). The transdiaphragmatic pressure (P_{di}) is then given by $P_{ab} - P_{pl}$. The standing pressure in normal subjects is usually between 10 and 15 cm H_2O. Measurements of P_{di} may be reported during maximum static inspiratory efforts at various lung volumes or alternatively the change in P_{di} (ΔP_{di}) between FRC and TLC during a full inspiration has been recommended as a useful clinical measurement (Newsom Davis et al., 1976). Measurements of transdiaphragmatic pressure in clinical practice are indicated in cases of suspected weakness or paralysis of the diaphragm; in patients with diaphragmatic paralysis no pressure is generated across the diaphragm either during a maximum static effort or a full voluntary inspiration but the values in diaphragmatic weakness rather than complete paralysis are not clearly established.

References

Agostoni, E. (1970). In "The Respiratory Muscles", (Eds, E. J. M. Campbell, E. Agostoni and J. Newsom Davis) pp. 48–79. Lloyd Luke, London.

Agostoni, E. and Mead, J. (1964). In "Handbook of Physiology. Section 3, Respiration". (W. O. Fenn and H. Rahn, Eds), Vol. 1, pp. 387–409. American Physiological Society, Washington D.C.

Agostoni, E. and Rahn, H. (1960). J. appl. Physiol. 15, 1087–1092.

American Thoracic Society (1979). Am. Rev. resp. Dis. 119, 831–838.

Bachofen, H. and Scherrer, M. (1970). In "Airway Dynamics", (Ed., A. Bouhuys), pp. 123–134. Thomas, Springfield, Illinois.

Caro, C. G. and DuBois, A. B. (1961). Thorax 16, 282–290.

Clements, J. A., Sharp, J. T., Johnson, R. P. and Elam, J. O. (1959). J. clin. Invest. 38, 1262–1270.

Cook, C. D., Mead, J. and Orzalesi, M. M. (1964). J. appl. Physiol. 19, 1016–1022.

DuBois, A. B., Botelho, S. Y., Bedell, C. N., Marshall, R. and Comroe, J. H. (1956a). J. clin. Invest. 35, 322–326.

DuBois, A. B., Botelho, S. Y. and Comroe, J. H. (1956b). J. clin. Invest. 35, 327–335.

Ferris, B. G. (1978). *Am. Rev. resp. Dis.* **118** (No. 6 part 2), 55–88.

Fry, D. L. and Hyatt, R. E. (1960). *Am. J. Med.* **29**, 672–689.

Gibson, G. J. and Pride, N. B. (1976). *Br. J. Dis. Chest* **70**, 143–184.

Gibson, G. J. and Pride, N. B. (1977). *Am. Rev. resp. Dis.* **116**, 637–647.

Gibson, G. J., Pride, N. B., Newsom Davis, J. and Loh, L. C. (1977). *Am. Rev. resp. Dis.* **115**, 389–395.

Gibson, G. J., Pride, N. B., Davis, J. and Schroter, R. C. (1979). *Am. Rev. resp. Dis.* **120**, 799–811.

Glaister, D. H., Schroter, R. C., Sudlow, M. F. and Milic Emili, J. (1973). *Resp. Physiol.* **17**, 347–364.

Goldman, M., Knudson, R. J. and Mead, J. (1970). *J. appl. Physiol.* **28**, 113–116.

Habib, M. P. and Engel, L. A. (1978). *Am. Rev. resp. Dis.* **117**, 265–271.

Heaf, P. J. D. and Prime, F. J. (1956). *Clin. Sci.* **15**, 319–327.

Ingram, R. H., O'Cain, C. F. and Fridy, W. W. (1974). *J. appl. Physiol.* **36**, 135–141.

Ingram, R. H. and Schilder, D. P. (1966). *Am. Rev. resp. Dis.* **94**, 56–63.

Jaeger, M. J. and Bouhuys, A. (1969). *Prog. Resp. Res.* **4**, 116–130.

Leith, D. E. and Mead, J. (1974). "Principles of Body Plethysmography". National Heart and Lung Institute, Division of Lung Diseases, Bethesda, Maryland.

Leuallen, E. C. and Fowler, W. S. (1955). *Am. Rev. Tub.* **72**, 783–800.

Macklem, P. T. (1974). "Procedures for Standardized Measurements of Lung Mechanics". National Heart and Lung Institute, Division of Lung Diseases, Bethesda, Maryland.

Macklem, P. T. and Roussos, C. S. (1977). *Clin. Sci.* **53**, 419–422.

Mead, J. (1960). *J. appl. Physiol.* **15**, 736–740.

Mead, J. (1961). *Physiol. Rev.* **41**, 281–330.

Mead, J., Turner, J. M., Macklem, P. T. and Little, J. B. (1967). *J. appl. Physiol.* **22**, 95–108.

Mead, J. and Whittenberger, J. L. (1953). *J. appl. Physiol.* **5**, 779–796.

Meneeley, G. R. and Kaltreider, N. L. (1949). *J. clin. Invest.* **28**, 129–139.

Milic Emili, J., Mead, J., Turner, J. M. and Glauser, E. M. (1964). *J. appl. Physiol.* **19**, 207–211.

Miller, R. D. and Hyatt, R. E. (1973). *Am. Rev. resp. Dis.* **108**, 475–481.

Newsom Davis, J., Goldman, M., Loh, L. and Casson, M. (1976). *Q. J. Med.* **45**, 87–100.

Peslin, R., Bohadana, A., Hannhart, B. and Jardin, P. (1979). *Am. Rev. resp. Dis.* **119**, 271–277.

Pride, N. B. (1971). *Br. J. Dis. Chest* **65**, 135–169.

Ringqvist, T. (1966). *Scand. J. clin. lab. Invest.* **18**, suppl. 88.

Salazar, E. and Knowles, J. H. (1964). *J. appl. Physiol.* **19**, 97–104.

Tockman, M., Menkes, H., Cohen, B., Permutt, S., Benjamin, J., Ball, W. C. and Tonascia, J. (1976). *Am. Rev. resp. Dis.* **114**, 711–722.

Trop, D., Peeters, R. and van de Woestijne, K. P. (1970). *J. appl. Physiol.* **29**, 283–287.

van de Woestijne, K. P. and Bouhuys, A. (1969). *Prog. Resp. Res.* **4**, 64–74.

Zapletal, A., Paul, T. and Samanek, M. (1976). *J. appl. Physiol.* **40**, 953–961.

H

10. INTRAPULMONARY DISTRIBUTION OF INSOLUBLE GASES

Keith Prowse

City General Hospital, Stoke-on-Trent, U.K.

When air is breathed in it flows down the major airways of the lung by convective, or bulk, flow. It must then mix with the gas already present in the lung which is mainly in the alveoli. These are so small that convective flow cannot occur and gas-mixing at this level takes place by molecular diffusion. Some gas-mixing occurs within the airways and the change from convective flow to diffusion mixing is not abrupt so that in the small airways the two processes occur simultaneously, with diffusion becoming more important as the alveoli are reached. Any condition which interferes with diffusive mixing, for example by increasing the distance across which the mixing must take place as happens in centrilobular emphysema, will impair lung function and interfere with the transport of oxygen to the gas/blood interface. The process will also be affected by any regional maldistribution of inspired gas within the lung such as may occur in those diseases which affect the bronchi or small airways.

Tests which purport to indicate the efficacy of intrapulmonary gas-mixing by diffusion must be interpreted with caution as they are also influenced by changes in distribution of ventilation.

The tests available fall conveniently into two groups: those carried out on a single breath and those involving multiple breath techniques. Relatively insoluble and physiologically inert gases are usually used because both oxygen and carbon dioxide continue to be exchanged across the alveolar membrane during the performance of the test and hence complicate further the interpretation of results.

SINGLE BREATH NITROGEN TEST

This is performed by measuring the expired concentration of nitrogen after the inhalation of an appropriate test gas such as oxygen. Other tests may be interpreted in a similar way. Alternative combinations are to measure the expired helium concentration after inspiration of 80% helium in oxygen or to measure expired carbon dioxide after breathing in air although the latter usually gives less good results.

Method

The apparatus required is a 3- or 4-way tap with mouthpiece; a nitrogen meter (rapid nitrogen analyser) or mass spectrometer set to read over mass peak 28; a volume measuring device with electronic output such as a spirometer or a pneumotachograph with electronic integration; and a recording instrument which is usually a twin coordinate (XY) chart recorder or a storage oscilloscope.

One limb of the 4-way tap connects to a Douglas bag containing oxygen. The bag should be flushed out several times with oxygen to ensure that it contains no residual nitrogen before it is filled for the procedure. The head of the nitrogen meter is interposed between the mouthpiece and the 4-way tap. This allows the concentration of nitrogen in the "oxygen bag" to be checked for each recording. The spirometer should be used over the middle of its range and the calibration of the volume axis (X axis) of the XY recorder is best done directly by volume. Although many dry spirometers have an electronic calibration facility they are not always linear, especially if the spirometer starts from zero (empty). Careful calibration of the recorder for both volume and nitrogen concentration (Y axis) is essential and this should be checked regularly. The pen of the recorder must be adjusted so that it does not give excess pressure on the chart as this will have a damping effect on the resultant record. The dead-space of the mouthpiece, tap and tubing should be kept to a minimum.

Procedure

The test is performed under quiet resting conditions with the subject seated. The subject is allowed to settle to the apparatus and mouthpiece by breathing through the 4-way tap to room air. A nasal clip is used to prevent gas flow through the nose. The subject then exhales to residual volume. The 4-way tap is switched to the oxygen bag and he inspires slowly and steadily to total lung capacity. The inspiratory flow rate should be less than 0.5 l s^{-1}. The subject then immediately exhales at the same rate into the spirometer until he reaches residual volume. The expired gas volume and nitrogen concentration are recorded simultaneously on the XY recorder. If a 3-way tap is used the expiratory port must be connected to the spirometer whilst the subject breathes in oxygen.

A typical normal expired nitrogen curve is shown in Fig. 1. The shape of the resultant curve can be divided into 4 phases. In phase 1, the gas sampled at the beginning of the expirate contains no nitrogen since it comes from the nasopharynx and large airways. In phase 2, the expired nitrogen concentration rises rapidly, and then reaches a steady but slowly rising concentration which is phase 3. In some subjects, as residual volume is reached, there may be an upturn in the expired nitrogen concentration which signals the beginning of phase 4. The rapid rise in gas concentration during phase 2 is due to the mixture of an increasing amount of alveolar gas with a diminishing amount of gas which is still coming from the large airways. The steady concentration of gas in phase 3 is called the "alveolar plateau". In an ideal lung with perfect gas mixing this would be horizontal but in practice, in normal subjects, it rises slowly, reflecting the net result of differing nitrogen concentrations in the alveoli caused by variations in gas-mixing and ventilation, and by continued gas exchange for oxygen during the procedure. Phase 4 denotes the beginning of airway narrowing or closure in the dependent parts of the lung and is discussed further under the section on closing volume. In subjects with chronic lung disease, such as chronic bronchitis and emphysema, the expired nitrogen trace

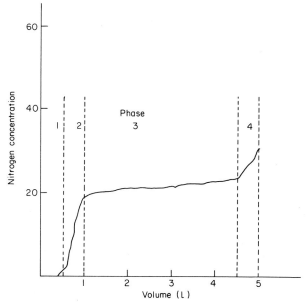

Fig. 1. The single breath nitrogen curve.

often follows a gradual curve with no clear division into the three main phases.

If the resultant curve does not show the first 3 phases clearly as in Fig. 1, first check the calibration of the spirometer and nitrogen meter, and then check the concentration of nitrogen in the inspired oxygen bag. Check the system for leaks and check the sensitivity of the XY recorder. Theoretically, the placement of the nitrogen meter before the mouthpiece means that the gas which it takes for measurement is lost to the volume measurement but this is of little practical importance for the single breath nitrogen index and is relevant only if precise estimation of anatomical dead-space is being attempted.

Anatomical Dead-Space (Fowler, 1952)

The final part of the inhalation of oxygen is called wasted gas because it remains within the large airways and plays no part in gas exchange.

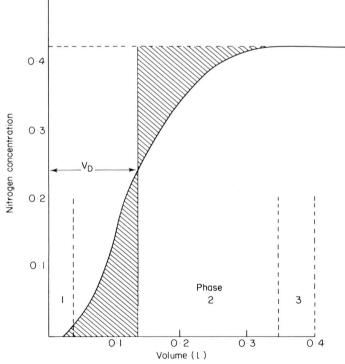

FIG. 2. Graphical calculation of anatomical dead-space from the single breath nitrogen curve. The vertical line is drawn so that the two shaded areas are equal. V_D = anatomical dead-space.

This volume of gas is the anatomical dead-space. It may be calculated from the curve by a simple graphical construction (Fig. 2). If no gas-mixing occurred within the airways there would be no phase 2 on the expired nitrogen curve but there would be an abrupt rise in concentration from zero to the level of the alveolar plateau. The volume exhaled up to this point would be the anatomical dead-space. Since, in practice, there is a gradual, though rapid, change in concentration the purpose of the graphical method is to find the position which the square wave would adopt if the ideal situation obtained. In Fig. 2, the anatomical dead-space is obtained by bisecting the steeply rising phase 2 of the curve in such a way that the two shaded areas are equal. In obtaining the initial curve the instruments should have a response time of less than 0.1 s and the records of volume and of concentration must be synchronous. In normal subjects the anatomical dead-space is about 120–150 ml, depending on the lung volume at which it is measured, i.e. at which the inspiration of oxygen is begun and on age and sex.

Single Breath Nitrogen Index

The slope of the alveolar plateau (phase 3) may be used to calculate the single breath index of uneven ventilation. This is taken arbitrarily as the change in nitrogen concentration between 750 ml and 1250 ml after the start of expiration. It will be seen from Fig. 1 that the alveolar plateau shows a series of peaks and troughs. These are the cardiogenic oscillations, the peaks corresponding to the cardiac systole. They make accurate measurement from the trace difficult. In practice it is best to draw by eye the "best-fit" straight line through the alveolar plateau and to derive the index by measurement of the slope of this line. In any given subject several traces (3–5) should be measured, preferably by two independent observers. The mean value is then taken as the single breath nitrogen index.

In normal subjects an average value is 0.5–1% per 500 ml expired gas. The index increases with age, reaching about 3% by the age of 70. In subjects with uneven gas-mixing, whether due to uneven distribution of inspired gas (regional inhomogeneity) or to diffusion problems giving an in-series dead-space (stratified inhomogeneity), the index may rise as high as 10%. For a discussion of the contribution of diffusion to the alveolar plateau the reader is referred to Cumming *et al.* (1967).

CLOSING VOLUME (Collins, 1973)

Closing volume is defined as that lung volume at which airways begin to close in the dependent parts of the lung. It is indicated by phase 4 of the single breath nitrogen curve. Closing capacity is the sum of closing volume and residual volume.

Closing volume may be measured by the single breath nitrogen test described above but is open to the objection that the changes in expired nitrogen concentration may be independent of airway closure. Methods using a bolus of test gas such as argon or helium are preferable (Linn and Hackney, 1973).

Method

The technique is similar to that described for single breath nitrogen but a bolus of test gas is inhaled initially followed by room air in place of the oxygen. The test gas used is either argon or helium and the appropriate analyser is used in place of the rapid nitrogen analyser.

The subject exhales to residual volume (RV) and is then connected to the spirometer which contains room air. A bolus of helium or argon (usually 300 ml) is injected into the mouthpiece at the beginning of inspiration and the subject breathes in slowly to total lung capacity (TLC). The effect of this is to distribute the helium or argon preferentially to the upper zones of the lung (Dollfuss *et al.*, 1967). The subject then exhales slowly to RV and the expired concentration of the marker gas is recorded continuously at the mouth as for nitrogen and plotted against expired gas volume (Fig. 3).

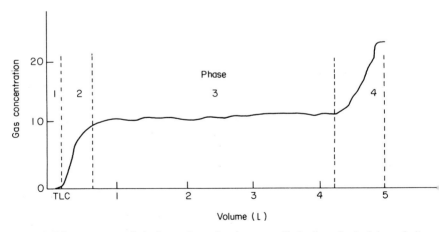

FIG. 3. Measurement of closing volume by the argon "bolus" method. A best-fit line drawn through phase 3 (the alveolar plateau) permits identification of the beginning of phase 4. The volume of phase 4 equals closing volume. Closing capacity = closing volume + residual volume.

The onset of phase 4 of the expired curve indicates the point at which the basal airways begin to close so that the expirate comes mainly from the upper regions of the lung where the concentration of argon or helium is relatively high. It may be difficult to identify the start of phase 4 because of the cardiogenic oscillations, the unevenness of the alveolar plateau or of curvilinear take-off. A best-fit line is drawn through the alveolar plateau and the beginning of phase 4 is taken at the point where the recorded tracing leaves this line permanently. Closing volume is then the expired volume between this point and RV. It should be noted that phase 4 cannot always be demonstrated in normal subjects. In patients with lung disease the slope of the alveolar plateau may be such as to make identification of phase 4 impossible.

The first description of measurement of closing volume involved the use of Xenon[133] which gives a better trace, permitting easier definition of the beginning of phase 4 (Dollfuss et al., 1967).

Whatever the method used measurements should be taken from 3–5 traces and the traces should ideally be read independently by two observers. Using this technique the coefficient of variation in healthy subjects is about 10% (Collins et al., 1973).

The use of the single-breath nitrogen curve for the determination of closing volume is similar. However, the subject inhales a full inspiration of oxygen and not a bolus. During the full inspiration more oxygen goes to the bases of the lung than to the apices and so the nitrogen concentration at the apices is relatively higher. In practice, the results obtained by the bolus method and the nitrogen method are similar.

Factors Affecting Closing Volume

The bolus of inspired test gas is distributed preferentially to the upper zones of the lung, because at and just above residual volume the airways in the dependent zones of the lung are narrowed or closed. This gives a concentration gradient of marker gas down the lung, the highest concentration being in the upper zones. If inspiration is too rapid, gas distribution is more even throughout the lung and the identification of phase 4 is more difficult. Where the inspiratory flow rate is low, e.g. $0.2–0.3 \text{ l s}^{-1}$, the concentration gradient between upper and lower zones may be as high as 10:1 but at flow rates of $3–5 \text{ l s}^{-1}$ this gradient is reduced to 2:1. If expiratory flow is too fast, phase 4 may be abolished.

Closing volume is also affected by gravity, and hence by the position of the patient. It increases with age and is abnormally large in obese individuals as well as in various forms of lung disease.

Early studies of closing volume suggested that it may give a valuable indication of uneven ventilation caused by small airway disease (McCarthy *et al.*, 1972) but it is not clear how it is influenced by diffusion abnormalities. There are technical difficulties in obtaining traces which are both good and reproducible in a given subject, and it may be variable even in normal subjects so that its use is now declining.

MULTIPLE BREATH INDICES

Multiple breath tests involve chiefly the washout of nitrogen from the lung during oxygen breathing. Like the single breath tests they are affected by diffusion abnormalities as well as by uneven distribution of ventilation, and the effects of the two are difficult to distinguish. Technically they are difficult and time-consuming to perform and have little, if any, place in routine lung function testing. Only an outline of the tests will be given here and for further details the reader is referred to the more detailed texts and papers.

Closed Circuit Methods

When residual volume is measured by helium dilution a crude measurement of evenness and efficiency of the distribution of ventilation may be obtained by measuring the number of breaths, or the time, taken for the concentration of helium in the spirometer to fall to within 10% of its equilibration value. Although easy to obtain, the index is of little clinical use because it is crude. It is affected by the volume of gas in the spirometer, the volume of dead-space of the apparatus, the efficiency of gas-mixing in the spirometer, the accuracy and stability of the helium analyser and the lung volume and tidal volume of the subject (Bates and Christie, 1950).

In normal subjects the fall of helium concentration to within 10% of equilibration value occurs in about 15–30 breaths depending on tidal volume and lung volume. Alternatively equilibration occurs in roughly 3 min, but up to 5 min is not uncommon in normal subjects. An abnormally long equilibration time or a large number of breaths to reach the selected limit are therefore indicators of considerable unevenness of lung ventilation but conversely marked abnormality may be present with a normal equilibration time.

Open-Circuit Methods

Open-circuit methods study the washout of nitrogen from the lung during the course of oxygen breathing, and most tests are performed using 100% oxygen. As this may itself affect ventilation a better nitrogen-free gas mixture for inspiration is a mixture of 79% argon and 21% oxygen. In principle the subject breathes normally and the expired gas volume and its end-tidal nitrogen concentration are measured breath by breath or cumulatively over several series of consecutive breaths.

In the simplest method the oxygen is inspired from a large Douglas bag and expired air is collected. Nitrogen concentration is measured at the mouth using a rapid nitrogen analyser. When the end-tidal nitrogen concentration falls to 2%, either the time, the number of breaths or total expired gas volume is recorded. Alternatively, the volume of oxygen inspired may be measured. Subjects with uneven ventilation will take longer, and will require a greater volume of gas to achieve an end-tidal nitrogen concentration of 2% than will normal subjects. Perhaps the best way of expressing the data is the Lung Clearance Index (LCI) originally proposed by Becklake (1952) and modified by Bouhuys (1963). This index is the volume of oxygen which will lower the end-tidal concentration of nitrogen to 2%, and is expressed as a multiple of functional residual capacity. In healthy young adults the normal range of LCI is 5.0–9.0.

More complex nitrogen washout tests involve the plotting graphically of end-tidal nitrogen concentration against number of breaths or against volume of gas inspired. When concentration is plotted on a logarithmic scale against the number of breaths a perfect mixing system gives a straight line whilst in normal subjects a slightly curved line is obtained. The line plotted from subjects with chronic lung disease shows a greater degree of curvature. These methods, and the advantages of plotting mixed-expired nitrogen concentration over end-tidal concentration are described by Cumming and Jones (1966) and Cumming (1967). These tests are of limited value in routine testing. Cumming (1967) proposed the lung nitrogen decay curve, which plots the decline in nitrogen volume in one litre of lung volume against expired gas volume represented as a cumulative fraction of lung volume (one turnover = one volume of gas expired equivalent to lung volume). This test has the advantage of plotting directly measurable quantities and permits comparison between patients. It is also possible to separate graphically the abnormality due to stratified inhomogeneity and regional inhomogeneity. It is of value as a research tool and for details the reader is referred to Cumming (1967) and Prowse and Cumming (1973).

Regional and Stratified Inhomogeneity

Abnormality of all the tests described may arise because there is variation in the distribution of inspired gas to different parts of the lung.

This is known as "regional inhomogeneity" and usually occurs as a result of variations in airways resistance in different parts of the lung.

Any factor which increases the path length over which gaseous diffusion must occur will also lead to abnormal results. This is known as stratified inhomogeneity from its effects on gas concentration within the lung. Thus in centrilobular emphysema there is dilatation of the respiratory bronchioles which form a series mixing chamber and increase the distance for diffusion whilst in panacinar emphysema the distal dilatation also increases the distance over which diffusive mixing must occur. A similar situation will arise if some airways are severely obstructed so that ventilation of the terminal units occurs through collateral pathways, again increasing the distance required for diffusion.

Both mechanisms are important in chronic lung disease and stratified inhomogeneity is an important cause of impaired gas mixing in chronic bronchitis. Only the lung nitrogen decay curve permits some indication of the relative importance of the two types of abnormality in a given subject. All of the other single and multiple breath tests are influenced by both regional and stratified abnormalities, underlining the difficulty of assessing accurately gas mixing by diffusion in the pulmonary function laboratory. A detailed discussion of gaseous diffusion in the lung is given by Horsfield (1980).

References

Bates, D. V. and Christie, R. V. (1950). *Clin. Sci.* **9**, 17–27.

Becklake, M. R. (1952). *Thorax* **7**, 111–116.

Bouhuys, A. (1963). *J. appl. Physiol.* **18**, 297–300.

Collins, J. V. (1973). *Br. J. dis. Chest* **67**, 1–18.

Collins, J. V., Clark, T. J. H., McHardy-Young, S., Cochrane, G. M. and Crawley, J. (1973). *Br. J. dis. Chest* **67**, 19–27.

Cumming, G. (1967). *Resp. Physiol.* **2**, 213–224.

Cumming, G., Horsfield, K., Jones, J. G. and Muir, D. C. F. (1967). *Resp. Physiol.* **2**, 386–392.

Cumming, G. and Jones, J. G. (1966). *Resp. Physiol.* **1**, 238–248.

Dollfuss, R. E., Milic-Emeli, J. and Bates, D. V. (1967). *Resp. Physiol.* **2**, 234.

Fowler, W. S. (1952). *Physiol. Rev.* **32**, 1–20.

Horsfield, K. (1980). *Brit. J. dis. Chest.* **74**, 99–120.

Linn, W. S. and Hackney, J. D. (1973). *J. appl. Physiol.* **34**, 396–399.

McCarthy, D. S., Spencer, R., Greene, R. and Milic-Emeli, J. (1972). *Amer. J. Med.* **52**, 747–753.

Prowse, K. and Cumming, G. (1973). *J. appl. Physiol.* **34**, 23–33.

Saunders, K. B. (1977). *In* "Clinical Physiology of the Lung", Chapt. 3, pp. 78–94. Blackwell Scientific Publications, Oxford.

11. MEASUREMENT OF CARBON MONOXIDE TRANSFER

Patricia M. Warren

City Hospital, Edinburgh, U.K.

THEORY

Gas exchange between alveolus and capillary occurs by diffusion. Various tests have been devised in an attempt to quantify this process. Intuitively it would seem that any pathological alteration to the alveolar–capillary membrane, in particular an increased thickness, might impair the rate of diffusion and consequently lead to hypoxaemia and carbon dioxide retention. However, the methods used clinically to assess pulmonary diffusion rates involve various assumptions which result in many factors influencing the result as well as the properties of the alveolar–capillary membrane.

In 1914, Krogh first used the term diffusing capacity (D) which she defined as:

$$D = \frac{\dot{V}}{P_A - P_c} \tag{1}$$

where $\dot{V}$ is the rate of gas uptake and P_A and P_c alveolar and capillary partial pressures respectively. Thus a value for diffusing capacity for the lungs can be obtained from a knowledge of the rate of gas uptake and the partial pressures of the gas in the alveoli and capillaries. This equation forms the basis of the clinical assessment of the ability of the lungs to transfer gas across the alveolar–capillary membrane by diffusion. This diffusing capacity is not a physical rate constant but includes factors for lung geometry and chemical interaction. Cotes (1979) suggested that the term "transfer factor for the lung" should be used instead of "diffusing capacity". This new term is used extensively in Britain and Europe but has not been adopted in North America where it is still referred to as the diffusing capacity.

Diffusing Capacity for Oxygen (D_LO_2)

The rate of diffusion of oxygen is obviously of major theoretical interest. According to eqn (1), in order to calculate D_LO_2, values are required for:

(1) Rate of oxygen uptake. This is the rate of oxygen consumption, $\dot{V}O_2$.

(2) Mean alveolar oxygen tension (P_AO_2). This can be calculated using the alveolar air equation if arterial carbon dioxide tension, the respiratory gradient and respiratory oxygen tension are known.

(3) Mean capillary oxygen tension ($P_{\bar{c}}O_2$).

The difficulties in calculating D_LO_2 arise because this variable cannot be measured but has to be estimated, the method for which was first described by Bohr (1909). It is based on the assumption that the rate of diffusion across the membrane is proportional to the alveolar–capillary oxygen tension difference at that point. A curve is constructed of the rate of change of capillary oxygen tension with time along the capillary. Capillary transit time is assumed to be 0.75 s. To construct the curve, values must be assigned to:

(a) Alveolar oxygen tension (P_AO_2) which can be calculated (see above).

(b) Mixed venous oxygen tension ($P_{\bar{v}}O_2$) which can be measured by sampling blood from a catheter placed in the pulmonary artery.

(c) The oxyhaemoglobin dissociation curve which can be obtained from published tables.

(d) The end-capillary oxygen tension ($P_c{}'O_2$) which has to be estimated. Because of venous admixture, $P_c{}'O_2$ is not equal to arterial oxygen tension (P_aO_2). A method for determining $P_c{}'O_2$ was described by Riley and colleagues (1951) which involves two assumptions. First, that at a low oxygen tension the contribution of venous admixture to the P_AO_2–$P_c{}'O_2$ difference is negligible and secondly that D_LO_2 is independent of oxygen tension. In practice measurements of P_AO_2, P_aO_2, $P_{\bar{v}}O_2$ and $\dot{V}O_2$ are made with the subject breathing first air and then a 12% oxygen mixture. The value for the percentage shunt obtained when breathing air is used to calculate $P_c{}'O_2$ when breathing the low oxygen mixture using the shunt equation. Full details of the method are described elsewhere (Comroe et al., 1962).

Once the curve has been constructed, the $P_{\bar{c}}O_2$ is obtained by integration. Graphically it is given by the intercept on the y-axis of a horizontal line at a level at which the areas bordered by the curve above and below the line are equal. Unfortunately, many of the assumptions in estimating $P_{\bar{c}}O_2$ are invalid. The rate of reaction of oxygen with haemoglobin is dependent on the number of molecules already bound to the haemoglobin molecule. As blood passes through the pulmonary capillary the rate of combination of oxygen with haemoglobin will decrease as the numbers of bound molecules increases. Therefore the contribution of the rate of chemical reaction to diffusion will vary with distance along the capillary thus invalidating Bohr's original assumption. In addition, true values for $P_c'O_2$ cannot be obtained using the two levels of inspired oxygen for several reasons. The breathing of low oxygen concentration mixtures does not eliminate the contribution of venous admixture to the $P_AO_2-P_c'O_2$ difference. Also the D_LO_2 cannot be assumed to be equal at the two levels of oxygen as the rate of combination of oxygen with haemoglobin will be greater in the hypoxaemic state (see above). In addition, true values for $P_c'O_2$, cannot be obtained using the two levels of inspired oxygen for several reasons. The breathing of low oxygen mixtures does not eliminate the contribution of venous admixture to the $P_AO_2-P_c'O_2$ difference. Also D_LO_2 cannot be assumed to be the same at the two levels of oxygen concentration because of the effect on the rate of combination of oxygen with haemoglobin. In addition, it is likely that the percentage shunt will differ on air and 12% oxygen. Finally, a capillary transit time of 0.75 s cannot be assumed as values as low as 0.1 s have been suggested (McHardy, 1972).

No adequate method of estimating $P_c'O_2$ is currently available. Since the construction of the $P_c'O_2$/transit time curve is critically dependent on the value assigned to the the $P_c'O_2$, any subsequent estimation of D_LO_2 will be questionable. Measurement of D_LO_2 is therefore neither practical nor meaningful using these techniques.

Diffusing Capacity for Carbon Monoxide (D_LCO)

Because of the difficulties in estimating D_LO_2, measurement of the diffusing capacity for carbon monoxide has become the routine test in clinical practice. Since the endogenous levels of carboxyhaemoglobin (COHb) are low and the affinity of haemoglobin for carbon monoxide is high it was thought that the capillary carbon monoxide tension (P_cCO) would remain negligible throughout the capillary and could be ignored. The equation for diffusing capacity for carbon monoxide therefore simplifies to:

$$D_LCO = \frac{\dot{V}CO}{P_ACO} \qquad (2)$$

Once again, the assumptions are probably invalid. The rate of combination of carbon monoxide with haemoglobin does take a finite time and may influence the diffusion rate. Also, in heavy smokers, the baseline level of COHb will not be negligible for which a correction should be made. However, measurement of the diffusing capacity, or transfer factor for carbon monoxide, is relatively simple and, if the limitations of interpretation are borne in mind, can be a useful index of the efficiency of gas exchange.

METHODS OF MEASURING THE TRANSFER FACTOR FOR CARBON MONOXIDE ($T_L$co)

Various tests have been devised for estimating $T_L$co (Bates, Macklem and Christie, 1971). Only the methods most commonly used will be described here.

Single Breath Method

The technique currently used is a modification (Ogilvie *et al.*, 1956) of the method originally described by Krogh (1914). A single vital capacity breath of a mixture of known concentration of CO is inhaled and the breath held for approximately 10 s at total lung capacity. The diffusing capacity is calculated from the rate of disappearance of CO from the alveoli per unit time.

The quantity of CO passing from alveolus to capillary can be expressed as the product of the volume of alveolar gas (V_A) and the fractional alveolar concentration of CO ($F_A$co). Since $P_A$co is equal to the product of fractional concentration and total gas pressure, we can write:

$$\frac{V_A F_A \, (co)}{t} = -T_L co \cdot F_A co \, (Pb - 47) \qquad (3)$$

where $(Pb - 47)$ is the barometric pressure minus the pressure exerted by water vapour in the lungs. The rate of change of alveolar CO concentration with time can be expressed as:

$$\frac{dF_A co}{dt} = -\frac{T_L co \, (Pb - 47) \, F_A co}{V_A} \qquad (4)$$

Integration of eqn (4) with respect to time gives:

$$F_A co(t) = F_A co(0) \exp \left[-\frac{T_L co(Pb - 47)t}{V_A} \right] \qquad (5)$$

where $F_A co(0)$ and $F_A co(t)$ are the alveolar concentration of CO at times zero and "t" respectively. Thus the exponential fall in alveolar CO

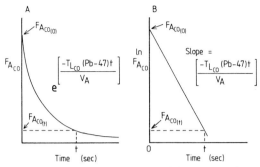

FIG. 1. Diagram of the rate of change of alveolar CO concentration ($F_A co$) with time showing (a) the exponential fall and (b) the linear change when expressed as ln $F_A co$.

concentration with time (Fig. 1a) is a function of the diffusing capacity. If the alveolar concentrations are expressed in logarithmic form, eqn (5) becomes:

$$\ln \frac{F_A co(t)}{F_A co(0)} = - \frac{T_L co(Pb - 47)t}{V_A} \qquad (6)$$

Graphically this is given by a straight line (Fig. 1b) with intercept on the y-axis of ln $F_A co(0)$ and a slope of $- \dfrac{T_L co(Pb - 47)}{V_A}$. By rearranging eqn (6), an expression is derived for $T_L co$:

$$T_L co = \frac{V_A}{(Pb - 47)t} \ln \frac{F_A co(0)}{F_A co(t)} \qquad (7)$$

The equation in this form is used to calculate $T_L co$ when the single breath method is used and values for V_A, $F_A co(0)$, $F_A co(t)$ and "t" must therefore be determined.

Technique and Measurements

The subject exhales to residual volume and then inhales a vital capacity breath of a gas mixture containing approximately 0.3% CO, 10% helium (He), 21% oxygen with balance of nitrogen (Fig. 2). The inspired volume is recorded. When total lung capacity (TLC) is reached, the breath is held for approximately 10 s and the subject then exhales. The initial part of the expiratory breath (usually 700–800 ml) is discarded. This allows for complete flushing of the respiratory dead-space in which no gas exchange has occurred. Thereafter a sample of expired gas is collected. This should be of adequate volume to allow for

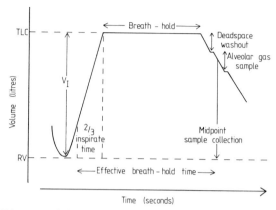

FIG. 2. Diagram of the single breath manoeuvre for measuring $T_L co$.

accurate analysis for gas composition, which, with modern analysers again usually needs to be about 700 ml. After completion of the manoeuvre, the expired gas and a sample of the inspirate mixture are analysed for CO and He concentrations.

(1) Measurement of V_A. Alveolar volume can be computed in two ways:

(a) Total alveolar volume: the volume initially inspired is added to a value for residual volume obtained using other methods.

(b) Effective alveolar volume: the inhaled CO and He are assumed to be diluted to a similar extent within the lungs. Since He is inert and does not pass across the alveolar-capillar membrane, the alveolar volume involved in gas exchange can therefore be calculated from the dilution of the He as follows:

$$V_A = V_I \times \frac{F_I \, He}{F_E \, He} \tag{8}$$

where V_I is the volume inspired and F_I He and F_E He are the inspiratory and expiratory fractional concentrations of He respectively. For eqn (7) to be valid, alveolar volume is assumed to remain constant throughout the breath-hold period. It is therefore important to ensure that no gas is inhaled or exhaled during that period.

(2) Measurement of $F_A co(0)$. Since the initial dilution of CO and He are assumed to be equal, alveolar concentration at time zero can be computed from the concentration of CO in the inspired gas ($F_I co$) and

the dilution of He:

$$F_A co(0) = F_I co \times \frac{F_E He}{F_I He} \qquad (9)$$

(3) Measurement of $F_A co(t)$. The concentration of CO in the inspired sample is assumed to represent the alveolar concentration at time "*t*".

(4) Measurement of effective breath-hold time. The length of time during which gas exchange occurs was initially taken as the length of the breath-holding period. However, this was shown to underestimate the contact time between alveolar gas and capillary blood and it was therefore suggested by Jones and Meade (1964) that the effective breath-hold time should be calculated as the sum of two-thirds inspirate time, breath-holding time and expirate time to the midpoint of the sample collection (Fig. 2).

Calculations

In practice, eqn (7) has been further modified (Cotes, 1979) for use in the routine clinical situation. Since the effective breath-hold period is measured in seconds but $T_L co$ is conveniently expressed as gas exchange per minute, a conversion factor of 60 must be included. Also for convenience, $\log_{10}$ are used instead of natural logarithms and barometric pressure is assumed to be 760 mmHg. Finally in Britain and Europe, $T_L co$ is now expressed in SI units of mmol $min^{-1} kPa^{-1}$ (= 0.335 ml min^{-1} mmHg, standard units). Combination of eqns (7) and (9) with inclusion of the appropriate factors gives:

$$T_L co = \frac{53.6 \, V_A}{t} \log \left[\frac{F_I \, CO}{F_E \, CO} \times \frac{F_E \, He}{F_I \, He} \right] \qquad (10)$$

where V_A is the alveolar volume measured in litres BTPS, *t* is effective breath-hold time in seconds F_I(co, He) and F_E(co, He) are the inspirate and expirate concentrations (fraction or percentage) of CO and He.

Technical Notes

(1) Validity of the alveolar sample. A major assumption of the techniques is that the concentration of gases in the sample collected during expiration is equivalent to the mean alveolar concentration at that time. In a normal subject, the initial 150–200 ml of gas exhaled come from the

dead-space and have a gas composition equal to that of the inspirate mixture. As expiration continues, the concentration of CO falls rapidly as a mixture of gas from the dead-space and alveoli is exhaled. Finally, the concentration reaches a plateau and mixed alveolar gas is exhaled during which the expirate sample should be collected. However, in the presence of severe ventilation/perfusion ($\dot{V}/\dot{Q}$) imbalance, no plateau of expiratory concentration is achieved as emptying alveoli of varying $\dot{V}/\dot{Q}$ ratios contribute to the expiratory gas mixture. It is therefore difficult to obtain a sample representative of overall gas composition.

(2) Reproducibility of inspirate volume. The value obtained for $T_L co$ is dependent on the lung volume at which it is measured (see later). Care should therefore be taken to ensure that the inspired volume is equal to the vital capacity measured independently.

(3) Estimation of effective breath-holding time. Most modern commercially available instruments for measuring the single breath $T_L co$ record a value for the effective breath-hold time. To achieve this, timing usually commences when a volume equal to the pre-set expiratory washout volume has been inhaled. Thus the value for effective breath-hold time will be affected by the rate of inspiration. However, the discrepancy probably only influences $T_L co$ significantly if inspiration is excessively slow.

Disadvantages of the Single Breath Method

(1) Measurement at TLC. Since the measurement is made with the lungs statically inflated to TLC, the measurement is non-physiological and the value obtained does not reflect gas exchange capabilities during tidal breathing.

(2) Patient co-operation. Performance of the test requires a high degree of patient co-operation both in terms of ability to follow a series of instructions and in being able to breath-hold at TLC for 10 s. The latter usually depends on the degree of respiratory disability of the patient. Many patients who have an $FEV_{1.0}$ below 1.0 l are too dyspnoeic to be able to hold their breath for the required length of time. Some commercial instruments have the facility for reducing the time for actual breath-holding. However there is evidence that $T_L co$ may decrease with decreasing breath-hold time (Magnussen *et al.*, 1979) with the effect being accentuated in the presence of airway obstruction. Use of a

reduced breath-hold time may therefore make comparison with predicted values (made with a 10-second breath-hold time) more difficult. However, provided a consistent breath-hold time was used it woud be possible to compare serial values in an individual.

(3) Minimum vital capacity. Performance of the test is also limited by a minimum vital capacity of approximately 1.5 l as the expiratory capacity must be sufficient to allow for adequate clearance of the respiratory dead-space and for the collection of an expiratory sample which can be analysed accurately. This latter requirement will be dependent on the analyser dead-space and response time.

(4) Diffusion during exercise. Because of the need to breath-hold at TLC, the single breath method is not suitable for use during exercise.

Advantages of the Single Breath Method

(1) Standardization of the measurement. In an individual subject, by carefully monitoring the inspirate volume, the lung volume at which the measurement is made can be standardized thus eliminating one of the major sources of variation in results obtained with other techniques.

(2) Back-pressure of COHb. The single breath estimation is less affected by the back-pressure of CO in the alveolar capillaries because of the relatively high concentration of CO in the inspirate mixture which maintains a large alveolar–capillary pressure gradient throughout the test and also because of the limited time for CO uptake. Therefore the error incurred by assuming capillary Pco to be zero is reduced. However, recent work suggests that, in certain circumstances, correction should be made for COHb (see later).

STEADY STATE METHOD

The steady state method involves measuring the rate of uptake of CO during steady state tidal breathing over a given period of time and a value for $T_L co$ calculated using eqn (2).

Techniques and Measurements

The subject breathes a mixture of a known concentration of CO containing approximately 0.1% CO in air for 6 min through a one-way valve. During the last minute, expired gas is collected and analysed for volume and mixed expired concentrations of CO, O_2 and CO_2, in addition, either a continuous expiratory record of CO concentration is made (Cotes, 1979) or breath-by-breath end-tidal samples are analysed for CO concentration (Bates *et al.*, 1955).

(1) Measurement of $\dot{V}co$. The uptake of CO is the difference between inspiratory and expiratory volumes of CO;

$$\dot{V}co = F_Ico \cdot \dot{V}_I - F_Eco\dot{V}_E \qquad (11)$$

where F_Ico is the fractional concentration of CO in the inspirate mixture which is known: F_Eco is the measured fractional concentration of CO in the expirate gas obtained by analysis; $\dot{V}_E$ is the measured expiratory volume; $\dot{V}_I$ is the inspiratory minute ventilation which can be calculated according to the formula:

$$\dot{V}_I = \dot{V}_E \left[\frac{1 - F_EO_2 - F_ECO_2 - F_ECO}{1 - F_IO_2 - F_ICO_2 - F_ICO} \right] \qquad (12)$$

where F_EO_2, CO_2, CO and F_IO_2, CO_2, CO are the mixed expired and inspired concentrations of O_2, CO_2 and CO respectively.

(2) Measurement of P_Aco. As in the single breath method, the plateau concentration of CO achieved during expiration is assumed to represent alveolar concentration. In the steady state method, this can either be

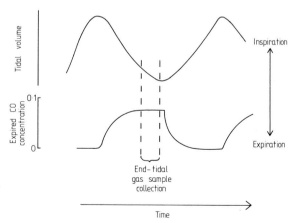

FIG. 3. Diagram of tidal volume and expiratory CO concentration recordings during a steady state. T_Lco manoeuvre showing the plateau of CO concentration at the end of expiration.

obtained by analysing the continuous record of expired CO concentration or by taking an average of the CO concentration from the breath-by-breath end-tidal samples (Fig. 3).

Calculations

In order to obtain $T_L co$ in mmol $min^{-1}kPa^{-1}$, eqn (2) becomes:

$$T_L co = \frac{0.335 \, \dot{V}co}{F_{ET}co \, (Pb - 47)} \tag{13}$$

where $\dot{V}co$ is the CO uptake in ml min^{-1} (STPD); $F_{ET}co$ is the fractional concentration of CO in the end-tidal (plateau) sample.

Technical Note

Validity of the alveolar sample. As with the single breath method, the assumption that end-tidal is equivalent to alveolar concentration is invalid in the presence of severe airway obstruction as gas concentrations do not plateau. In addition, if the end-tidal sampling method is used, tidal volume must be adequate to expel the dead-space gas before sampling. This is not usually a problem on exercise but may influence measurements made at rest.

Disadvantages of the Steady State Method

(1) Pattern of breathing. The measurement is influenced by the rate and depth of breathing. Consequently the test is difficult to standardize even within the individual.

(2) Back-pressure of CO. Because the CO mixture is breathed for 6 min, the increase in $P_c co$ may influence the results to a greater extent than with other methods.

Advantages of the Steady State Method

(1) Measurement during normal respiration. Since the measurement is made during the tidal breathing it may give a more physiological representation of gas exchange than is obtained using other methods. Measurements can also be made during exercise.

(2) Patient co-operation. The test requires minimal patient co-operation other than the wearing of a noseclip and mouthpiece.

REBREATHING METHOD

A rebreathing technique for measuring T_Lco using stable CO was first described by Lewis and colleagues (1959). More recently, modifications suitable for use either in the laboratory utilizing already available single breath apparatus (Marshall, 1977) or at the bedside (Clark *et al.*, 1978) have been described. The patient rebreathes from a bag containing a known concentration of CO for less than one minute and the rate of uptake is calculated from the change in CO concentration in the bag during the rebreathing period. As with the single breath method the rate of disappearance of CO from the rebreathing circuit after the initial dilution into the residual volume is exponential (Fig. 4) and an equation similar to eqn (7) is used to calculate T_Lco.

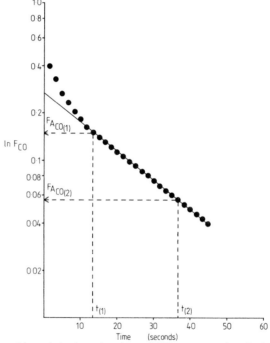

FIG. 4. Diagram of breath-by-breath values of CO concentration during a rebreathing manoeuvre showing the initial non-linear fall in concentration followed by the linear change during which period the initial $F_Aco(1)$ and final $F_Aco(2)$ CO concentrations are taken.

Technique and Measurement

The method given here is that of Lewis and colleagues (1959) and describes the basic principles of the method. The original papers should be consulted for details of the various modifications. A bag is filled with a volume equal to the patient's $FEV_{1.0}$ of a mixture of known concentrations of approximately 0.3% CO, 10% He with the remainder O_2 enriched air to prevent hypoxia developing during the rebreathing period. After exhaling to residual volume, the patient is connected to the bag and rebreathes the mixture for 30–45 s at a regular rate (approximately 30 breaths per minute) emptying the bag with each breath and ending the manoeuvre with an exhalation into the bag. The gas mixture in the bag is then analysed for He concentration. In addition, the CO concentration of the bag is recorded continuously (or at frequent regular intervals such as 5 s) throughout the rebreathing period.

(1) Measurement of VA. The alveolar volume involved in gas exchange is calculated as for the effective alveolar volume in the single breath method:

$$V_A = \frac{V_b\, F_b\, He(0)}{F_b\, He(t)} \qquad (14)$$

where V_b is the initial bag volume and is equivalent to the inspired volume of the single breath method. It can be obtained either by filling the bag with a known volume or by using a bag-in-box system and recording bag volume on a spirogram. $F_b\, He(0)$, $F_b\, He(t)$ are the fractional concentrations of He in the bag before and after rebreathing.

(2) Measurement of $F_A co(1)$ *and* $F_A co(2)$. The initial fall in CO concentration is due to the dilution of the mixture into the residual volume. By plotting the fall in CO concentration during rebreathing on semilogarithmic graph paper (Fig. 4), this is seen as an initial non-linear change. The exponential fall in concentration due to diffusion is described by the following linear portion. The concentrations of $F_A co(1)$ and $F_A co(2)$ are taken at any convenient points on the latter section.

(3) Measurement of time. This is the period in minutes between the points selected as (1) and (2):

Calculation

The equation used is in the form:

$$T_{L}co = \frac{0.335\, V_A}{(Pb - 47)\,(t(1) - t(2))} \ln \frac{F_A co(1)}{F_A co(2)} \qquad (15)$$

to give a value for $T_L co$ in mmol min^{-1} kPa^{-1}. Lung volume was conventionally expressed at STPD although routine measurements are now usually made at BTPS.

Technical Note

Bag volume. The bag volume should be at least 80% of the vital capacity and the patient encouraged to empty the bag with each breath since decreasing the bag volume has been shown to reduce the value obtained for $T_L co$ (Lewis *et al.*, 1959) presumably due to a reduced lung volume at which the measurement is then made.

Disadvantages of the Rebreathing Method

(1) Predicted Values. There are no predicted values made using this technique although those for the single breath method could be used as close correlations have been shown between results obtained with the two methods (Lewis *et al.*, 1959; Marshall, 1977).

(2) Patient Co-operation. Although the degree of co-operation is less than for the single breath method, dyspnoeic patients may still find the technique difficult to perform.

Advantages of the Rebreathing Method

(1) Bedside use. A modified form has been described for use at the bedside (Clarke *et al.*, 1978) which might be valuable in monitoring severely ill patients such as those with recurrent intrapulmonary haemorrhage (see later) who cannot be brought to the laboratory.

(2) Minimum volume. The rebreathing technique is not limited by either minimum inspiratory capacity as in the single breath method or a minimum tidal volume as required for the steady state measurement.

(3) Availability of equipment. Most routine laboratories use the single breath method. However, since a proportion of patients are unable to perform the single breath manoeuvre, the availability of a second technique may be desirable. The rebreathing method can be performed without any additional equipment other than that required for the single breath method (Marshall, 1977).

MEASUREMENT OF MEMBRANE DIFFUSING CAPACITY (D_m) AND CAPILLARY BLOOD VOLUME (V_c)

As described above, diffusion across the alveolar–capillary membrane and chemical reaction in the blood both contribute to the transfer factor for carbon monoxide. These two components can be described mathematically (Roughton and Forster, 1957). If diffusion across the alveolar–capillary membrane (membrane diffusing capacity, D_m) alone is considered, eqn (1) can be written in the form:

$$\frac{\Delta Qco}{\Delta t} = D_m (P_A co - P_c co) \qquad (16)$$

where ΔQco is the amount of CO passing across the membrane in the time Δt. However, the amount of CO combining with the available haemoglobin in the blood in time "t" is given by:

$$\frac{\Delta Qco}{\Delta t} = \Theta V_c \cdot P_c co \qquad (17)$$

where Θ is the reaction rate constant for the combination of CO and haemoglobin in mmol min^{-1} kPa^{-1} l^{-1} blood and includes a term for the rate of diffusion across the red cell membrane, and V_c is the pulmonary capillary blood volume. Since 99% of the CO entering the capillary combines with haemoglobin, eqns (16) and (17) can be considered equal and an expression for $P_c co$ is obtained

$$P_c co = P_A co/(1 + \Theta V_c/D_m) \qquad (18)$$

Substitution for $P_c co$ in eqn (16) gives

$$\Delta Qco/\Delta t = D_m \left[P_A - \frac{P_A co}{1 + \Theta V_c/D_m} \right] \qquad (19)$$

and combination of eqns (2) and (19) results in the following expression for the components of $T_L co$:

$$1/T_L co = 1/D_m co + 1/\Theta co V_c \qquad (20)$$

Since CO and O_2 compete for the same binding sites on the haemoglobin molecule, the rate of reaction of CO with haemoglobin is inversely related to the P_{O_2}. Thus, Θ and consequently $T_L co$ will vary with the P_{O_2} at which the estimation is made. However, $D_m co$ and V_c are independent of P_{O_2}. Therefore by measuring $T_L co$ at two or more levels of oxygen, eqn (2) can be solved to give D_m and V_c. The test is not used routinely but is of interest as a research tool.

Techniques and Measurements

Conventionally, measurements of the single breath $T_L co$ are made at two levels of oxygen, 100% and 21% (air).

$T_L co$ *at high* Po_2. The subject breathes 100% of O_2 for 10 min to wash out nitrogen from the alveoli. When $T_L co$ is measured at raised levels of Po_2, correction must be made for the back pressure of CO in the capillary. This can be done by connecting the subject at the end of the washout period to a rebreathing circuit consisting of a 5 l bag initially filled with 100% O_2 and a CO_2 absorber. The subject rebreathes for four minutes after which the rebreathing bag and alveolar concentrations will be in equilibrium. The single breath $T_L co$ is then measured in the standard manner using an inspiratory mixture of approximately 0.3% CO, 10% He with the remainder O_2. At the end of the manoeuvre, the expirate sample is analysed for O_2 concentration in addition to CO and He concentrations.

$T_L co$ *at low* Po_2. The subject breathes air for 10 min to flush out the O_2. The $T_L co$ is then measured using an inspiratory mixture of approximately 0.3% CO, 10% He, 21% O_2 with balance N_2 and the expired gas is again analysed for CO, He and O_2 concentrations.

Calculations

The $T_L co$ at high and low O_2 concentrations are calculated as described earlier with the following correction for CO back-pressure at the high Po_2. Capillary Pco is described by the following relationship (Cotes, 1979):

$$P_c co = P_c o_2 \times \frac{Fco}{Fo_2} \qquad (21)$$

where $P_c co$, $P_c o_2$ are the capillary CO and O_2 tensions, Fco, Fo$_2$ are the fractional concentrations of CO and O_2 in the bag at the end of the rebreathing period.

$P_c co$ can be estimated using the relationship

$$P_c o_2 = P_A o_2 - \frac{\dot{V}o_2}{1.23\ T_L co} \qquad (22)$$

where $\dot{V}o_2$ is the basal O_2 consumption either measured or estimated from a nomogram; $T_L co$ is the transfer factor for CO in air. $P_A o_2$ is calculated from the equilibration concentration. To correct for the CO back-pressure, $P_c co$ is converted to a concentration and this value subtracted from the estimated CO concentration at time "0" and "t". The linear relationship between Θ and Po_2 is described by the equation

$$\frac{1}{\Theta} = \frac{a + b \ P_c o_2}{[Hb]/14.9} \qquad (23)$$

where a and b are constants determined by the permeability of the red cell membrane to CO. Classically, values of 0.33 and 0.0057 are assigned to a and b respectively (Roughton and Forster, 1957) but other figures are quoted in the literature (Cotes, 1979). $P_c o_2$ is estimated as described above with $P_A o_2$ calculated from the expired concentration. [Hb] is the measured haemoglobin concentration in gm dl^{-1} and corrects for deviation from the standard value of 14.9 gm dl^{-1} at which the constants were determined *in vitro*.

D_m *and* V_c. Values for D_m and V_c can be attained graphically by plotting against $1/\Theta$ (Fig. 5). The slope of the line joining the two points is $1/V_c$ and the intercept on the y-axis is $1/D_m$. Alternatively, eqn (20) can be solved algebraically (Cotes, 1979).

The values obtained for D_m and V_c are very sensitive to small changes in slope and intercept. A more reliable estimate for both these variables is therefore obtained by estimating T_Lco at several levels of oxygen and constructing a regression line through the points using the least-squares method.

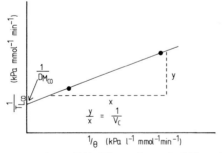

FIG. 5. Graphical solution of eqn (20). The reciprocal of T_Lco is plotted against the reciprocal of Θ. The slope of the line joining the points is $1/V_c$ and the intercept on the y-axis is $1/D_m$.

FACTORS AFFECTING T_Lco

Many physiological variables influence T_Lco. These can be considered in terms of those factors which alter lung geometry (chiefly due to a change in the surface area for gas exchange) and which principally affect

D_m and those causing changes in the blood component either due to alteration in Θ or V_c. The $T_L co$ is also affected by the inter-relationships of alveolar ventilation and perfusion and diffusion.

Lung Geometry

Lung volume. The $T_L co$ increases with increasing lung volume both in terms of the total lung capacity and of the degree of inflation. The former is a function of stature as is seen from population studies and is reflected in the predicted normal values (see below). In addition, $T_L co$ rises as the lung volume at which the measurement is made increases. Values of 0.8 mmol min^{-1} kPa^{-1} l^{-1} (Hamer, 1963) and 1.19 mmol min^{-1} kPa^{-1} l^{-1} (Rose *et al.*, 1979) for the single breath method and 1.11 mmol min^{-1} kPa^{-1} l^{-1} (Rose *et al.*, 1979) for the rebreathing method have been reported for increases in lung volume above functional residual capacity. The increase is chiefly due to a rise in D_m (Hamer, 1963) with V_c tending to fall as the lungs inflate. This increase in $T_L co$ is thought to be due to an increase in the effective surface area for gas exchange resulting from an expansion of the alveoli and the unfolding of the alveolar walls. This effect of lung volume partially accounts for the difference in values obtained for $T_L co$ by the different methods. The change in $T_L co$ with lung volume has two practical implications. Firstly, as was stressed above, care should be taken to ensure maximal inspiration when using the single breath technique so that $T_L co$ is consistently measured at total lung capacity. Secondly, if total lung capacity is varying with the course of the disease it may be necessary to express the $T_L co$ per litre lung volume ($T_L co/V_A$) in order to compare serial results in the same patient. This variable is termed the transfer coefficient (*k*co) and has the units mmol min^{-1} kPa^{-1} l^{-1}.

Blood Component

Haemoglobin Concentration

Since the rate of uptake of CO from the alveoli is influenced by the rate of combination with haemoglobin, $T_L co$ is dependent on the haemoglobin concentration in the pulmonary capillaries. Thus, $T_L co$ has been shown to be reduced in anaemia (Guleria *et al.*, 1971) and elevated in polycythaemia rubra vera (Burgess and Bishop, 1963). In practical terms for clinical measurement this has two consequences.

(i) Correction for haemoglobin concentration in anaemia. In some clinical conditions, for example in patients undergoing renal dialysis which may cause anaemia due to haemodialysis, failure to correct for the haemoglobin concentration will result in a falsely low value for $T_{L}co$. Two groups (Dinkara *et al.*, 1979; Cotes *et al.*, 1972) have derived correction equations for the single breath estimation which are, respectively:

$$T_{L}co(c) = T_{L}co(m)/0.06965 \, [Hb] \qquad (24)$$

$$T_{L}co(c) = T_{L}co(m) \, (14.6a + [Hb]/(1 + a) \, [Hb] \qquad (25)$$

where $T_{L}co$ (C) and $T_{L}co$ (M) are the corrected and measured values for $T_{L}co$ respectively; [Hb] is the concentration of haemoglobin in ml dl^{-1}; *a* is the D_{m}/V_{C} ratio.

The equation of Dinkara and colleagues was derived using data from a cross-sectional study of patients with varying degrees of anaemia from a variety of causes. The factor obtained corrects the observed values for $T_{L}co$ to the mean predicted value for that individual. Thus the corrected $T_{L}co$ is standardized to an expected value and not to a given level of haemoglobin. This gives a linear relationship between corrected $T_{L}co$ and haemoglobin concentration. In the study by Cotes and co-workers, the effect on $T_{L}co$ of increasing haemoglobin concentration by iron replacement therapy in healthy young women suffering from iron deficiency anaemia was measured. The results were found to fit the theoretical curve predicted by the equation of Roughton and Forster (1957; eqn 20). The equation was therefore derived to correct the observed $T_{L}co$ to a standard haemoglobin concentration of 14.6 gm dl^{-1}, assuming a D_{m}/V_{C} ratio of 0.7 in accordance with the predicted values reported and a value for Θ when breathing air of 1. This gives a curvilinear relationship between corrected $T_{L}co$ and haemoglobin concentration. The equation derived by Dinkara and colleagues produces a greater correction in $T_{L}co$ which becomes more pronounced as the haemoglobin concentration falls than is given by the equation of Cotes and co-workers. Both equations have limitations. Since the correction factor of Dinkara and colleagues was not calculated from a direct change in haemoglobin concentration but assumed that the reduction in $T_{L}co$ in their patients was entirely due to the effect of anaemia, their equation may overestimate the correction required. However, the equation derived by Cotes and colleagues was based on the change in $T_{L}co$ with increase in haemoglobin concentration, standardized to give a haemoglobin concentration and has a theoretical basis. It is therefore probably the best equation currently available.

(ii) Detection of intrapulmonary haemorrhage. The increase in $T_L co$ in the presence of a raised level of haemoglobin has been found to be a useful indicator of the occurrence of bleeding into the alveoli which occurs in various immunologically mediated disorders such as Goodpasture's syndrome or pulmonary haemosiderosis. Such episodes may be difficult to detect using other conventional tests such as the chest radiograph (Greening and Hughes, 1981). By using a radioactive isotope ($C^{15}0$), Ewan and colleagues (1976) showed that when an episode of bleeding occurred, there was an increase in kCO but that the clearance of radioactivity from the lung was reduced, implying that the increased uptake of CO was due to combination with the haemoglobin in the fresh uncoagulated blood which had pooled in the alveoli. Greening and Hughes (1981) using the single breath method showed that a rise of kCO and to a lesser extent $T_L co$ (*after correction for haemoglobin concentration*) using the formula of Cotes *et al.* of 50% or more above baseline value (*not* the patient's predicted value) is indicative of recent intra-pulmonary haemorrhage. Since the extravasated blood will rapidly denature and the haemoglobin no longer combine with CO, it is essential that $T_L co$ is measured frequently in patients in whom intrapulmonary haemorrhage is suspected. Greening and Hughes report a minimum half-time for decline of kCO and $T_L co$ of 1.7 days and they therefore recommend that serial measurements of $T_L co$ should be made at intervals of not more than 3 days and preferably daily in these patients. Frequent measurements are also required to establish a baseline level for the individual. Such measurements of $T_L co$, in conjunction with traditional methods (chest radiograph, fall in haemoglobin concentration, haemoptysis) can be helpful in these patients by monitoring intrapulmonary haemorrhage (Greening and Hughes, 1981).

Carboxyhaemoglobin (COHb)

Back-pressure of CO is usually considered negligible in the estimation of $T_L co$. However, this assumption may be invalid in heavy smokers in whom COHb levels as high as 20% may occur. In addition, the combination of CO with haemoglobin produces a functional anaemia by reducing the amount of available haemoglobin and consequently reduces Θ. Although correction for back-pressure and the percentage of COHb is not currently standard in routine laboratories, the advent of facilities for rapid and simple measurement of venous COHb in conjunction with many commercial blood-gas analysers (see Chapter 6), routine correction for both back-pressure (calculated from COHb%

and the CO dissociation curve) and COHb% itself should perhaps be considered in smokers. A correction factor for the single breath $T_L co$ using healthy non-smoking subjects has been derived by relating the measured $T_L co$ to the COHb% produced by acute inhalation of low concentration CO gas mixtures (Mohsenifar and Tashkin, 1979) where:

$$\text{Percent reduction } T_L co = -0.97 \text{ COHb\%} + 0.33 \qquad (26)$$

However, correction for back-pressure and COHb% does not entirely account for the reduced $T_L co$ in smokers since for a given level of COHb, the reduction in $T_L co$ is greater than predicted from the above equation and D_m is less than in non-smokers (Frans *et al.*, 1975). These observations suggest smoking causes some structural lung damage.

Capillary Blood Volume (V_c)

(i) Effect of exercise. In normal subjects, exercise increases $T_L co$. If a steady state technique is used to measure $T_L co$ part of this increase is the result of exercise hyperpnoea increasing lung volume (Anderson and Shepherd, 1968). However, if lung volume is kept constant by measuring $T_L co$ by the single breath method, the rise on exercise has been shown to be due to an increase in V_c (Danzer *et al.*, 1968). The linear increase in $T_L co$ with work rate at low levels of exercise is attributed to capillary recruitment due to perfusion of the lung apices. At higher levels of exercise, the less steep rise in $T_L co$ with further increases in work rate is probably due to dilatation of blood vessels after maximum recruitment has been reached (Stokes *et al.*, 1981).

(ii) Disorders of the pulmonary circulation. The variation in $T_L co$ in disorders of the pulmonary circulation (in the presence of otherwise normal lung function) have been shown to result from the alterations in V_c produced by changes in inflow (pulmonary arterial) and outflow (pulmonary venous) pressures (Burgess, 1974). Thus conditions in which there is an obstruction of the inflow of blood to the lungs (for example by pulmonary emboli), V_c is reduced and $T_L co$ falls. Conversely, conditions which are characterized by a low pulmonary vascular resistance with an increase in pulmonary blood flow (as in the presence of left-to-right shunts), V_c is increased and $T_L co$ elevated above normal.

J

Influence of Regional Distribution of Ventilation and Perfusion

Uneven distribution of ventilation and perfusion throughout the lungs has relatively little effect on T_Lco measured by either the single breath or rebreathing methods but will influence steady state estimates especially at rest (Bates *et al.*, 1971). Theoretical calculations have also shown that inequalities of ventilation–diffusion and diffusion–perfusion ratios will cause underestimation of T_Lco both by steady state (Chinet *et al.*, 1971) and single breath (Piiper and Sikand, 1966) methods.

PREDICTED NORMAL VALUES

Many population studies have been reported in which predicted normal values have been derived. In general, T_Lco and its subdivisions D_m and V_c positively correlate with height and age, with kco correlating with age alone. Reference to these studies with details of the prediction equations are given elsewhere (Cotes and Hall, 1970; Bates *et al.*, 1971; Cotes, 1979). However, many of these studies have been done using mixed populations of smokers and non-smokers. A recent study in which 96% of the subjects were lifetime non-smokers reported predicted values for T_Lco and kco which for men were greater than other reported values and for women were among the highest previously reported(Crapo *et al.*, 1981). In view of these findings and the observations that T_Lco and D_m are reduced in smokers, the values used for predicting normality should be based on data from a population of non-smokers only.

References

Anderson, T. W. and Shephard, R. J. (1969). *Respiration* **26**, 102–115.
Bates, D. V., Boucot, N. G. and Dormer, A. E. (1975). *J. Physiol.* **129**, 237–252.
Bates, D. V., Macklem, P. T. and Christie, R. V. (1971). *In* "Respiratory Function in Disease", 2nd Edn, pp. 10–95. W. B. Saunders Co., Philadelphia.
Bohr, C. (1909). *Skand. Arch. Physiol.* **22**, 221–280.
Burgess, J. H. (1974). *Circulation* **49**, 541–550.
Burgess, J. H. and Bishop, J. M. (1963). *J. Clin. Invest.* **42**, 997–1006.
Chinet, A., Micheli, J. L. and Haab, P. (1971). *Respir. Physiol.* **13**, 1–22.
Clarke, E. H., Jones, H. A. and Hughes, J. M. B. (1978). *Lancet* **i**, 791–793.
Comroe, J. H., Forster, R. E., Dubois, A. B., Briscoe, W. A. and Carlsen, E. (1962). *In* "The Lung", pp. 111–139. Year Book Medical Publishers Inc., Chicago.
Cotes, J. E. (1979). *In* "Lung Function", 4th Edn, pp. 238–259; 340–395. Blackwell Scientific Publications, Oxford.
Cotes, J. E., Dabbs, J. M., Elwood, P. C., Hall, A. M., McDonald, A. and Saunders, M. J. (1972). *Clinc. Sci.* **42**, 325–335.

Cotes, J. E. and Hall, A. M. (1970). *In* "Normal Values for Respiratory Function in Man", pp. 327–343. Panminerva Medica, Torino.

Crapo, R. O. and Morris, A. H. (1981). *Am. Rev. resp. Dis.* **123**, 185–189.

Danzer, L. A., Cohn, J. E. and Zechman, F. W. (1968). *Respir. Physiol.* **5**, 250–258.

Dinkara, P., Blumenthal, W. S., Johnston, R. F., Kauffman, L. A. and Solnick, P. B. (1970). *Am. Rev. resp. Dis.* **102**, 965–969.

Ewan, P. W., Jones, H. A., Rhodes, C. G. and Hughes, J. M. B. (1976). *N. Engl. J. Med.* **295**, 1391–1396.

Frans, A., Stanescu, D. C., Veriter, C., Clerbaux, T. and Brasseur, L. (1975). *Scand. J. Resp. Dis.* **56**, 165–183.

Greening, A. P. and Hughes, J. M. B. (1981). *Clin. Sci.* **60**, 507–512.

Guleria, J. S., Pande, J. N., Sethi, P. K. and Roy, S. B. (1971). *J. appl. Physiol.* **31**, 536–543.

Hamer, N. A. (1963). *Clin. Sci.* **24**, 275–285.

Jones, R. S. and Meade, F. (1961). *Quart. J. exp. Physiol.* **46**, 131–143.

Krogh, M. (1914). *J. Physiol.* **49**, 271–300.

Lewis, B. M., Lin, T-H., Noe, F. E. and Hayford-Welsing, E. J. (1959). *J. clin. Invest.* **38**, 2073–2086.

Magnussen, H., Holle, J. P., Hartmann, V. and Schoenen, J. D. (1979). *Respiration* **37**, 177–184.

Marshall, R. (1977). *Am. Rev. resp. Dis.* **115**, 537–539.

McHardy, G. J. R. (1972). *Br. J. dis. Chest.* **66**, 1–20.

Mohsenifar, Z. and Tashkin, D. P. (1979). *Respiration* **37**, 185–191.

Ogilvie, C. M., Forster, R. E., Blakemore, W. S. and Morton, J. W. (1956). *J. clin. Invest.* **36**, 1–17.

Piiper, J. and Sikand, R. S. (1966). *Respir. Physiol.* **1**, 75–87.

Riley, R. L., Cournand, A. and Donald, K. W. (1951). *J. appl. Physiol.* **4**, 102–120.

Rose, G. L., Cassidy, S. S. and Johnson, R. L. (1979). *J. appl. Physiol.* **47**, 32–37.

Roughton, F. J. W. and Forster, R. E. (1957). *J. appl. Physiol.* **11**, 290–302.

Stokes, D. L., MacIntyre, N. R. and Nadel, J. A. (1981). *J. appl. Physiol.* **51**, 858–863.

12. ASSESSMENT OF THE CONTROL OF BREATHING AND MONITORING DURING SLEEP

A. Gordon Leitch

City Hospital, Edinburgh, U.K.

CONTROL OF BREATHING

Haldane (1935) demonstrated the remarkable stability of alveolar Pco_2 in man and showed that elevation of alveolar Pco_2 produced by inhaling carbon dioxide resulted in striking increases in ventilation leading to the conclusion that the "respiratory centre" was exquisitely sensitive to changes in arterial Pco_2. Many years later animal experiments established the presence of chemoreceptive areas in the lateral medulla oblongata which were sensitive to local changes in Pco_2 or (H^+) (Mitchell, 1963); stimulation of these areas increased ventilation (Mitchell *et al.*, 1963; Loeschke, 1974). These chemosensitive areas, now labelled the Central Chemoreceptors, are considered to mediate most of the ventilatory response to changes in arterial Pco_2 by influencing respiratory neurones in the brain stem.

The ventilatory response to inhaled CO_2, now known to be genetically determined (Leitch *et al.*, 1975; Leitch, 1976b) and age related (Kronenberg and Drage, 1973) has a wide range of normal values from 4.3–$61.3\,1\,1\,min^{-1}\,kPa^{-1}\,Pco_2$ (Rebuck and Read, 1971; Hirschman *et al.*, 1975). It may be high in sprint athletes (Rebuck and Read, 1971) and head injury (Moss *et al.*, 1974) and is reduced in sleep (Bulow, 1963), acute asthma (Rebuck and Read, 1971) and severe chronic bronchitis and emphysema with CO_2 retention (Flenley and Millar, 1967) as well as in some apparently normal people and endurance athletes (Rebuck and Read, 1971). Induced metabolic acid-base changes alter the ventilatory response to CO_2. Acidosis lowers the intercept of the $\dot{V}/Pco_2$ line on the Pco_2 axis and alkalosis increases it, neither condition producing a change in slope (Cunningham *et al.*, 1961; Goldring *et al.*, 1968).

Haldane was also aware that hypoxia stimulated ventilation although the effect was less striking than that produced by increases in P_{CO_2} (Boycott and Haldane, 1908). The carotid and aortic chemoreceptors, first studied by Heymans and Heymans (1926) were shown to discharge, with resulting increases in ventilation, in response to lowered P_aO_2 (Hornbein *et al.*, 1961) and increases in P_aCO_2 and H^+ (Lahiri and Delaney, 1975a and b). The effect of changes in P_{CO_2} or H^+ is most marked at low P_{O_2} and in normoxic man the peripheral chemoreceptor probably mediates only 15–20% of the ventilatory response to inhaled CO_2 (Cunningham *et al.*, 1964; Wade *et al.*, 1970), this component being abolished at P_{O_2} above 30 kPa (Dejours, 1962). The principal function of these *Peripheral Chemoreceptors* is to sense changes in arterial P_{O_2} and from studies in patients who have undergone bilateral carotid body resections, we know that this is mediated almost entirely by the carotid bodies (Lugliani *et al.*, 1971).

The ventilatory response to hypoxia is genetically determined (Leitch *et al.*, 1975; Leitch, 1976b); decreases with age (Kronenberg and Drage, 1973) and shows a wide range of values in normal man (Hirschman *et al.*, 1975). The response is decreased in high altitude residents (Sorensen and Severinghaus, 1968a), cyanotic congenital heart disease (Sorensen and Severinghaus, 1968b), the obesity-alveolar hypoventilation syndrome (Sutton *et al.*, 1976) and in some patients with severe chronic bronchitis and emphysema (Flenley *et al.*, 1970) and may be increased in patients with severe head injury (Leitch *et al.*, 1980).

The aim of the next section is to outline available methods for measuring these ventilatory responses to carbon dioxide and hypoxia.

MEASUREMENT OF CHEMICAL CONTROL OF BREATHING

Apparatus

A system which is suitable for measurement of both ventilatory response to carbon dioxide and hypoxia is described below.

Supply of inspired gases

Gas mixtures are conveniently delivered from a rotameter assembly (Fig. 1) with a minimum of three rotameters: rotameter (1) giving a

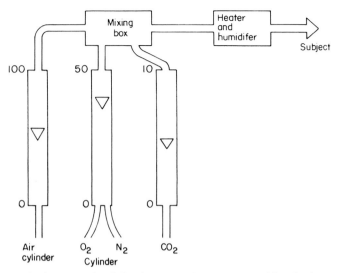

FIG. 1. A system for delivering a continuous range of inspired gas.

flow of up to 100 l min^{-1} air, rotameter (2) giving a flow of up to 50 l min^{-1} of nitrogen or oxygen, and rotameter (3) giving a flow of up to 10 l min^{-1} of carbon dioxide. Alterations in flow rates of different gases allow preparation of the complete range of hypoxic, hyperoxic, and hypercapnic gas mixtures. The gases may come directly from cylinders, but a cheap alternative system for air is a rheostat controlled vacuum cleaner. The gases from the rotameters (total flow rate conveniently 100 l min^{-1}) should pass into and through a mixing box and then be warmed and humidified prior to delivery to the breathing circuit through low resistance respiratory tubing (Fig. 1).

Circuitry (Fig. 2)

The valve box is connected to the gas supply tubing via a T-tube of similar dimensions. Non inspired gases are conducted in respiratory tubing to a reservoir which may be open or closed, preferably the latter. With a closed, compliant reservoir (a rubber concertina suspended on springs) with an adjustable exhaust system (a vacuum cleaner again) a floppy balloon (condom latex or Paul's tubing) attached to the reservoir allows the operator to adjust pressure fluctuations in the system occasioned by ventilation to oscillate around atmospheric pressure. A continuous positive pressure in the circuit, indicated by erect Paul's tubing, can be avoided with this system and thus leakage of the gas supply

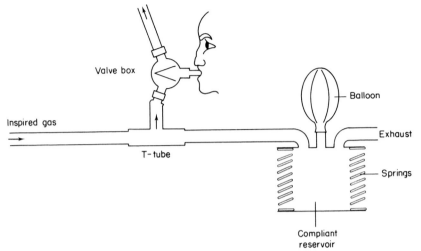

Valve box

Balloon

Inspired gas

Exhaust

T-tube

Springs

Compliant
reservoir

FIG. 2. Arrangements of apparatus on inspiratory side of valve box.

through the T-tube and the inspiratory valve flaps with the resultant errors in measurement of ventilation avoided.

Valve Box

A low resistance, low dead space valve box is desirable for ventilation which may range from 10–60 l min^{-1} in studies on healthy subjects. An Otis–McKerrow valve is suitable and can be simply modified for sampling of respiratory gases near the lips. Expired gas should always pass through low resistance tubing.

Measurement of Ventilation

Expired minute ventilation can be measured in a number of ways:

(a) By timed collections in Haldane bags or spirometer.
(b) Using a dry gas meter after the expired gas has been passed through a condenser to dry it. The volumes may be read directly from the meter or from an electronically produced digital output (a photoelectric cell placed under the dial).
(c) With a heated pneumotachograph (e.g. Fleisch No. 3) on the expiratory side of the valve and electronic integration of flow to give volume.

The advantage of the first two methods lies in their simplicity, the disadvantage is that only *minute* ventilation (and frequency) can be measured. Advantages of the pneumotachograph include the ability to produce breath by breath values for instantaneous minute ventilation (VE,INST) (VE,INST = $V_T \times 60/t$, where V_T = tidal volume and t = breath duration), as well as values for tidal volume, frequency and inspiratory and expiratory times. Disadvantages of the pneumotachograph include its propensity to change calibration factor in the course of an experiment and the need to ensure that the pneumotachograph output for a given flow is unaffected by changes in gas composition (unlikely to be a problem below 30% oxygen mixtures).

The pneumotachograph is particularly suited to circuits employing computers for analogue to digital conversion and display of respiratory variables (see below).

Measures of Po_2, Pco_2 *and* S_aO_2

In normal subjects Po_2 and Pco_2 at the lips can be continuously sampled using either fast-response CO_2 and O_2 analysers or a respiratory mass spectrometer previously calibrated with gases of known composition analysed with the Lloyd–Haldane apparatus. In such normal subjects the end-tidal values for Pco_2 and Po_2 are considered to reflect arterial values.

In subjects with disordered lungs, direct expired gas samples do not reflect arterial blood-gas tensions which must be estimated directly in blood obtained from a radial or brachial arterial catheter. In such subjects, the effect of changing the inspired gas composition must be monitored closely with frequent arterial blood gas estimations.

The Hewlett-Packard ear oximeter is a reliable and non-invasive method of monitoring oxygenation (Douglas *et al.*, 1980).

Recording

Outputs such as Po_2, Pco_2, V_T and V_E can be recorded on a chart recorder such as a Mingograph (Eleina-Schonander) for subsequent calculation by hand utilising appropriate calibrations or if off-line computer facilities are available on magnetic tape for subsequent analysis. Online computer facilities are ideal but expensive.

The Ventilatory Response to Carbon Dioxide

This measurement, made under hyperoxic conditions ($P_aO_2 > 30$ kPa) is believed to reflect the sensitivity of the central chemoreceptor to CO_2. As with other measurements made at rest it is essential for the subject to

256 A. G. LEITCH

be comfortable and to be remote from visual, auditory and tactile stimuli which may influence ventilation. Soothing music supplied by earphones is desirable and if manipulations near the subject are necessary during the experiment it is best for the subject to be blindfolded. The relation between ventilation and P_{CO_2} at a given P_{O_2} is linear above resting P_{CO_2} and is described by the equation: $\dot{V}_E = S(P_{CO_2} - B)$ where S is the slope of the line in $1 \ min^{-1} \ kPa^{-1}$ and B (kPa) is the intercept on the x axis. Two methods of measurement are currently employed.

The Steady State Method

On exposure of a subject to a given concentration of CO_2 in inspired air it takes approximately 6 or 7 minutes before minute ventilation and arterial or end-tidal P_{CO_2} stabilize. Measurements made after this (e.g. between 7–10 min are "steady-state" measurements of ventilation and P_{CO_2}. Determination of three such points of the $\dot{V}_E/P_{CO_2}$ line following sequential inhalations of 2%, 4% and 6% CO_2 in hyperoxic gas mixtures allow determination of the slope (S) and intercept (B) of the CO_2 response line. Where measurements of the CO_2 response line are being made at many different P_{O_2} levels (see later) two points on each line may suffice, the determination of more points unnecessarily prolonging an already lengthy experiment.

The Rebreathing Method

First developed by and theoretically justified by Read (1966; Read and Leigh, 1967) the rebreathing method allows the measurement of the hyperoxic CO_2 response in a few minutes. Measurement of slope (S) of the CO_2 response line by this method correlates well with steady state methods except in metabolic disturbances of acid-base balance (Cameron et al., 1972). The intercept (B) of the CO_2 response line is higher by 0.8 kPa on average with this method for reasons discussed by Read and Leigh (1967).

The simplest methodology employs a bag-in-box technique where the subject rebreathes from a 6 l bag containing 7% CO_2 93% O_2. P_{CO_2} is monitored at the mouth; ventilation is measured either by a pneumotachograph connected to the box or by a spirometer or dry gas meter connected to the box by a breathing valve (Fig. 3).

Volume and P_{CO_2} are averaged over 15 or 30 s intervals after the first 30 s of the record have been discarded. A plot of $\dot{V}_E$ against P_{CO_2} will give the hyperoxic CO_2 response line. Alternatively, breath by breath values for $\dot{V}_E$ and P_{CO_2} can be plotted if these are available.

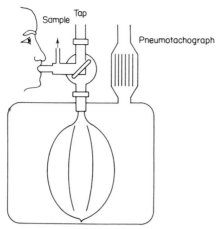

FIG. 3. Bag in box circuit.

The Ventilatory Response to Hypoxia

As a general rule it is unwise to lower Po_2 below 5 kPa for any length of time when studying normal subjects.

The Steady State Response

This classical method (Lloyd *et al.*, 1958) involves determination of the ventilatory response to CO_2 during hyperoxia as well as at one or more reduced levels of Po_2. For most purposes determination of S at Po_2 equal to 6.7 kPa and 30 kPa will suffice (Leitch *et al.*, 1974; Leitch *et al.*, 1976b). Such a study takes one hour consisting of 5 periods each of 10 min breathing the following gas mixtures:

(1) air breathing for acclimatization
(2) 2% CO_2 at PO_2 = 30 kPa
(3) 2% CO_2 at PO_2 = 6.7 kPa
(4) 5% CO_2 at PO_2 = 30 kPa
(5) 5% CO_2 at PO_2 = 6.7 kPa

Measurements of $\dot{V}_E$, end tidal Pco_2 and Po_2 are made in the last three minutes of each 10 minute period. A typical response from a study is shown in Fig. 4. Hypoxic drive can be expressed as the ratio of the slopes of the two lines or alternatively as the increment in ventilation occurring at resting Pco_2 when Po_2 falls from 30 to 6.7 kPa (Sorensen and Severinghaus, 1968).

If several CO_2 response lines at different Po_2 s (e.g. 30, 12, 9, 7, 6 and 5 kPa) are measured, and this is a lengthy experiment, then a more

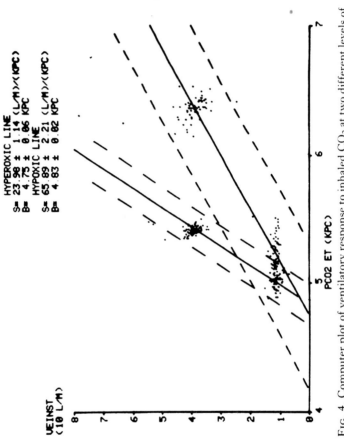

Fig. 4. Computer plot of ventilatory response to inhaled CO_2 at two different levels of P_{O_2} (30 kPa and 6.7 kPa, hyperoxic and hypoxic lines respectively). The slopes of the CO_2 response lines with their 95% confidence limits are shown.

sophisticated analysis, well described by Cunningham (Lloyd and Cunningham, 1963), is possible. Readers are referred to this paper for further details but warned that determination of hypoxic sensitivity by this method is less reproducible, perhaps because of the duration of the experiment, than with other methods (Leitch *et al.*, 1976b).

Progressive, Isocapnic Hypoxia

First described by Weil *et al.* (1970) this method involves recording breath by breath values for instantaneous minute ventilation while arterial Po_2 is lowered from 13 to 5 kPa over 12–15 minutes either by the addition of nitrogen to the inspired air or by the use of a rebreathing circuit where Po_2 falls as the result of metabolic utilization of oxygen (Rebuck and Campbell, 1974). Pco_2 is kept constant at resting levels in the first method by addition of CO_2 to the inspired gases and in the second by absorption with a "scrubber" circuit.

The relationship between ventilation and Po_2 is curvilinear (Fig. 5) and hypoxic sensitivity can be expressed by the shape parameter of the curve A when $\dot{V}_E = \dot{V}_o + [A/(P_{AO_2} - 4)]$, [4] representing the Po_2 in kPa at which the slope of the $\dot{V}_E/Po_2$ curve approaches infinity.

Curve fitting facilities are not essential if an ear-oximeter is used (Rebuck and Campbell, 1974) for then the relationship between $\dot{V}_E$ and S_aO_2 is linear, the slope of the line representing hypoxic sensitivity.

Transient Hypoxia during Exercise

Dejours (Dejours *et al.*, 1958; Dejours, 1962) was the first to explore the effects of transient changes in Po_2 on ventilation and his methods have since been employed in a number of situations (Edelman *et al.* 1973). Exposure of a normal subject to three breaths of nitrogen during mild exercise (3 mph on a level treadmill) produces transient hypoxaemia and a transient hyperventilation (Fig. 6). This test has been used as a screening test for reduced hypoxic sensitivity in normal man and a wide range of responses expressed as $\dot{V}_E/S_aO_2$ has been detected (Leitch, 1981). The test is recommended for its simplicity.

Transient Hyperoxia

Exposure to a few breaths of 100% oxygen effectively abolishes the peripheral chemoreceptor contribution to ventilation at rest or on exercise (Dejours, 1962) representing 10–20% of total ventilation

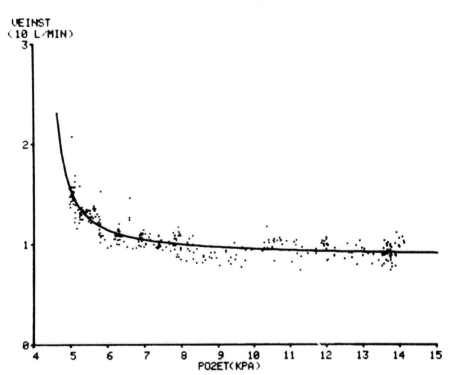

FIG. 5. Computer plot of ventilatory response to progressive isocapnic hypoxia in one subject at rest. Each point represents one breath.

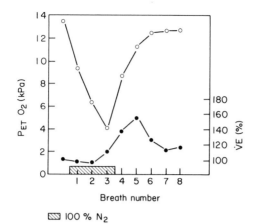

Breath number

☒ 100 % N₂

FIG. 6. Transient hypoxia on exercise. Changes in P_{O_2} end-tidal and $\dot{V}_E$ following three breaths of 100% nitrogen.

(Lambertson *et al.*, 1963) in normal man. This test has been used in patients with chronic bronchitis (Lee and Bishop, 1974), interstitial lung disease (Stockley and Lee, 1976) thyroid disease (Stockley, 1976) and in patients with head injury (Leitch *et al.*, 1980) and is particularly useful for detecting increased peripheral chemoreceptor contributions such as occur in head injury (Fig. 7).

Measurement of Occlusion Pressure

In the methods described above minute ventilation has been used as the indicator of respiratory centre output in response to chemical stimuli. Although this is acceptable for studies in normal subjects, the altered resistance and compliance of the lungs and chest wall found in disease may make ventilation an unreliable indicator of the output of the respiratory centre.

Whitelaw and colleagues (1975) have described an alternative measure of respiratory drive in conscious man—the occlusion pressure. This is the pressure recorded at the mouth 0.1 s after occlusion of the inspiratory side of a breathing circuit while the subject is at end-expiration or functional residual capacity. The apparatus required is simple and the only precaution to be stressed is that it should be silent and that the subject should be unaware of impending occlusion. A tap or shutter on the inspiratory side of a non-rebreathing valve is closed during an expiration and the measurement made during the subsequent inspiration. One measurement can be made every ten breaths. The

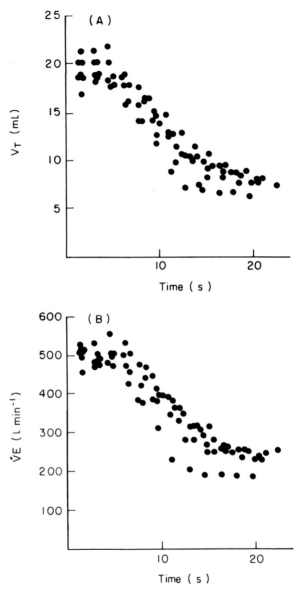

FIG. 7. Changes in instantaneous minute ventilation and tidal volume following seven breaths of 100% oxygen in a head-injured patient.

occlusion pressure or $P_{0.1}$ correlates well with the electrical activity in the phrenic nerve (Lourenco *et al.*, 1966). Since it is measured in the absence of air, flow is independent of lung and chest wall compliance and airway resistance.

In the presence of respiratory loads the $P_{0.1}$ response to progressive hypoxia or CO_2 rebreathing can increase even when the ventilatory response is restricted indicating an increase in respiratory centre output in response to the load even although appropriate increases in ventilation are restricted by the load (Lopata *et al.*, 1977).

It would therefore seem sensible in studies on subjects with lung disease to measure both the ventilatory and $P_{0.1}$ responses to chemical stimuli.

SLEEP STUDIES

Ventilatory responses to carbon dioxide and hypoxia (particulary the former) are decreased during sleep (Phillipson, 1978) and both hypercapnia and hypoxia occur during sleep in normal man as well as worsening during sleep in patients with cor pulmonale (Leitch *et al.*, 1976a). Recently, application of the methods outlined below have resulted in a marked increase in understanding of the changes in respiratory variables which may occur during sleep.

Methods and Apparatus

Sleep studies are best performed in a sleep laboratory so designed as to exclude the monitoring equipment from the subject's immediate environment. However, any quiet area, suitably sound-proofed and provided with a comfortable bed will do. Subjects should ideally have two and certainly one night sleeping in this environment to accustom themselves to the situation and the many attachments to their body necessary for full monitoring.

Sleep Staging

Electroencephalogram (EEG), electromyogram (EMG) and electro-oculogram (EOG) recording throughout the night by standard methods (Rechtschaffen and Kales, 1968) allows subsequent scoring of sleep stages into stages 1–4 and rapid eye movement or REM sleep.

Air Flow

Air flow can be monitored at both nostrils and the mouth by suitable placed thermistors or thermocouples. More recently, a microphone, placed over the sternal notch, to record breath sounds has been used to indicate the presence or absence of air flow (Krumpe and Cunningham, 1980). All of these methods are qualitative, not quantitative.

Chest Wall Movement

Movements of the chest wall can be recorded qualitatively by a pneumogram, an impedance stethogram, magnetometers or by a "respiratory vest" (Sackner, 1980).

Arterial Oxygen Saturation

Ear oxygen saturation can be recorded using the Hewlett-Packard ear oximeter (Douglas *et al.*, 1980).

Other Measurements

Heart rate can be recorded using chest wall ECG electrodes. In special cases it may be useful to record pulmonary arterial pressure from an indwelling right heart catheter or arterial blood gas tensions on samples from an indwelling arterial catheter (Douglas *et al.*, 1979). Endoesophageal pressure can be recorded from a transducer tipped catheter inserted through the nasopharynx into the oesophagus to supplement other methods of measuring respiratory excursions.

Recording and Analysis

EEG, EMG and EOG are recorded on one paper chart recorder. Other variables are usually recorded on a separate chart recorder. Subsequent analysis is facilitated if a time signal generator is used to mark both charts thus allowing matching of changes in respiratory variables to sleep stage. Alternatively respiratory variables can be recorded (with a time signal) on magnetic tape for subsequent analysis off-line by computer (Loudon *et al.*, 1980) or they can be recorded directly by computer.

Applications

Recent investigations with the above methods have revealed profound falls in arterial oxygen saturation in patients with chronic respiratory failure and cor pulmonale secondary to chronic bronchitis and

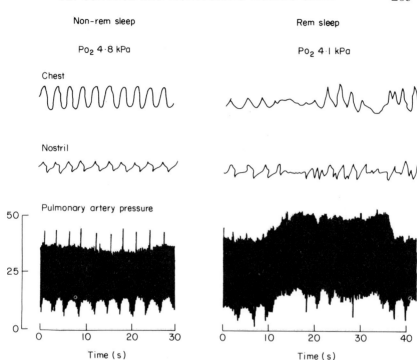

FIG. 8. Nasal airflow, chest-wall movement and pulmonary artery pressure in non-REM sleep and during a hypoxic episode of REM sleep.

emphysema (Wynne *et al.*, 1979; Douglas *et al.*, 1979). These hypox-aemic episodes usually occur in REM sleep, are associated with disordered breathing patterns and are associated with worsening of pulmonary arterial hypertension (Fig. 8). Similar, but less striking, changes may be seen in patients with asthma (Catterall *et al.*, 1982).

Monitoring of respiratory variables has also provided insight into the hypersomnia syndromes frequently associated with obesity in which hypersomnia and snoring are associated with respiratory failure and, often, right heart failure (Guillemenault and Dement, 1978). In these syndromes monitoring of nasal and oral as well as respiratory movements has revealed episodes of apnoea (defined as cessation of airflow for greater than 10 s) which are associated with hypoxaemia, pulmonary artery hypertension and, in some cases, cardiac arrhythmias. The apnoeic episodes may be central (absence of airflow and respiratory movements), obstructive (absence of airflow with respiratory movements) or mixed where the two are combined (Fig. 9). The central form of apnoea may be amenable to respiratory stimulants such as progester-

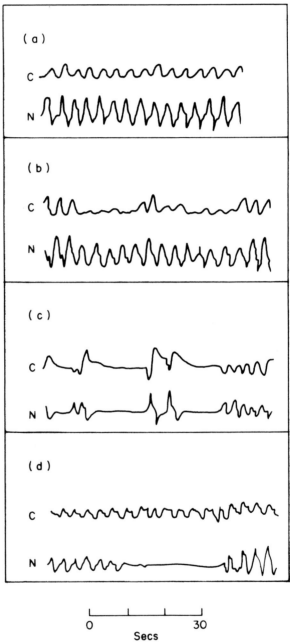

FIG. 9. Records of nasal airflow and chest-wall movement during normal breathing, hypopnoea, central apnoea and obstructive apnoea.

one (Sutton *et al.*, 1975). The obstructive form of apnoea with obstruction occurring at the level of the oropharynx is probably due to a combination of anatomical and physiological abnormalities (Remmers *et al.*, 1978) and may ultimately require treatment by tracheostomy (Coccagna *et al.*, 1972).

References

Boycott, A. E. and Haldane, J. S. (1908). *J. Physiol.* **37**, 355–372.

Bulow, K. (1963). *Acta Physiol. Scand.* **59**, Suppl. 209.

Cameron, I. R., Davies, R. J., Linton, R. A. F. and Poole-Wilson, P. A. (1972). *J. Physiol.* **226**, 56P.

Catterall, J. R., Douglas, N. J., Calverley, P. M. A., Brash, H. M., Brezinova, V., Shapiro, C. M. and Flenley, D. A. (1982). *Lancet* **i**, 305–307.

Coccagna, G., Mantovan, M., Brignani, F., Parchi, C. and Lugaresi, E. (1972). *Bull de Physiopath. Respiratoire* **8**, 1217–1227.

Cunningham, D. J. C., Shaw, D. G., Lahiri, S. and Lloyd, B. B. (1961). *Quart. J. exp. Physiol.* **46**, 323–330.

Cunningham, D. J. C., Patrick, J. M. and Lloyd, B. B. (1964). *In* "Oxygen in the Animal Organism" (Eds F. Dickens and E. Neil) p. 277. Pergamon, Oxford.

DeJours, P. (1962). *Physiol. Rev.* **42**, 335–350.

DeJours, P., Labrousse, Y., Raynaud, J., Girard, P. and Teillac, A. (1958). *Rev. fr. Etud. clin. biol.* **3**, 105–116.

Douglas, N. J., Calverley, P. M., Leggett, R. J. E., Brash, H. M., Flenley, D. C. and Brezinova, V. (1979). *Lancet* **i**, 1–4.

Douglas, N. J., Brash, H. M., Wraith, P. K., Calverley, P. M., Leggett, R. J. E., McElderry, L. and Flenley, D. C. (1980). *Am. Rev. resp. Dis.* **119**, 311–313.

Edelman, N. H., Epstein, P., Lahiri, S. and Cherniack, N. S. (1973). *Resp. Physiol.* **17**, 302–314.

Flenley, D. C. and Millar, J. S. (1967). *Clin. Sci.* **33**, 319–334.

Flenley, D. C., Franklin, D. H. and Millar, J. S. (1970). *Clin. Sci.* **38**, 503–518.

Goldring, R. M., Cannon, P. J., Heinemann, H. O. and Fishman, A. P. (1968). *J. Clin. Invest.* **47**, 188–202.

Guillemenault, C. and Dement, W. C. (eds.) (1978). "Sleep Apnea Syndromes". Liss, New York.

Haldane, J. S. and Priestley, J. G. (1935). "Respiration". O.U.P., London.

Heymans, J. F. and Heymans, C. (1926). *C. R. Soc. Biol. (Paris)* **94**, 399–407.

Hirschman, C. A., McCullough, R. E. and Weil, J. V. (1975). *J. appl. Physiol.* **38**, 1095–1098.

Hornbein, T. F., Griffo, Z. J. and Roos, A. (1961). *J. Neurophysiol.* **24**, 561–579.

Kronenberg, R. S. and Drage, C. W. (1973). *J. Clin. Invest.* **52**, 1812–1819.

Krumpe, P. E. and Cummiskey, J. M. (1980). *Am. Rev. resp. Dis.* **122**, 797–801.

Lahiri, S. and Delaney, R. G. (1975a). *Resp. Physiol.* **24**, 249–266.

Lahiri, S. and Delaney, R. G. (1975b). *Resp. Physiol.* **24**, 267–286.

Lambertson, C. J., Hall, P., Wollman, H. and Goodman, M. W. (1963). *Ann. N.Y. Acad. Sci.* **109**, 731–742.

Lee, K. D. and Bishop, J. M. (1974). *Clin. Sci. Mol. Med.* **46**, 347–356.

Leitch, A. G. (1981). *Lancet* **i**, 428–430.

Leitch, A. G. (1976a). "The Hypoxic Drive to Breathing in Normal Man". PhD Thesis. University of Edinburgh.

Leitch, A. G. (1976b). *Ann. Hum. Biol.* **3**, 447–454.

Leitch, A. G., Clancy, L. J. and Flenley, D. C. (1974). *Clin. Sci. Mol. Med.* **47**, 377–385.

Leitch, A. G., Clancy, L. J. and Flenley, D. C. (1975). *Clin. Sci. Mol. Med.* **48**, 235–238.

Leitch, A. G., Clancy, L. J., Costello, J. F. and Flenley, D. C. (1976a). *Brit. Med. J.* **1**, 365–367.

Leitch, A. G., Clancy, L. J. and Flenley, D. C. (1976b). *Clin. Sci. Mol. Med.* **51**, 12P.

Leitch, A. G., Clancy, L. J., Leggett, R. J. E., Tweeddale, P., Dawson, P. and Evans, J. I. (1976c). *Thorax* **33**, 711–713.

Leitch, A. G., Balkenhol, S., McLennan, J. E., McLaurin, R. L. and Loudon, R. G. (1980). *J. appl. Physiol.* **49**, 52–58.

Lloyd, B. B., Jukes, M. G. M. and Cunningham, D. J. C. (1958). *Quart. J. Exp. Physiol.* **43**, 214–227.

Lloyd, B. B. and Cunningham, D. J. C. (1963). *In* "Regulation of Human Respiration" (Eds B. B. Lloyd and D. J. C. Cunningham), pp. 331–342. Blackwell, Oxford.

Loeschke, H. H. (1974). *In* MTP International Review of Science. Physiology Series 1. Vol. 2. "Respiratory Physiology" (Eds A. C. Guyton and J. G. Widdicombe). Butterworths, London.

Lopata, M., Evanich, M. J. and Lourenco, R. V. (1977). *Amer. Rev. resp. Dis.* **116**, 449–456.

Loudon, R. G., Leitch, A. G., Walsh, J. F., Kramer, H. and Ridgway, T. H. (1980). *Abs. Pap. A.C.S.* **180**, 60.

Lourenco, R. V., Cherniack, N. S., Malm, J. C. and Fisherman, A. P. (1966). *J. appl. Physiol.* **21**, 527–533.

Lugliani, R., Whipp, B. J., Seard, C. and Wasserman, K. (1971). *New Eng. J. Med.* **285**, 1105–1108.

Mitchell, R. A., Loeschke, H. H., Massion, W. H. and Severinghaus, J. W. (1963). *J. appl. Physiol.* **18**, 523–533.

Moss, I. R. A., Wald, A. and Ransohoff, J. (1974). *Amer. Rev. resp. Dis.* **109**, 205–215.

Phillipson, E. A. (1978). *Amer. Rev. resp. Dis.* **118**, 909–940.

Read, D. J. C. (1966). *Australas. Ann. Med.* **16**, 20–32.

Read, D. J. C. and Leigh, J. (1967). *J. appl. Physiol.* **23**, 53–70.

Rebuck, A. S. and Read, J. (1971). *Clin. Sci.* **41**, 13–21.

Rebuck, A. S. and Campbell, E. J. M. (1974). *Amer. Rev. resp. Dis.* **109**, 345–350.

Rechtschaffen, A. and Kales, A. (1968). Manual of standardised terminology, technique and scoring system for sleep stages of human subjects. N.I.N.D.B. Bethesda, Maryland.

Remmers, J. E., Degroot, W. J., Sauerlan, E. K. and Anch, A. M. (1978). *J. appl. Physiol.* **44**, 931–938.

Sackner, M. A. (1980). In Diagnostic Techniques in Pulmonary Disease. (Ed. M. A. Sackner, Part I), New York, Marcel Dekker.

Sorensen, S. C. and Severinghaus, J. W. (1968a). *J. appl. Physiol.* **25**, 217–220.

Sorensen, S. C. and Severinghaus, J. W. (1968b). *J. appl. Physiol.* **25**, 221–224.

Stockley, R. A. (1976). *Clin. Sci. Mol. Med.* **51**, 12P.

Stockley, R. A. and Lee, K. D. (1976). *Clin. Sci. Mol. Med.* **50**, 109–114.

Sutton, F. D., Zwillich, C. W., Creagh, C. E., Pearson, D. J. and Weil, J. V. (1976). *Ann. intern. Med.* **83**, 476–479.

Wade, J. G., Larson, C. P., Hickey, R. F., Ehrenfeld, W. K. and Severinghaus, J. W. (1970). *New Engl. J. Med.* **282**, 823–825.

Weil, J. V., Byrne-Quinn, E., Sodal, I. E., Friesen, W. O., Underhill, B., Filley, G. F. and Grover, R. F. (1970). *J. Clin. Invest.* **49**, 1061–1065.

Whitelaw, W. A., Derenne, J. P. and Milic Emili, J. (1975). *Resp. Physiol.* **23**, 181–199.

Wynne, J. W., Block, A. J., Hemenway, J., Hunt, L. A., Shaw, D. and Flick, M. R. (1978). *Chest* **73** (Suppl.) 301.

13. EXERCISE TESTING

G. Laszlo and G. J. R. McHardy

Bristol Royal Infirmary, Bristol, U.K.
City Hospital, Edinburgh, U.K.

CLINICAL AND PHYSIOLOGICAL PRINCIPLES

Exercise tests are useful in the investigation of the function of the heart and lungs. Like any system, faults may appear under stress which are not apparent during quiet operation. In practice, exercise tests are carried out for the following reasons:

(1) To determine maximum exercise performance.
(2) To uncover physiological abnormalities which may not be present at rest.
(3) To investigate the mechanisms of adaptation to exercise in health and disease and their modification by therapeutic intervention.

The principles and practice of exercise testing have been well reviewed and the reader is referred to specialized works (Godfrey (1974), Jones *et al.* (1975), Wasserman and Whipp (1975) and Spiro (1977) for the respiratory tests, Boyle (1981) for a description of exercise testing in ischaemic heart disease).

Muscular exercise increases the requirement of the body for oxygen and the output of carbon dioxide. Muscles are adapted to function over a wide range of tissue Po_2 and Pco_2, therefore an increased delivery of oxygen to the tissues does not require a proportional increase in the output of the heart. Other organs do not increase their metabolic requirement during exercise but they are poorly tolerant of variations in Po_2 and chemical milieu. Therefore, an important aspect of adaptation to exercise is the maintenance of constant blood-gas pressures in the blood leaving the lungs (the arterial blood). Pulmonary ventilation therefore increases proportionately to the metabolic demand. Imperfections in the distribution of ventilation and perfusion within the lungs result in inefficiency of pulmonary gas exchange and therefore an increased ventilatory requirement and low arterial P_{O_2}. These respiratory abnormalities may be detected during sub-maximal tests.

Exercise itself may induce decreases of bronchial calibre in patients with bronchial asthma. This may occur during prolonged exercise but usually *after* six to eight minutes of intensive exercise. Simple measurements of peak flow rate or FEV_1 before and at intervals after a period of maximum exercise are diagnostic.

When the coronary arteries are narrowed, the blood supply to the exercising heart may be insufficient for its needs. A reduced oxygen supply to heart muscle with the consequent liberation of the products of anaerobic metabolism, may result in chest pain, which is usually relieved by up to five minutes' rest. Such pain usually causes depression of the ST segments of the 12-lead electrocardiograph over the appropriate area; the changes are transient and their severity and extent correlated with the severity of the impairment of the coronary circulation. Maximal exercise tests are required to demonstrate this phenomenon which may be of diagnostic value in cases of unusual chest pain or of prognostic value when considering surgical intervention.

DURATION AND TYPE OF TESTS

No single test provides a complete diagnostic assessment to cover all clinical situations, so most laboratories select one of a number of standard protocols to meet the individual need. Table I lists some of the alternatives.

TABLE I

Alternative protocols in exercise testing

Measurements:	Simple	Complex
Equipment?:	Free walking or running	Stationary ergometer
Ergometer:	Cycle	Treadmill
Protocol:	Fixed load	Incremental load
Duration:	Unsteady state	Steady state
End point:	Submaximal	Maximal

MEASUREMENTS

The respiratory physiologist is interested mainly in the relationship of the rate and depth of breathing, the carbon dioxide output and the oxygen uptake in relation to the physical work performed. Heart-rate and electrocardiographic monitoring are essential adjuncts. The maintenance of a normal arterial P_{CO_2} implies intact ventilatory control mechanisms, while the presence of a normal arterial P_{O_2} or oxygen saturation is a *sine qua non* of normal pulmonary gas exchange. Heart-rate and electrocardiographic monitoring are necessary. Knowledge of the cardiac output is helpful in defining the normal cardiovascular response to exercise and for the interpretation of blood gas abnormalities which may be compounded by poor tissue perfusion as well as the impairment of the gas exchanging mechanism of the lungs. Specialized measurements such as carbon monoxide uptake (diffusing capacity) may also be undertaken during exercise for particular purposes. The remainder of this chapter is concerned with some of the problems of measurement and will not deal further with interpretation of the results.

Ventilation, Oxygen Consumption and Carbon Dioxide Output

The formula for oxygen consumption is:

$$\dot{V}_{O_2} = \dot{V}_I \cdot F_{I O_2} - \dot{V}_E \cdot F_{E O_2}$$

That for CO_2 output is:

$$\dot{V}_{CO_2} = \dot{V}_E \cdot F_{E CO_2} - \dot{V}_I \cdot F_{I CO_2}$$

In a well ventilated room, $F_{I CO_2}$ is 0.03% and usually ignored. The formula therefore simplifies to:

$$\dot{V}_{CO_2} = \dot{V}_E \cdot F_{E CO_2}$$

The classical method of calculating ventilation and gas exchange is sufficient for most purposes, but it depends on the assumption that there is a steady state of carbon dioxide and oxygen exchange. In this situation, the volume of the nitrogen inspired is equal to that expired, the difference between $\dot{V}_I$ and $\dot{V}_E$ being accounted for entirely by differences between $\dot{V}_{O_2}$ and $\dot{V}_{CO_2}$. $\dot{V}_I$ may then be calculated from $\dot{V}_E$ and vice versa from the formula:

$$\dot{V}_I \cdot F_{I N_2} = \dot{V}_E \cdot F_{E N_2}$$

$F_{E N_2}$ may be calculated from the formula:

$$F_{E N_2} = 1 - (F_{E O_2} + F_{E CO_2})$$

In this context $F_{I N_2} = .7904$ which actually includes argon and other trace gases but not carbon dioxide.

For a rigorously accurate analysis of oxygen consumption when steady state conditions are not present, it is necessary to measure both inspired and expired ventilation. The subject may breathe in from one spirometer and out into another. Analysis is performed on the expired gas. Alternatively, a pneumotachograph may be placed on the inspired and the expired lines. This also permits analysis of the inspiratory and expiratory flow patterns. Calibration of these devices must be rigorous, if such measurements are to achieve the highest degree of accuracy. The pneumotachograph on the inspired line must be calibrated with room air at room temperature while that on the expired line should be heated and calibrated with a moistened mixture of 4% carbon dioxide, 16% oxygen, balance nitrogen.

Circuits for the Measurement of Ventilation

The essential ingredient is a non rebreathing valve with equal resistance on both sides which should not exceed 0.5 cm $H_2O/l. \sec^{-1}$. Table II lists a few of the devices available for measuring ventilation and collecting expired gas.

TABLE II

Choice of equipment for the construction of exercise circuits

	Inspired	Expired
Ventilation	Dry gas meter Pneumotachograph Anemometer	100–150 l capacity Spirometer
Gas collection		PVC bag Mixing chamber Spirometer (100–150 l capacity)

A non-rebreathing valve is necessary to separate the inspired and expired flow of air. This should have as low as possible dead-space and resistance. The requirements for physiological studies of high endurance in healthy individuals are different from those involving patients with respiratory limitations who cannot achieve high air flows. In the latter case, a robust value of three-quarter inch (2 cm) diameter with mica spring loaded one-way valves suffices. This device has a dead-space of approximately 60 ml. The Lloyd valve (Cunningham et al., 1965) achieves a much lower resistance for the same dead-space. It is made of perspex and the flap valves are returned to position under the influence of gravity. These valves must be kept scrupulously clean and all traces of saliva removed, the final rinse being with distilled water. These valves are more likely to stick and to give trouble.

For most ordinary purposes, a reasonable compromise may be achieved by using a larger version of the first valve, available commercially with a dead-space of 100 ml and diameter of one inch (2.5 cm). The additional dead-space results in a significant increase in the ventilatory requirement and allowance must be made for normal values. The valve has a sufficiently low resistance in the range required for most clinical exercise tests.

For accurate measurements of ventilation, tidal volume and inspiratory and expiratory flow rates, high quality perspex valves are an essential investment. Low resistance is paramount when air flow rates are to be studied. Low dead-space is important when a rapid shallow breathing patterns are adopted. Choice of valve therefore remains a compromise in each case.

For measurements in the steady state, a 100–150 l, water filled spirometer (Tissot, Chapter 2) is the best reservoir for the collection of expired gas which can be circulated within it by means of a fan. It is necessary to flush out the dead-space with expired gas for a considerable period of time. 100 or 150 l plastic bags with suitable ports, also flushed out for a period, form an adequate substitute when inspired ventilation is to be measured. Reservoirs of expired air may be emptied rapidly by means of a small vacuum cleaner motor. Mixed expired gas may be analysed continuously at the distal end of a suitable mixing chamber (Fig. 1). A minimum volume of 3 l is required with suitable baffles.

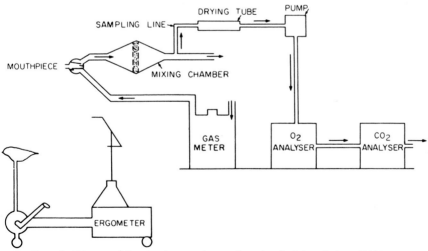

FIG. 1. Diagram of a simple exercise testing circuit (after Spiro, 1977).

Devices incorporating a mixing chamber on the expired side and the pneumotachograph or rotating vein anemometer have become much more accurate with the availability of inexpensive microcomputing techniques. Continuous sampling of mixed expired gas by means of rapidly responding analysers with automated averaging techniques yields identical results to those obtained by analysis of mixed expired gases. Moreover, the availability of stable integrators and the possibility of performing integration after recording of the flow rates within the computer, has greatly simplified the measurement of ventilation by this means. However, the electronic measurement of inspired ventilation by means of potentiometers attached to the dial of a gas meter or the pulley of a Tissot spirometer is extremely accurate, needing no recalibration provided that the power source is stable (Spiro, 1977).

Analysis of Expired and Inspired Gases at the Mouth

Rapid continuous tidal gas analysis at the mouth provides valuable information and continuous monitoring of the respiratory pattern. Carbon dioxide is usually displayed during the test. The tidal oscillations of CO_2 indicate stability of breathing pattern and provide an early warning of malfunctioning of the expired valve flap when CO_2 fails to fall to zero concentration during inspiration.

Rapid continuous gas analysis, for example, by mass spectrometry, permits other measurements to be made by respiratory means. When the lungs are healthy, the gas pressures in the blood leaving the lungs bear a close relationship to the mean P_{CO_2} at the mouth (after allowance is made for wash out of the gas in the valve box and the mouth and upper airways where no gas exchange takes place). This mean value bears a predictable relationship to the "end-tidal" point when allowance is made for the rate and depth of breathing (Bradley et $al.$, 1976). In the presence of severe ventilation–perfusion mismatching, the end-tidal point and the mean expired P_{CO_2} cannot be used to predict arterial P_{CO_2}. Analysis of the changes of expired gas concentrations after changes are made in the composition of the inspired gases may be used to derive information about a number of cardio respiratory functions. A chapter has been devoted to carbon monoxide uptake which is limited by intrapulmonary gas distribution and diffusion from the alveoli into the red cells. Carbon monoxide is uniquely suitable for this purpose because of its very high chemical affinity for haemoglobin and its relatively low solubility in water and lung tissues. The uptake of other gases of moderate solubility is limited by the rate at which the lungs are perfused, relatively simple and accurate measurements of cardiac output may be obtained employing these gases (Cander and Forster, 1959; Sackner *et al.*, 1975; see also p. 158).

Oxygenated, mixed venous P_{CO_2} may be determined simply by rebreathing mixtures of carbon dioxide, oxygen and nitrogen for ten seconds. The method is described in detail by Jones *et al.* (1967 and 1975).

The reader is referred elsewhere for a detailed description of these techniques which are mentioned here because they require the facility of rapid switching from one respiratory circuit to another, without change of the position of the mouthpiece. Figure 2 illustrates two methods of achieving this. In one, two or more circuits can be brought in front of the mouthpiece at the cost of little additional dead-space by having the circuits moveable. This is necessarily cumbersome. If the circuits are to remain fixed in position, additional dead-space is required for a pneumatically operated valve to switch the conducting passage from one circuit to another. Much ingenuity has been expended in the design of these circuits, none of which is ideal.

Other Possible Modifications to the Respiratory Circuit

(1) Measurement of expired ventilation may be obviated by the introduction of a carefully measured bias flow of an insoluble foreign gas into the inspired air ($\dot{V}_{bias}/\dot{V}_E = F_E$ gas).

(2) The resistance of the valve box may be overcome by the addition of a bias flow of large volumes of air. Measurements of expired gas concentrations will then differ only slightly from those of the inspired gas with consequent loss of accuracy.

(3) Measurements of expired gas concentrations may be made from tidal sampling at the mouth, provided that there is an accurate device for sensing the onset and cessation of expiratory flow and provided that careful allowance is made for the delay between sampling and analysis in the mass spectrometer or rapid analysers.

Measurement of Ventilation Without a Mouthpiece

Changes in the rate and depth of breathing may readily be determined by strapping devices onto the chest wall which give signals as a result of displacement. The simplest is the old fashioned mercury strain gauge which was strapped round the chest and offered some resistance to breathing. Magnetometers placed on the chest wall give a deflection proportional to the distance between them. Simple systems are quite

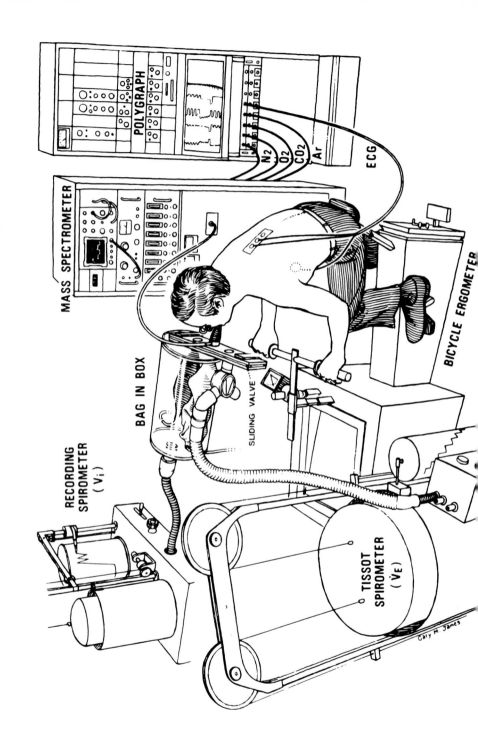

POLYGRAPH

N₂
O₂
CO₂
Ar

ECG

MASS SPECTROMETER

BICYCLE ERGOMETER

BAG IN BOX

SLIDING VALVE

RECORDING
SPIROMETER
(V̇ᵢ)

TISSOT
SPIROMETER
(V̇ᴇ)

Gary M. James

From
Solenoid 2

Gas port 1   Gas port 2

O-
rings

From
Solenoid 1

Plastic
piston
valve

Rubber piston seals

Mouthpiece

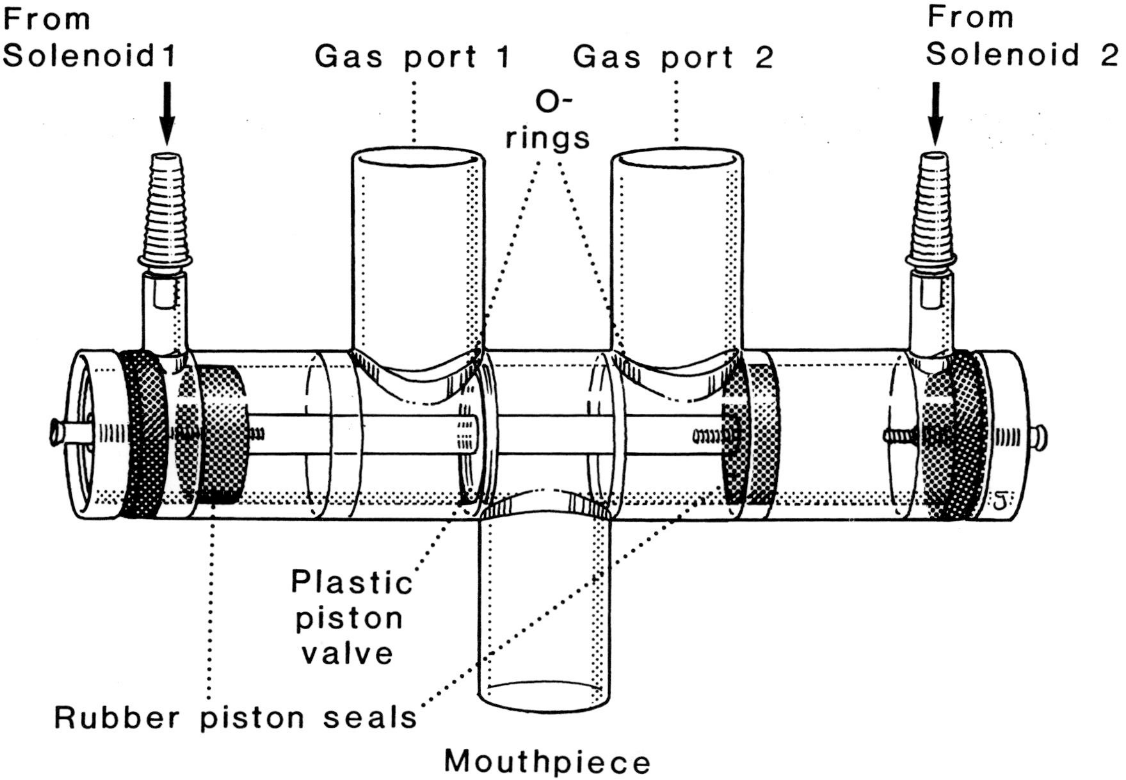

Fig. 2. Two methods of changing rapidly from one circuit to another. (a) Fixed mouthpiece and moveable circuits (designed by G. T. R. Lewis). (b) A pneumatic tap which selects one of two outlets (designed by Dr Norman L. Jones).

(b)

K

alinear and unsuitable for quantitative analysis of respiratory volumes as opposed to deformation of the thoracic cage.

The inductance plethysmograph (Cohn *et al.*, 1975) has been described in Chapter 2. The sensors are attached like a cuirass to the chest wall. The device may be calibrated at various tidal volumes and breathing frequencies to yield reliable estimates of ventilation to a relatively high degree of accuracy. The calibration of the device changes with posture but, for the purposes of exercise test on a static ergometer, this does not introduce a problem. The problem of measuring respiratory gas exchange non-invasively has not yet been solved.

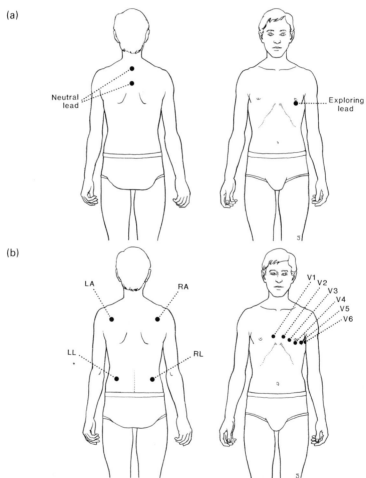

FIG. 3. Position of electrocardiograph leads (a) simulated V4; (b) 12: lead electrocardiograph.

Heart-Rate

This may be measured simply by counting off on an electrocardiograph. Heart-rate meters are readily available and easily constructed which identify and count the R waves. For this purpose, a simulated V4 is most likely to give a tall R wave, permitting a deflection meter to count these and ignore the P and T waves. In patients with right ventricular hypertrophy, it may be necessary to place the exploring electrode more laterally on the chest wall (V5 or V6) and to increase the amplification. For the purposes of identifying rhythm changes and heart-rate, a simulated V4 is sufficient. A simple, three-lead system attached to lead 1 of the bi-polar electrodes will suffice (Fig. 3a).

For a full ECG recording, facilities for 12-lead electrocardiography are required, preferably recording three channels simultaneously. The leads are placed as in Fig. 3b, or wherever movement artefact is least.

For stable recordings, careful preparation and close apposition of the skin electrodes is necessary. We recommend cleaning with a mixture of acetone and ethyl acetate to remove grease from the skin and abrading slightly with a wooden spatula before applying the electrode jelly recommended for use with the electrodes chosen. Interference between the ergometer and the ECG channel is a common source of difficulty which has to be overcome by suitable earthing of the ergometer circuit.

Continuous monitoring of the electrocardiogram on an oscilloscope or continuously moving paper is mandatory during exercise testing.

Blood Pressure

This most basic of measurements is most difficult. Arterial blood pressure can only be measured accurately by means of an indwelling arterial catheter attached to a transducer. This is rarely justified in investigation of the respiratory system although it is standard procedure in cardiac laboratories, where investigations are being conducted in preparation for major surgical procedures. However, the failure of systolic pressure to rise in the normal manner is an important early warning of the presence of cardiac disease and blood pressure monitoring is an essential adjunct to the performance of maximal exercise testing in patients with ischaemic heart disease. No satisfactory method yet exists. Most units, therefore, adopt the simplest method which is to measure the systolic pressure with the aid of a standard sphygmomanometer stethoscope or by palpation from time to time during the exercise test. During exercise, systolic pressure rises and diastolic pressure falls. The latter cannot be determined by auscultation of the Korotkov sounds. Commercially available systems which automatically inflate the cuff and auscultate by Doppler techniques (Hill and Dolan, 1976) are not reliable in exercise.

Changes in blood pressure can be monitored in the resting individual by means of finger pulse sensors. However, these are not accurate during exercise tests. The circulatory adjustment to severe exercise consists in part of a redistribution of blood flow from organs where it is not critical; to exercising muscle. Intense vasoconstriction of the skin is therefore the rule and this alters the impulses from the digital pulp.

Pulmonary Artery Pressure

In patients without myocardial disease, pulmonary artery pressure may safely be measured in the upright position by means of a fine catheter floated into the pulmonary artery.

Cardiac Output

Reference has already been made to indirect methods of assessing pulmonary blood flow by means of the uptake and excretion of foreign gases whose absorption is limited by the circulation, as compared with insoluble gases which act as markers for the intrapulmonary distribution of inspired gas. These methods are not readily applicable to those with severe lung disease, when the wash-in of all gases, whether insoluble or insoluble, into the alveoli, is very slow, or when a significant proportion of the blood flow is distributed to very poorly ventilated alveoli. There is no way of measuring blood flow to unventilated portions of the lung by measurements made exclusively in respired gases.

The most accurate reference method for determination of pulmonary blood flow is by the direct Fick principle.

The following is a mass equation for oxygen uptake, permitting the calculation of cardiac output if oxygen uptake and arterial and venous oxygen contents are analysed simultaneously.

$$\text{Cardiac output} = \frac{O_2 \text{ consumption}}{\text{arterial } O_2 \text{ content} - \text{venous } O_2 \text{ content}}$$

The patient must be in steady state of oxygen uptake and measurements made simultaneously. The technique, therefore, requires the simultaneous sampling of mixed venous blood from the pulmonary artery catheter, arterial blood and accurate assessment of oxygen uptake, traditionally by the collection of mixed expired gas in a Tissot spirometer. Such measurements are accurate at rest and under all conditions of steady state exercise, but require cardiac catheterization and arterial blood sampling.

The accuracy of the method depends partly on the fact that quite wide variations of pulmonary ventilation cause very little change in oxygen uptake because of the shape of the oxygen dissociation curve. (Chapter 4).

In theory, it should be possible to obtain the same results, substituting CO_2 for oxygen in the equation. In practice this is very difficult because it is hard to achieve a steady state of CO_2 output. The CO_2 dissociation curve (the relationship between CO_2 pressure and CO_2 content of arterial blood) is very steep in the range of pressures found within the lungs. The result of this is that minor changes in the pattern of breathing produce quite large oscillations of arterial CO_2 content. In exercise, when the turnover of CO_2 is greatly increased, these swings are proportionately less important. Oxygenated mixed venous P_{CO_2} may be estimated by rebreathing and arterial P_{CO_2} obtained by direct sampling from an artery. With some loss of accuracy, capillary samples may be used. The veno–arterial content difference for CO_2 may be determined from partial pressure measurements by the knowledge of the CO_2 dissociation slope. This is predictable from the knowledge of haemoglobin concentration, pH of the blood and P_{O_2}. (McHardy, 1967). It should, however, be admitted that the formulae are derived from analyses on very small numbers of blood samples obtained in the early days of blood gas chemistry. Ideally, the CO_2 dissociation slope of an individual patient's blood should be determined at each session by tonometry, but the art of analysis of CO_2 content in whole blood is largely lost and unskilled measurements are likely to introduce more error than the use of published nomograms.

Some uncertainty exists about the significance of rebreathing methods of estimating oxygenated mixed venous P_{CO_2} during exercise. (Jones et al., 1967). The choice of indirect methods for the estimation of cardiac output is adequate for most purposes. Most methods agree with direct Fick measurements, when careful comparisons are made to within 10% in grouped mean data, and have a coefficient of variation of around 20%.

Non-Respiratory Measurement of Cardiac Output

The impedance cardiogram is a device which measures alterations in transthoracic impedance, correcting for respiratory oscillations. It reflects changes in pulmonary blood flow and, assuming these are uniformly distributed across the lungs, may be calibrated in any position to yield accurate measurements of cardiac output. It is a useful device when exact numerical values are not required. Claims for its simplicity and accuracy are exaggerated and it seems to be more difficult to obtain meaningful results than when it is being tested under ideal experimental conditions in normal subjects. It is probably most useful in intensive care wards as a semi-qualitative monitor of change. For detailed account of the measurement of cardiac output by indicator dye dilution and thoracic impedance, the reader is referred to Hill and Dolan (1976).

Blood Gas Measurements

Repeated direct sampling of arterial blood requires the insertion of an indwelling arterial catheter. In the majority of cases, adequate information may be obtained by indirect means, usually involving arterializing the capillaries of the skin. Arterialization of capillary blood implies increasing the blood flow to an area of skin to such an extent that the oxygen consumption there is low in relation to blood flow. Little gas exchange takes place in any given unit of capillary blood which then approximates closely to arterial blood. Arterialization may be achieved by heating the skin and by rubbing on rubifacients such as Algipan, or similar proprietry preparations of capsicum or thurfyl nicotinate cream.

Arterialized Capillary Blood Sampling

Modern micro-electrodes are capable of accurate analysis of Pco_2 and Po_2 in samples of 50 μl or less. The ear lobe is the favoured site for arterialized capillary sampling, although finger pulp may be equally accurate. Rubifacient creams cause no serious discomfort when applied to the ear lobe and the patient is unable to see the sampling process which is quick and almost painless. A modification of the method described by Godfrey et al. (1971) is recommended (Spiro and Dowdeswell, 1976). A rubifacient is rubbed onto the surface of the ear lobe. A no. 11 fine scalpel blade is used to make a slash of about 3 mm depth across the tip of the ear lobe onto a sterilized rubber bung which prevents accidental cuts being made elsewhere. The lobe should drip blood profusely at rest because the blood flow falls in exercise. A heparinized swab may be clamped to the ear with a clip and should be released frequently and the ear lobe rubbed to maintain blood flow throughout the test. Commercially available sampling capillaries as appropriate to the micro blood gas analyser, primed with heparin, may be used to collect the samples, rather than the expensive method recommended by Godfrey of using an intravenous cannula with a luer fitting. Blood should be collected directly into the capillary tube by inserting it into the slit to ensure anaerobic sampling. The blood should not be massaged directly into the tube because this alters its pH, but such massage is recommended between samples to maintain vasodilation. One operator is generally required to look after the blood sampling process. It is possible to acquire the knack of filling the capillary tube over a period of time to obtain simultaneous arterial and expired gas samples for determining the degree of imperfection of pulmonary gas exchange and for use in the indirect Fick equation for calculation of cardiac output.

Ear Lobe Oximetry

The oximeter is described elsewhere (Chapter 5). It is suitable for the identification of arterial desaturation during exercise. The high cost of this instrument makes it less available than it should be, but several studies bear witness to its accuracy, especially when arterial saturation is above 50%.

Other Measurements

For accurate interpretation of blood gas measurements, a knowledge of body temperature is required. Alveolar temperature lies closer to core temperature than to mouth temperature, the latter is most accurately assessed by the insertion of a thermistor probe into the rectum. When this is considered undesirable, the external auditory meatus of the ear or the skin of the groin under clothing may be used to monitor changes in body temperature. In general, skin temperature does not reflect changes in core temperature during exercise. The subject is discussed fully by Harris *et al.* (1978). Measurement of changes in body temperature are necessary if subtle analyses of the changes in blood Pco_2, pH and Po_2 are to be made, since these measurements are dependent for their accuracy on a knowledge of the temperature of the blood *in vivo*, as well as in the recording electrodes. During heavy exercise, body temperature may rise by 1°C changing Po_2 and Pco_2 by 5% and 4% respectively (Chapter 4).

PROTOCOL

Incremental loads of 1 or 4 min duration (Jones *et al.*, 1975) are most commonly used, in steps of 25 or 50 watts. Fixed single loads are useful when a series of complex measurements are to be made or when comparisons are made before and after some form of therapy or intervention. In the latter case, rehearsal effect should be taken into account. Performance with a fixed load test on two or three consecutive days may result in improvement between the first and the second, but usually there is little difference between the second and the third. By contrast, physical training may improve performance more gradually over a period of time, and this effect is soon lost if training is discontinued.

Standardized fixed load tests which cover all eventualities have necessarily to be very light for all patients to be able to tolerate them. However, in certain circumstances, a load corresponding to a given percentage of an individual's maximum may be selected for a serial study.

Steady State

After a change of workload, one to two minutes is required for full adjustment of the physiological variables, ventilation, heart rate, oxygen consumption and CO_2 output. Speed of adjustment is a function of physical fitness. From the third to the fourth minute after the onset of exercise, most subjects achieve a quasi-steady state in which pulmonary oxygen and carbon dioxide exchange reflect tissue metabolism. If exercise is prolonged, subtle alterations take place in the proportion of fat to carbohydrate metabolized, resulting in the gradual fall of the products of anaerobic metabolism.

Submaximal and Maximal Tests

Maximal exercise tests imply that the subject is to exercise either to exhaustion or to some pre-determined physiological limit identified by the operator. The hazard of such procedures is necessarily greater than that of submaximal testing.

The following end points may be identified.

Cardiovascular Limitation.

Maximum heart rate is achieved. Above a certain heart rate, the output of the heart falls because insufficient time is available for the chambers to fill during diastole (relaxation). Maximum heart rate is a function of age, the formula most commonly used being

210 − 0.8 × age (Astrand formula in Spiro *et al*., 1977). The operator should stop the test at this point.

Severe chest pain. The patient is usually instructed to stop when this occurs. Ischaemic heart pain, *angina pectoris*, is typically central and may also be felt in the throat, jaws, back or down the arms. Characteristically, it is accompanied by electrocardiographic changes, but these may be most easily detected when the patient lies down after the test.

Systolic blood pressure ceases to rise incrementally. This is generally an indication of impending myocardial insufficiency.

The appearance of exhaustion, profuse sweating, pallor or an ashen complexion with blue lips and ears. These are signs of impending cardiovascular collapse or inadequate oxygenation and call for immediate termination of the test.

The development of multiple ventricular extra systoles (VES). There is no general agreement on what frequency is acceptable. Ten VES per minute, not occurring at rest but developing during exercise, is probably the safe limit and the test should be terminated if there are runs of ventricular tachyarrhythmia, or two or more VES occur consecutively.

Faintness (syncope). Faintness or dizziness may be caused by inadequate cardiac output to the brain. The cause may be failure of the heart to pump, obstruction to the circulation or transient fall of cerebral blood flow caused by overbreathing with fall of arterial Pco_2 and consequent respiratory alkalosis. The latter condition is usually recognizable as the patient is normally visably overbreathing. A history of effort syncope will normally have been obtained and maximal exercise tests should not normally be carried out in such patients.

Fall of arterial Po_2 may also cause faintness and dizziness. This symptom may occur when there is failure of the apparatus with the resultant inadvertent rebreathing. All breathing circuits must be checked before the test.

Respiratory Limitation

Patients may safely be asked to exercise until they are too short of breath to carry on, provided that the above cardiovascular reasons for stopping the test do not occur. The majority of patients with lung disease will be limited by shortness of breath.

Weakness or Aching of the Legs

Most normal subjects carrying out unfamiliar exercise such as cycling will be limited by the power of untrained muscles as much as by cardiovascular or respiratory factors. Those with severe hip disease or with poor circulation to the lower limbs are normally limited by these factors, and maximal stress to the cardiovascular respiratory system is usually not possible. Other muscle groups may be exercised, for example, hand grip may be tested but only in trained subjects is exercise by small muscle groups limited by cardio respiratory factors rather than by pain or weakness.

CONDUCT OF A CYCLE ERGOMETER

Preparation

Patients visiting the exercise laboratory for the first time may be somewhat alarmed by the apparatus and by the thought of what is in store. Our practice is therefore to show the patient around the laboratory and show them how they are merely required to perform breathing tests similar to those already carried out at rest, under conditions of exercise.

The patient is then asked to change or to strip to the waist. Patients should be warned beforehand of the need to bring suitable clothing and shoes. The electrodes are placed in position in the changing room, while the calibration process is completed, preferably in the patient's absence.

The equipment should be in working order and all checks completed before the patient is invited to mount the ergometer, after which the test should proceed with as little delay as possible.

If samples are to be obtained at rest, these should ideally be measured seated in a comfortable chair. When severely disabled patients are to be studied, there is some advantage to be gained in making all the measurements in a dental chair or equivalent seat, the pedals of the cycle ergometer being operated in the semi-recumbent position. Most patients will be able to tolerate the saddle of a normal cycle ergometer though they will require some practice in turning the pedals if they have not previously ridden a bicycle. It is difficult to obtain true resting conditions when perched on a saddle for five minutes at a time, and values for oxygen consumption and carbon dioxide output will be considerably greater than those obtained when seated in comfort. Five minutes of acclimatization are required to obtain steady resting samples. Since resting ventilation is only $5-10$ 1 min^{-1}, considerable time is required to wash out the expired tubing before measurements of expired gases are made.

Nervous individuals who overbreathe easily may become dizzy perching on the saddle at rest. Such subjects are better studied in exercise immediately as overbreathing is much less likely to cause rapid falls of arterial Pco_2 because of the higher CO_2 turnover rate.

When the subject is comfortable and not unduly anxious, the heart rate falls to 80 beats per minute, when measurements of ventilation and oxygen consumption will probably reflect a true resting condition.

Comfort

It is essential that the subject should be seated comfortably and that the mouthpiece should be in the correct position. Numerous ways exist of mounting the mouthpiece. Slight mobility of this may be an advantage but a fixed device is quite acceptable, provided that it can be adjusted readily, should the patient adopt a different position of his head and neck during heavy exercise than at rest when the initial adjustment was made. The subject should be leaning forward slightly in the position adopted by most amateur cyclists on an upright bicycle. Experienced cyclists should have the saddle placed high enough for the legs to be almost, but not quite, extended on to the lower pedal. Those who have not cycled before may require a lower saddle position, enabling them to apply pressure with the instep rather than with the toe. Under these conditions, exercise is likely to be limited by fatigue of the legs or inability to turn the pedals, rather than by cardiac or respiratory limitation.

Starting and Stopping

Usually, one operator will attend to the patient, the mouthpiece and the blood sampling while the second operator watches the machines and the monitors, performing calibrations as and when necessary.

On a cycle ergometer, a short warm-up period at light workloads to build up the speed to the usual 60 r/min, is desirable. The protocol is then followed as rigidly as possible.

Problems may occur with excessive salivation. Most test protocols allow for occasional removal of the mouth from the mouthpiece to deal with excessive salivation. This is an important precaution as Lloyd valves in particular function badly when wet. The nose clip may be released at the same time as negative pressure effects may occur in the inner ears as a result of repeated swallowing with the nose occluded.

When the test is to be concluded, the patient may continue to turn the pedals against a much reduced or zero load as this minimizes the risk of rebound hyperventilation and subsequent aching of the limbs. Pulse rate should be monitored until it has almost settled down.

Peak flow is measured before, and five minutes and ten minutes after cessation of exercise and the patient observed for a possible development of exercise-induced bronchial asthma.

Safety

The electrocardiogram must be monitored continuously throughout the test. The indications for stopping the exercise have been enumerated above. It is also desirable to monitor CO_2 continuously at the mouth, to identify rapid changes in breathing patterns or malfunctioning of the valve. The identification of the end point of a maximal exercise test is described on p. 286.

The patient is instructed to discontinue exercise and take the mouth off the mouthpiece, should there be pain in the chest or any part of the body, any feeling of dizziness or faintness or any sensation of obstruction to the breathing. It is safe to continue a test until the patient is too short of breath to continue. The test must be stopped if any other limiting factor supervenes.

Resuscitation facilities with a functioning telephone should be available very close to the testing procedure. Two operators should always be present in the room. Medical supervision is required under the following conditions:

(1) all patients over the age of 40;
(2) all patients with known cardiac disease;
(3) any patient with bronchial asthma whose resting pulmonary function is abnormal.

Properly conducted exercise tests are safe and the rare event of ventricular fibrillation (two occurrences out of 17 000 tests in one series), successful resuscitation is usual. Patients with pulmonary hypertensive disorders are particularly prone to unexpected death within 48 h of unusual exercise and should be tested only when the indications are very clear.

Occasionally, a patient will attend for an exercise study who has taken very little exercise for a number of years, but who will conceal the extent to which the experience is new. Usually, such patients develop inappropriate tachycardia and the exercise test is terminated for that reason, but the appearance of pallor or inappropriate sweating, or the development of a bluish tinge of the face, ears or lips calls for the immediate discontinuation of the test. From time to time, patients will have a myocardial infarct within a short period of the test which would have occurred in any case. This will happen only rarely if patients are examined when in their normal state of health. The operator should ascertain that there has been no deterioration since the test was planned and that he is not suffering from any infectious disorder. The test should be cancelled if there is any suspicion of acute illness.

In general, patients who exert to breathlessness or angina every day may safely be studied in the laboratory to the same degree of breathlessness or chest pain, provided that the test is conducted in such a way that no undue terror is evoked by the unfamiliar surroundings. Patients who react to disability by becoming immobile are very difficult to study and useful information is not normally obtained, since the test usually has to be terminated before abnormal changes of ECG, ventilation or heart rate are seen. Such patients, if incommoded by their disability, may usefully be retrained by repeated exercise procedures, employing simple electrocardiographic monitoring. Such retraining may be beneficial to the patient's health and confidence, but a dramatic improvement of effort tolerance is not often achieved.

References

Boyle, R. M: (1981). *Brit. J. Hosp. Med.* **25**, 8–14.

Bradley, C. A., Harris, E. A., Seelye, E. R. and Whitlock, R. M. L. (1976). *Clin. Sci. Mol. Med.* **51**, 323–333.

Cander, L. and Forster, R. E. (1959). *J. appl. Physiol.* **14**, 541–551.

Cohn, M. A., Watson, H. L., Weisshut, R., Scott, F. and Sackner, M. A. (1975). *In* "Proceedings of the 2nd International Symposium on Ambulatory Monitoring" (Eds Scott, F. D. *et al.*). Academic Press, London and New York.

Cunningham, D. J. C., Elliott, D. H., Lloyd, B. B., Miller, J. P. and Young, J. M. (1965). *J. Physiol.* **179**, 498.

Godfrey, S. (1974). "Exercise Testing in Children". Saunders, London.

Godfrey, S., Wozniak, E. R., Courtenay Evans, R. J. and Samuels, C. S. (1971). *Brit. J. Dis. Chest* **65**, 58–64.

Harris, E. A., Seelye, R. and Whitlock, R. M. L. (1976). *Clin. Sci. Mol. Med.* **51**, 335–344.

Hill, D. W. and Dolan, A. M. (1976). "Intensive Care Monitoring". Academic Press, London.

Jones, N. L., Campbell, E. J. M., McHardy, G. J. R., Higgs, B. E. and Clode, M. (1967). *Clin. Sci.* **32**, 311–327.

Jones, N. L., Campbell, E. J. M., Edwards, R. H. T. and Robertson, D. G. (1975). "Clinical Exercise Testing". Saunders, Philadelphia and London.

McHardy, G. J. R. (1967). *Clin. Sci.* **32**, 299–309.

Sackner, M. A., Greeneltch, D., Heiman, M. S., Epstein, G. and Atkins, N. (1975). *Amer. Rev. Resp. Dis.* **111**, 157–165.

Spiro, S. G. (1977). *Brit. J. Dis. Chest* **71**, 145–172.

Spiro, S. G. and Dowdeswell, I. R. G. (1976). *Brit. J. Dis. Chest* **70**, 263.

Wasserman, K. and Whipp, B. J. (1975). *Amer. Rev. Resp. Dis.* **112**, 219–249.

14. RESPIRATORY FUNCTION TESTING IN INFANCY AND CHILDHOOD

M. Silverman

Hammersmith Hospital, London, U.K.

GENERAL PRINCIPLES

Those who have attempted to measure even the simplest aspects of lung function in young children will realize that art, as well as science, is involved in respiratory function testing in childhood. Special problems have to be overcome in dealing with infants, who cannot cooperate and who must be subjected to the least possible disturbance. In dealing with older pre-school children, the art of persuasion relies on an understanding of the relationship between parents and children; often a confident approach to children achieves results. Provided anxiety is allayed, the natural inquisitiveness and playfulness of children should be turned to advantage in the exciting environment of a lung function laboratory. Clearly, experience in dealing with children is essential and personnel with special training or a natural facility with children will be more successful in obtaining results.

While many aspects of lung function testing in adults and children, especially in older children, are identical, some tests have their major place in paediatrics. Such tests often require no cooperation from the subject (e.g. respiratory jacket; forced oscillation technique) or are non-invasive (e.g. peak flow rate measurement).

A decision to carry out lung function tests will generally have followed clinical assessment, ancillary radiology and biochemical and immunological tests. In most paediatric lung function laboratories, sweat testing, skin prick testing and bronchial reactivity testing will be performed by those responsible for the measurement of respiratory physiological function. The order in which these investigations are performed should be that which causes least disturbance to the child.

TABLE I
Frequency of measurement

Purpose	Frequency	Examples
Diagnosis	Single occasion	Bronchial reactivity
Progress of disease	Variable intervals, depending on course of disease	Chronic disease of airways, pulmonary fibrosis, disordered neuromuscular function
Pattern of disease	Frequently (often several times daily)	Asthma

As well as the choice of appropriate lung function tests, the frequency with which measurements are performed will depend on their purpose (Table I). In childhood in particular, lung function may change with great rapidity, so that more frequent testing may be required than in adult practice. A useful compendium of reference values for children is provided by Polgar and Promadhat (1970). The changing pattern of pulmonary physiology with age has been well summarized by Hodson *et al.* (1977) and by Godfrey (1981).

An ability to abandon a testing session when cooperation begins to fail is as important as a positive approach to lung function testing in childhood. Even if attempts are abandoned, fulsome praise should be lavished on parents and child, in the expectation that the next attempt will be more successful.

In this chapter, techniques will be described in detail only where their major application is in childhood, or where there are particular problems in the adaptation of equipment or the interpretation of results.

SPECIFIC PROBLEMS IN CHILDREN

Growth

Change in Body Size

Since lungs and body grow in unison, most parameters of lung function are closely related to height (or length, in infants who must be measured supine). There is a less good relationship with weight (especially in under- or overweight), while there is a poor correlation between lung function and age. Internal standards of lung function (i.e. ratios between measured variables) may be relatively independent of age and size (e.g. dynamic compliance vs thoracic gas volume (TGV); maximum expiratory flow (TLC/s) at 50% TLC). This only holds true where there is a linear relationship between the parameters, and where the intercept is close to zero. Where these restrictions do not hold true (e.g. for the relationship between airway conductance and TGV in childhood) normal values cannot be predicted from a ratio, but from a formula which takes account of the intercept (or from a plot of the two parameters concerned). In other instances, internal standards must also be related to age (e.g. closing volume as a proportion of vital capacity), indicating developmental changes in the lung which are independent of lung size.

There are two periods of especially rapid growth: infancy and puberty. Changes in lung mechanics and gas exchange over the first few days of life must be related not only to body size, but also to gestational age and postnatal age, to take account of state of development of the respiratory musculature, and the state of adaptation to extrauterine life (particularly the clearance of fetal lung fluid). Around puberty, sex differences become apparent and must be taken into account. As the lean body mass of adolescent boys is relatively greater than that of girls, those aspects of lung function which depend on muscle power (e.g. TLC) or endurance (e.g. maximal exercise performance), become relatively greater in boys. Thus the stage of puberty (indicated by the primary and secondary sexual characteristics) may be an important factor, together with an assessment of lean body mass.

Arm span in childhood is almost identical to height, and can be used as the standard against which to assess lung function in children who cannot stand (e.g. because of neuromuscular disease) or who are deformed by acquired disease (e.g. scoliosis) or congenital abnormality (e.g. spina bifida). Normal standards for childhood lung function in relation to height can be used, substituting arm span.

Where population standards of lung function are being assessed, or when lung function is being measured for research purposes, precise anthropometry should be aimed at (Buckler, 1979). As a simple means of reducing error, some care should be taken to standardize the measurement of height and weight.

Lung Growth and Development

Accompanying body growth, lung growth is reflected by changes in pulmonary function (Table II). Changes in the mechanical properties of the lungs and in gas exchange with age have been extensively

TABLE II
Lung growth†

	Increase from birth to adult
Respiratory airways	10 times
Alveolar diameter	5 times
Number of alveoli	12–15 times
Lung mass	15 times
Lung surface area	20–30 times

† From Dunnill (1962).

reviewed (Bryan *et al.*, 1977; Hodson *et al.*, 1977). Of more concern here are the practical implications of lung growth.

Apparatus dead-space must be kept to a minimum to prevent rebreathing. The anatomical dead-space throughout life is approximately 2.2 ml/kg body weight and the resting tidal volume approximately 7 ml/kg body weight. Thus, if MVV is measured with a spirometer, the tidal volume of a small child may be insufficient to clear the dead-space of the tubing. A compromise has to be reached between reduction of apparatus dead-space and consequent increase in apparatus resistance (van der Hardt, 1981) (MVV = maximum voluntary ventilation).

The small tidal volumes and respiratory flow rates of infants and young children mean either that electrical signals from measuring devices suitable for adults must be amplified, along with the "noise", or that appropriate measuring devices themselves are employed.

Thus smaller diameter pneumotachographs, and smaller volume whole body plethysmographs will improve the signal/noise ratio for paediatric use. Some standard measurements (e.g. single breath Kco) are impossible in young children, because their vital capacity is too low to allow adequate sampling, using standard equipment.

In young infants, or older children with restrictive lung disease, respiratory frequencies of up to 1–1.5 Hz are encountered. The frequency response of measuring equipment (e.g. transducers) and of recording equipment (e.g. *x–y* plotters) should be sufficient for these frequencies. Respiratory pressure waveforms include significant harmonics of 5 to 10 times the natural frequency. The frequency response of transducers for neonatal use should therefore be flat up to about 10 Hz. At high frequencies, the utmost care must also be taken to match the response times of all the equipment to avoid errors due to phase differences (Helms *et al.*, 1981).

Patient Cooperation

Over the age of 5–6 years, most children of normal intelligence can be cajoled into performing lung function tests. In early infancy, only indirect measurements of lung function are possible with the subject awake (apart from the measurement of crying vital capacity). However, during natural sleep (after a feed) or under the influence of a hypnotic drug (e.g. chloral hydrate 60 mg/kg body weight by mouth) a range of more invasive procedures can be performed, under medical supervision. Between the ages of 1 and 5 years, few direct lung function tests are possible.

Three criteria apply to the choice of lung function test in childhood.

(i) Discrimination, the ability of a test to identify a particular pathophysiological process;

(ii) Sensitivity, the precision with which minor degrees of abnormality can be identified;

(iii) Reproducibility, the ability to detect small changes within individual patients.

In paediatrics, it is the third of these criteria, reproducibility, which is usually the limiting factor, for two main reasons. First, the signal to noise ratio is usually smaller. Second, patient cooperation is generally less well maintained by children and may be influenced by such factors as mealtimes (or hunger), especially in infants, or by recent respiratory tract infections. These factors, as well as environmental antigen exposure in sensitive individuals, should all be considered.

In childhood, the most frequent role of lung function tests is to detect change within individual patients over periods of time. Hence the within-patient reproducibility is the most important criterion. Techniques for rendering tests non-effort-dependent have generally failed to achieve their objective of improving reproducibility (see p. 319). The within-patient reproducibility of some commonly used tests of lung function in adults and children, is given in Table III.

Posture and Sleep State

During infancy, lung function is measured with patients supine (or in right lateral position) and asleep, their most usual states of posture and wakefulness. The population standards have all been collected in the same way. Sleep state, because of its relationship to postural muscle tone, does influence lung function. In the newborn, thoracic gas volume may fall during the change from slow-wave sleep to rapid-eye-movement sleep (Henderson-Smart and Read, 1979), as intercostal

TABLE III

Reproducibility of lung function tests in normal children and adults: within-subject coefficient of variation†

Test		Coefficient of variation (%)	
		Children	Adults
Peak flow rate		4	—
FEV$_1$	: volume/time curve	5	3
FEF$_{25-75}$	: spirogram	8	8
FEF$_{25}$	: MEFV curve	14	12
FRC	: gas dilution	7	5
TLC	: plethysmograph	6	—
Rt	: forced oscillation	12	32
Raw	: plethysmograph	11	—
CV	: single breath test	24	21

† From various sources. For definitions see pp. 314–320.

muscle phasic activity and diaphragmatic tonic activity diminish. Inspection of the eyelids or a simple electro-oculogram, gives some idea of sleep state (Curzi-Dascalova, 1978; Hoffman *et al.*, 1977). The interpretation of the electro-encephalogram also used, is controversial, and probably no more precise than simple observation.

It may take two hours for an infant to settle down sufficiently for lung function testing. A feed and nappy change may help, as well as warmth (especially important for pre-term infants). A competent assistant must be in attendance whenever an infant is in the laboratory.

Older children are normally measured standing or seated. Supine, there is normally a fall of up to 10% in vital capacity, due probably to an increase in pulmonary capillary blood volume. This should be taken into account if measurements are made on supine patients (e.g. recovering from neuromuscular or surgical procedures).

Recording Equipment

Unless the operator is extremely experienced, it is important to display the physiological signals and not rely on computed results alone. Inconsistent results can then be more easily attributed to equipment failure or, as occurs more commonly, to errors in the performance of the test. Failure to deliver a full inspiration or expiration when required, leaks around the mouthpiece, tachypnoea at rest, swallowing and closure of the glottis frequently account for artefact and variable results. Observer error can be accounted for if the data are permanently recorded and available for repeated analysis.

Computer analysis should only be carried out on data which have been inspected by a competent operator (i.e. one who is capable of manual analysis of the results), so that artefact-free data are analysed. This approach has been shown to work in practice (Wong and Silverman, 1982).

INFANCY (BIRTH–12 MONTHS)

Tidal Ventilation (Flow and Volume)

Tidal volume may be measured for its intrinsic usefulness (e.g. during mechanical ventilation or intensive care) or during the course of the calculation of other parameters such as minute ventilation, (e.g. in studies of metabolism), or in the study of patterns of breathing (e.g. sleep studies). It may be measured directly, from measurements of airflow at the mouth or indirectly by quantitative analysis of thoraco-abdominal displacement. Most of the direct methods, although accurate, involve some degree of facial stimulation, which, by reflex pathways, may distort the pattern of breathing. Indirect methods, although less accurate, allow more natural breathing (see p. 303).

Direct Measurements

For the measurement of airflow, in infants, only the face mask meets requirements of low resistance, low dead-space and freedom from air leaks. The endotracheal tube may be adapted to measure flow during intensive care or resuscitation (Boon *et al.*, 1979) but is neither leak-free nor of low resistance. Nasal adaptors have been used (Radford, 1974) and are appropriate early in infancy when quiet breathing takes place through the nose. However, the nasal airways contribute about 50% of the total airways resistance in infancy (Stocks, 1977a and b), and this proportion must increase with the insertion of nasal cannulae which clearly provide a much greater resistance to airflow than does a face mask (Goldman *et al.*, 1979). Moreover, reflexes resulting from nasal stimulation may disturb breathing considerably. An ingenious flow system employing a double pneumotachograph with zero dead-space has been described (Ruttimann *et al.*, 1980).

Commercially available hard rubber face masks (Table IVa) can be used, sealed with silicone putty (e.g. Therapeutic Putty, Carters, Westbury, Wiltshire). A ring of putty is placed around the nose and

TABLE IVa

Guide to appropriate size of Rendell-Baker face mask for measurement of lung function in infants

Size of mask	Size of infant (kg)	Mask Volume (ml) (excluding pneumotachograph dead-space)	Infant tidal volume (ml)
0	1–4	12	10–30
1	3–6	22	20–50
2	5–10	33	30–75

(1) Variations in face size occur; black infants generally require a larger size than indicated.
(2) In use, the effective dead-space is lower than the figures given above, since the infant's face occupies part of the mask.

TABLE IVb

Guide to appropriate size of Fleisch pneumotachograph for infant lung function measurement

Size	Pneumotachograph Nominal maximum flow rate (l/min)	Dead-space (ml)	Infant size (kg)
00	4	1.7	1–3
0	20	4.7	2–10
1	60	15	>10

mouth, avoiding compression of the nasal passages, and a second ring on the mask (Fig. 1). As the mask is applied, the two layers of putty fuse. Because of its rigidity, the mask helps to support the cheeks during respiratory manoeuvres which alter mouth pressure. The resistance of a mask and attached tubing should be less than $0.1 \text{ cm } H_2O \, l^{-1} \, s^{-1}$. With attached recording apparatus a resistance of up to $4 \text{ cm } H_2O \, l^{-1} \, s^{-1}$ may be achieved.

Airflow is most commonly measured with a pneumotachograph and pressure transducer whose output is linear over the range of flow expected, and volume is derived by electronic integration of the flow signal. That part of the drift of the volume signal which is due to the respiratory exchange ratio can be eliminated using a one-way valve system (Radford, 1974), so that only inspired or expired air flow are measured. The pneumotachograph/pressure transducer system should be calibrated periodically (weekly) using an accurate flowmeter (e.g. Rotameter). The volume signal should be calibrated by hand- or

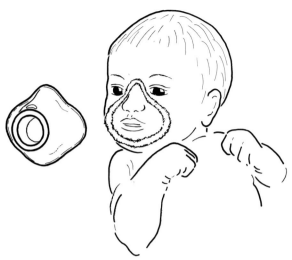

FIG. 1. Infant face mask.

machine-pumping a calibrated syringe, before each set of measurements. A guide to pneumotachograph sizes is given in Table IVb.

From the timed recording of flow and volume, it is a simple matter to calculate tidal volume and minute ventilation, allowing manually for integrator drift.

Alternative direct methods for measuring tidal breathing including wet and dry spirometry have been used. Rebreathing of expired gas is inevitable unless air is circulated within the system by means of a fan.

Plethysmographic Measurements

If the body is encased in a container (the plethysmograph), the head or face free, then changes in the volume of the thorax and abdomen during breathing cause changes in pressure within the container. Calibration, by pumping known volumes of air into the plethysmograph, must be carried out with the patient *in situ*. Then, changes in pressure may be converted into changes in volume. The rigid face-out plethysmograph designed by Cross (1949) may thus be used to measure tidal volume without the problem of drift encountered with flow integration. This advantage is outweighed by the rather complex procedure for preventing air leaks around the face.

The respiratory jacket (Milner, 1970) provides a novel and practical solution which requires no patient cooperation and which allows undisturbed breathing. This double-skinned latex rubber jerkin slips over

TABLE V
Respiratory jackets†

Size of subject (kg)	Size of jacket	Jacket dimensions Lengh (cm)	Circumference (cm)
2.5–5	AA	28	50
4–10	A	36	64
10–20	B	45	74
20–40	C	52	90
Adult female	D	63	100
Adult male	E	72	116

† Available from: (1) Fabrication Sales Department, Dunlop Limited, GRG Division, PO Box 151, Cambridge Street, Manchester M60 1PD, U.K.; or (2) Kastley Limited, PO Box 24, Blackburn, Lancashire, U.K.

the shoulders like a vest and covers the chest and abdomen (Table V). It is inflated to 3–4 cm H_2O, so that tidal breaths produce changes in pressure in the jacket of 1–2 cm H_2O. These pressures, produce little restriction, and only a small drop in resting lung volume. Calibration should be performed *in vivo* to demonstrate linearity over the range of volume changes expected.

Overheating (of the patient as well as the air in the jacket) does not seem to be a problem. Adiabatic effects are also minimal, producing a 10% pressure overswing at 180 cycles/min. Movement artefact and the need for re-calibration after movement are greater drawbacks. The jacket is equally effective in erect or supine posture.

The jacket itself exhibits hysteresis (Helms *et al.*, 1981). which means that pressure changes within it are out of phase with respiratory volume changes. This renders the signal valueless for dynamic measurements, although it is possible that by a subtraction technique, a signal could be obtained which was in phase with volume change, and from which, by differentiation, a flow signal could be derived. However, for measurement of undisturbed tidal volume alone over short periods of time, the method is almost ideal, and attempts to justify the dynamic use of the jacket have been made (Stokes *et al.*, 1981).

Respiratory inductance plethysmography provides another promising approach to body-surface monitoring of tidal volume in infancy (Dolfin *et al.*, 1982). Intermittent calibration by means of a face-mask and pneumotachograph is required. Barometric plethysmography (Haddad *et al.*, 1979) appears to be the only method which allows tidal volume determination without any interference whatever.

Respiratory Control

Pattern of Breathing

Wide, sometimes hazardous, variations in the depth and rate of breathing occur in premature infants and some children when they are asleep. This is a topic of great relevance to the investigation of apnoea of prematurity and of sudden infant death syndrome. Respiratory rhythm can be monitored by devices which detect changes in chest dimensions (magnetometers, circumferential strain gauges, inductance vests) or by transthoracic impedance. Some are used in apnoea monitors. If calibrated using measurements of airflow made at the mouth, the devices which measure change in dimensions may, over short periods of time, provide quantitative information. All the devices are easily displaced, and consequently require frequent calibration. No surface monitor will detect obstructive apnoea (the persistance of respiratory efforts against upper airway obstruction, e.g. closed glottis).

Thoracic impedance changes with airflow and blood flow within the chest. In infants, the cardiac signal may be relatively large, particularly during apnoeic spells. For quantitative work, a 4-electrode system is preferable to the unstable, position-sensitive 2-electrode devices used for simple respiratory monitoring. Such a system has been used successfully for the non-invasive detection of changes in lung volumes during sleep. The barometric method has been successfuly applied to the study of natural respiratory patterns in newborns (Haddad *et al.*, 1979).

Respiratory Muscle Function

From the pattern of chest and abdominal wall movement, much can be inferred about the action of the respiratory muscles in health (e.g. in relation to posture or sleep state in newborn) or disease (e.g. in neuromuscular disease). The relative contributions of diaphragm and chest wall to breathing may be studied indirectly with pairs of magnetometers on chest and abdomen or directly by surface electromyography (Muller *et al.*, 1979; Fleming *et al.*, 1979).

Magnetometer circuits should produce linear signals over the range of distances encountered in newborns (Stark *et al.*, 1979); equipment designed for older subjects may prove unsuitable. A quantitative analysis of contribution of ribcage and diaphragm to breathing in the newborn may be carried out by the method of Konno and Mead (1967), provided that the ribcage moves with a single degree of freedom. This approach has been little used in newborns (Stark *et al.*, 1979). Surface electromyography is fraught with artefact, but may have a place in the study of respiratory muscle fatigue in newborn babies (Muller *et al.*, 1979).

Chemical Control of Breathing

Chemical control of breathing in infants has been studied by measurements of the steady state ventilatory response to mild degrees of hypoxia (Rigatto *et al.*, 1975a) or hypercapnia (Rigatto *et al.*, 1975b). There are no standards for these procedures, which are all at the moment experimental.

Static Lung Volumes

The theoretical background to the two approaches to lung volume measurement, by plethysmography and inert gas dilution, has been described (Chapter 9). This section deals with the technical difficulties presented by the newborn, and their solution.

Plethysmography

A totally enclosed constant volume (Du Bois) box of 40–60 l capacity is generally used, for infants of 1.5–12 kg; the constant pressure (Mead) plethysmograph has found little application for the study of infants. The plethysmograph (box) should be almost airtight in use, a leak of 20–30 s half-life diminishing the box-pressure drift due to temperature change, without affecting important pressure signals. Before any measurements are made, however, thermal equilibrium must be reached. This takes up to 20 min. A rigid compensating chamber of similar volume connected to the plethysmograph via an adjustable needle valve provides a back-off pressure for the box pressure transducer to compensate for sudden changes in ambient temperature and pressure. TGV is derived from the box pressure to mouth pressure ratio during respiratory efforts against an occluded airway (Chapter 9). Successful measurements depend on a leak-proof mask and occluding valve.

A successful system is that described by Stocks *et al.* (1977). The mask and valve system has a dead-space of 12 ml, critical when the TGV of the subject may be only 50–60 ml. The valves must be of low dead-space, quiet (to avoid shock waves) and airtight as well as being easy to clean. The pneumatic system operating the conical aluminium

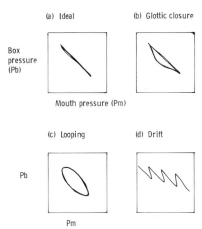

FIG. 2. Oscilloscope images of loops obtained during measurement of thoracic gas volume (a) ideal; (b) demonstrating glottic closure; (c) looping caused by phase lag; (d) thermal or instrumental drift.

valves described by Stocks *et al.* (1977) has functioned for several years with little trouble. The occluded face mask must be airtight (Fig. 1): failure to achieve this will produce "looping" of the mouth pressure vs box pressure signal during occlusion (Fig. 2).

Whether or not the results are analysed by computer (Wong, 1982), or simply based on the angle subtended by the box pressure and mouth pressure signals displayed on the 2 axes of an x-y oscilloscope (Fig. 2a), a permanent record should be kept, as a means of detecting artefacts which may not be otherwise apparent by inspection of the oscilloscope during occluded breathing.

Common problems in TGV measurement include:

(a) air leaks, either from box or mask, which produce "looping" (Fig. 2c);

(b) failure to occlude at end-expiration; this can be corrected for, along with apparatus dead-space, if tidal ventilation has been recorded for a few breaths prior to occlusion, so that the tidal volume included during occlusion can be measured;

(c) glottic closure; this results in an easily recognized pattern on the X-Y oscilloscope (Fig. 2b);

(d) thermal instability: there is box-pressure drift (Fig. 2d); if small this can be corrected for on the chart record;

(e) restlessness brought about by airway occlusion;

(f) apnoea induced by occlusion, a feature of very immature infants, and one which is potentially hazardous.

The box must be calibrated for each infant, using a hand-held syringe or pump operating at the infant's breathing frequency, to correct for adiabatic effects. Calibration is normally carried out without the child in the box, since *in vivo* calibration is technically difficult. A volume of non-compressible material equal to the child is placed in the box for calibration. A number of 500 ml bags of saline equal in weight to the infant may conveniently be used.

The plethysmographic technique has been used for many years with little variation in methodology and remarkably reproducible results for TGV, despite its cumbersome structure and its technical demands. Recently, theoretical problems have been recognized which cast doubt on the accuracy of the technique in some situations and the method requires further evaluation (Beardsmore *et al.*, 1982; Helms, 1982). Normal supine infants have a TGV of around 32 ml/kg (Stocks, 1977). Posture, anaesthesia, sleep state and recent milk intake, as well as disease, may all alter the resting TGV.

Inert Gas Dilution (FRC)

These techniques too, depend on achieving a gas-tight seal at the face-mask, nasal cannulae or endotracheal tube. Of the two methods most commonly available, nitrogen washout and helium dilution, the helium method is the most reliable, since even minimal contamination by air (79% N_2) will produce errors in the nitrogen technique.

The technique and calculations are adapted from adult methods (Krauss and Auld, 1971; Taussig *et al.*, 1977). The potential errors due to leaks, air contamination or failure of equilibration are similar. A method has recently been described whereby FRC can be measured through a leaky endotracheal tube, by measuring and allowing for leakage (Fox *et al.*, 1979). In normal infants FRC, at about 27 ml/kg (Stocks, 1977) is lower than the plethysmographic TGV.

The difference in value between FRC and TGV is greatest in the first days of life, and in the most immature infants (Krauss and Auld, 1971), as well, of course, as in lung disease. It has been suggested that gas dilution techniques may underestimate lung volume in early life (Stocks, 1977) because airway closure during expiration occurs within the tidal volume range (Mansell *et al.*, 1972).

Measurement of Oesophageal Pressure

Ideally, a measurement of pleural pressure change is required for the calculation of pulmonary compliance (C_l) and resistance (R_p). In prac-

TABLE VI

Techniques for measurement of oesophageal pressure in infancy

	Rubber balloon and air-filled catheter	Fluid-filled catheter	Miniature transducer
LIMITATIONS			
Frequency response	Adequate, if catheter >1.5 mm i.d.	May be inadequate at breathing rates over 60–80	Adequate
Working range	Depends on dimensions must be defined for each balloon	Depnds on perfusion rate	May be wide, as specified
Stability *in vitro*	Stable	Stable	Stable
Stability and accuracy *in vivo*	Pressure changes are reproducible but absolute pressures may vary during use; oesophageal hysteresis may occur	Subject to blockage by mucus, bubbles; absolute pressures affected by changes in posture	Affected by local factors within oesophagus; unreliable in infants
Cost	Cheap	Very cheap	Expensive
APPLICATIONS			
	For all routine measurement of lung mechanics	For measurements during intensive care, when a feeding catheter may be used to minimize disturbance	Inadequate for use in infancy

tice, it is accepted that changes in oesophageal pressure (P_{oes}) if accurately measured, reflect changes in mean pleural pressure. Some of the assumptions implied have been discussed in Chapter 9.

There are disadvantages in each of the three currently available techniques for measurement of oesophageal pressure (Table VI). Each may have a place in practice, although none is ideal.

Whichever technique is used, the catheter should be passed through the mouth. Since infants are obligate nose breathers, the added resistance imposed by a nasal catheter may affect pulmonary mechanics significantly (Stocks, 1980). By convention, the right lateral position is used, but although absolute oesophageal pressure is affected by posture, oesophageal pressure changes during breathing are similar in lateral and supine positions (Vanderghem *et al.*, 1983).

There appears to be no oesophageal pressure gradient in normal supine infants (Beardsmore *et al.*, 1981). The site in the oesophagus at which measurements may be made, may thus seem unimportant. In practice, the distal 2/3 of the oesophagus provides the most reproducible values, provided the cardiac sphincter and the site of the maximum cardiac artefact are both avoided (Beardsmore *et al.*, 1981).

Oesophageal Balloon

While the use of catheter-mounted, fine rubber balloons to measure oesophageal pressure in adults is a standard procedure (Chapters 1 and 9), there are no standards for their use in infants. A thorough description of the manufacture of balloons and the assessment of the physical characteristics of the balloon–catheter–pressure transducer system has been provided by Beardsmore *et al.* (1980), together with details of the *in vitro* and *in vivo* assessment of the balloons.

The smaller size (both length and diameter) of infant oesophageal balloons means that their working range, where compliance is infinite ("working range") is necessarily small. Great precision is required to ensure that in use, the working range is not exceeded, leading to damped signals. Damping of some of the higher harmonics of the fundamental respiratory frequency will also occur if the catheter to which the balloon is attached is smaller than 1.5 mm internal diameter. (The system should give a linear response up to ten times the fundamental frequency, i.e. 10 Hz in infancy.)

In vivo, the accuracy with which pressure changes are detected should always be measured by comparing simultaneous recordings of oesophageal and face mask ("mouth") pressure during respiratory efforts against an occluded airway, the "occlusion test" (Beardsmore *et al.*, 1980). Ideally the change in oesophageal pressure (ΔP_{oes}) should be equal to the change in mouth pressure (ΔP_m), since there is no gas flow, i.e. $\Delta P_{oes}/\Delta P_m = 1.00$. Ideally, values between 0.95 and 1.05 should be attained; a wider limit might sometimes be necessary although outside these limits, measurements of pulmonary resistance and compliance may be inaccurate. Values greater than 1.05 may indicate glottic closure or a mask leak during occlusion, while in certain types of patient (particularly children with neuromuscular disease and pre-term babies) oesophageal pressure may not reflect mean pleural pressure. On occasions, even a ratio of 1.00 may be misleading. An overfilled balloon can magnify cardiac artefact, converting a damped signal into an apparently accurate one.

In general, efforts should be made by adjusting the position and internal volume of the balloon to achieve a $\Delta P_{oes}/\Delta P_m$ ratio of 1.00 before starting measurements. The temptation to "correct" measurements of ΔP_{oes} using a correction factor derived from an unsatisfactory $\Delta P_{oes}/\Delta P_m$ ratio should be avoided: the error is unlikely to be consistent over the whole range of oesophageal pressures encountered.

With care in the measurement of oesophageal pressure, measurements of pulmonary resistance, hitherto a variable parameter of limited value, may be as accurate and reproducible as airways resistance measured in the plethysmograph.

Fluid Filled Oesophageal Catheter

Measurements of oesophageal pressure during intensive care may only be ethically justified via an existing gastric feeding tube. While important information may thus be obtained, the many drawbacks of the system must be accounted for (Table VI).

A comparison of fluid and air filled oesophageal catheters by Maxted *et al.* (1977) pointed out some of the following defects of fluid-filled systems: the hydrostatic pressure effect of alterations in the relative levels of catheter tip and transducer; the relatively poor frequency response in comparison with the air-filled balloon system; the need to flush with relatively large volumes of fluid, depending on the compliance of the catheter $(1–2 \text{ ml min}^{-1})$; the need to avoid a flushing system which will dampen the signal; the ease with which oesophageal debris partially occludes the holes and dampens the signal during use. The accuracy of a fluid-filled system is critically dependent on the characteristics of the catheter and transducer.

Miniature Catheter-Tip Transducer

The theoretical advantages of the precise measurement of local oesophageal pressure with a miniature pressure transducer should circumvent most of the problems listed above. However, in practice, despite excellent characteristics *in vitro*, the reproducibility of measurements *in vivo* is poor (Beardsmore *et al.*, 1982). This is probably because local factors (folds of oesophageal mucosa, bubbles of air in swallowed saliva) can have a large affect on the tiny, exposed diaphragm of the transducer. At the moment, miniature catheter tip transducers cannot be recommended for the measurement of lung mechanics in infants.

Pulmonary Compliance

Dynamic Compliance

The accurate measurement of dynamic compliance is technically difficult, and the interpretation of results, in the presence of airways disease, is difficult.

In the standard technique, the flow signal, (usually measured by a pneumotachograph, at a face mask), the volume signal (electronically integrated flow signal) and the oesophageal pressure are simultaneously recorded during quiet breathing. The dynamic compliance is the change in volume (ΔV) divided by the change in oesophageal pressure (ΔP_{oes}) between points of zero flow (i.e. the extremes of tidal volume). The prerequisites of an accurate result include: the accurate measurement of oesophageal pressure (see the above section); the trouble-free integration of the flow signal (correction for integrator drift is often required); the absence of phase differences between the various pressure sensitive transducers (i.e. those connected to the pneumotachograph and the oesophageal catheter). It is clear that small phase differences in the equipment may produce large errors (Helms *et al.*, 1981).

In the presence of lung disease, the value of dynamic compliance in infancy is likely to be affected by the high natural frequency of breathing, as well as by a variety of disease processes. The interpretation of a low value of compliance is therefore difficult. Nevertheless, population values for dynamic compliance in infancy are available (Stocks, 1977).

Static Compliance

The calculation of static compliance requires the accurate measurement of changes in lung volume over a greater range than the tidal volume used to measure dynamic compliance. This, as well as the need to measure the transpulmonary pressure under static conditions, presents particular problems in infants.

By assuming a very large value for chest wall compliance (a fair assumption during neuromuscular blockade), it may not even be necessary to measure oesophageal pressure: mouth pressure changes may be an adequate measure of transpulmonary pressure changes and therefore, total respiratory compliance may be close to lung compliance. Volume changes can simply be produced using a large syringe during airway occlusion.

During spontaneous breathing, a form of static compliance may be calculated by assuming that the end-expiratory transpulmonary pressure (at the point of zero air flow at the mouth) represents a static value.

This may be so in normal infants, but is unlikely to be true in the presence of lung disease. Changes in end expiratory lung volume can be produced using expiratory resistances or a pressure breathing (continuous positive airway pressure) system. Changes in end expiratory lung volume during a series of measurements are related to changes in transpulmonary pressure to produce a "static" pressure volume curve. The change in volume may be measured directly from the integrated flow signal (although over the time required for a set of measurements, electronic drift may be too great) or indirectly using a respiratory jacket.

A technique which permits the measurement of total respiratory compliance (or static lung compliance) during tidal breathing in newborn babies, has been described by Olinsky *et al.* (1976). This novel approach relies on the transient inhibition of breathing, induced by sudden airway occlusion during inspiration (Hering–Breuer reflex). This technique has not been thoroughly assessed.

These techniques are now experimental, but may supersede dynamic compliance measurements in the near future.

Airflow Resistance

Airways Resistance (Plethysmographic technique)

The calculation of airways resistance using the plethysmograph assumes that only those pressure changes needed to overcome the resistance of the airways to gas flow are recorded. If changes in temperature and humidity of respired gas occur, the results may be invalid. In adult practice, the panting manoeuvre overcomes the problem. In infancy, ideal conditions can only be obtained by providing a rebreath-bag of humidified air (or oxygen-enriched air) at 37°C, from which the patient breathes during the measurement of airways resistance. "Looping" of the pressure-flow plot, if it is due only to changes in temperature and humidity of respired gas, can be eliminated using such a system (Radford, 1974). The phase relationship between box pressure and flow may also be altered by mask leaks, box leaks and box pressure drift (due to alterations in environmental conditions or temperature).

Before measuring airways resistance in a supine, sleeping infant, it is necessary to be able to switch the infant into the rebreathing circuit using a valve system operated externally (e.g. Stocks *et al.*, 1977) and then to observe that the flow and box pressure signals displayed on an oscilloscope form a closed loop. When these conditions have been achieved, recordings of flow, box pressure and mask pressure can be

L

made. It is customary also to record tidal volume. After 5–10 satisfactory breaths, the airway may be occluded at end expiration for several breaths (see p. 304) while mask and box pressure are recorded, for thoracic gas volume measurement.

The relationship between box pressure and mask pressure (assumed to represent mean alveolar pressure) during airway occlusion, is required in the calculation of airways resistance. However, during occlusion, as well as the infants lung volume, apparatus dead-space is included in the total occluded volume. The size of the dead-space, in which adiabatic changes will occur during occluded respiratory efforts, will influence the accuracy of measurements of TGV and airways resistance. The ratio of the change in mouth pressure (ΔP_m) to box pressure (ΔP_b) during occlusion must be corrected by the apparatus dead-space, as well as the dead-space of the upper airways of the infant (approximately 0.5 × anatomical dead-space) before it can be used to convert box pressure into alveolar pressure during spontaneous breathing:

$$\text{alveolar pressure} = \frac{\Delta P_m}{\Delta P_b} \times \frac{\text{Total occluded gas volume (TOGV)}}{\text{TOGV} - \text{VD}_{\text{apparatus}} - 0.5 \times \text{VD}_{\text{anat}}}$$

For a full discussion, see Stocks (1977b).

Apparatus resistance at the flow rates recorded, must be subtracted from the final resistance value obtained, to give the true airways resistance. Carefully performed, the coefficient of variation of repeated measurements is low (less than 5%).

While in adults, it is customary to measure airways resistance at a fixed flow rate, it is obviously impossible to define a single equivalent value for all infants. The alternatives are to measure inspiratory resistance at a fixed proportion (e.g. 2/3) of the maximum inspiratory flow rate, or, as for pulmonary resistance, to measure between mid-(iso-) volume points. The former method, while giving a precise value for resistance over one small part of the respiratory cycle, is technically more demanding, since the flow rate is measured at a time when it is changing rapidly. The mid-volume resistance is a mean value, which however, does not avoid turbulance-dependent resistance changes at the extremes of inspiration and expiration. The argument is not resolved.

Normal values should be collected by each laboratory. Some standards have been collected by Stocks (1977a).

Using a microcomputer, Wong and Silverman (1982) have described a system which not only computes airways resistance automatically, but which, by providing a plot of box pressure against flow throughout the respiratory cycle, can provide detailed information about changes in resistance throughout the respiratory cycle. Thus, the site and pattern of airways obstruction can be accurately described.

Pulmonary Resistance

More easily available is the technically simpler method for pulmonary resistance, requiring only a means of measuring oesophageal pressure change, and flow at the mouth. Commonly, the measurement of dynamic pulmonary compliance is performed simultaneously from a volume signal.

Despite the defects of the supine posture for oesophageal pressure measurement (see p. 307), most pulmonary resistance measurements have been made in this position. If the oesophageal catheter is passed through the nose, the total airways resistance will be distorted; the oral route should be used. Meticulous attention to technical detail is required, since small phase differences may produce vast errors.

Pulmonary resistance is conventionally calculated as the pressure difference corresponding to the change in flow between points of equal lung volume: a mean value for inspiratory and expiratory resistance. This procedure minimizes the effect of lung volume (i.e. compliance) on oesophageal pressure, but may introduce an error due to lung hysteresis ("tissue resistance").

With careful measurement, airways resistance (in the plethysmograph) can be calculated over small sections of the respiratory cycle. This cannot easily be done for pulmonary resistance, since the oesophageal pressure changes *during* airflow are the result of elastic forces (plus hysteresis) as well as resistive forces. However with meticulous attention to the technique of oesophageal pressure measurement, values of pulmonary resistance are very close to equivalent values of airways resistance measured in the plethysmograph and as reproducible.

PRE-SCHOOL CHILDREN (1–5 YEARS)

Only the most precocious young children can participate actively in lung function testing. For the rest, a few techniques may be used which require a minimum of cooperation or which succeed despite open hostility.

The use of general anaesthesia (Doershuk, 1970) in order to measure lung function is rarely, if ever, justified. The relevance of measurements made under anaesthesia is dubious.

314   M. SILVERMAN

During acute respiratory illness, blood gas analysis may be the single most important clinical investigation. However, using the respiratory jacket to monitor tidal volume, and by attaching a pressure transducer to a saline filled feeding tube withdrawn so that its tip lay in the mid-oesophagus, Stokes *et al.*, (1981), have shown how to collect data ethically on young sick children, although the accuracy of such measurements is in doubt. Similar measurements could be made using the other forms of respiration monitor mentioned earlier (respiratory impedence, inductance or magnetometry).

Sleep Studies

Sleep studies are often more rewarding than daytime measurements in pre-school children (Hoffman *et al.*, 1977). Children can usually be moved around quite vigorously during their first hours of sleep without waking. Non-invasive monitoring of respiratory rate and depth (p. 303) should be combined with a measure of airflow at the mouth and nostrils (e.g. by thermistor), since obstructed breathing, in which chest wall movements may continue unchanged or even increased in amplitude, may be missed if an index of airflow is not available.

Arterial Po_2 (P_aO_2) may be monitored in infancy using a skin sensor (transcutaneous Po_2; $P_{tc}O_2$) at 44.5°C. The $P_{tc}O_2$ may be a useful index of change in P_aO_2 although absolute values are unreliable after the first year of life. The electrode position must be changed every 4 hours to prevent burns. Ear oximetry may soon be possible with a miniature sensor (Chapter 5).

For CO_2 monitoring, until the transcutaneous sensor is shown to be rapid and accurate in older children, end tidal Pco_2 ($P_{et}CO_2$) will continue to provide a close approximation to P_aCO_2 for children with normal lungs. $P_{et}CO_2$ is obtained by continuous sampling through a nasopharyngeal catheter, using an infra-red CO_2 analyser (Chapter 6). The analyser needs to be calibrated and used at a flow rate which does not exceed the patient's maximum expiratory flow rate at mid expiration. Nasal catheters frequently become obstructed. For this and many other technical reasons, an observer should be present throughout any sleep study.

Respiratory Resistance

Respiratory resistance is almost the only useful test of lung function which can be measured in wide awake pre-school children. There are two techniques.

Forced Oscillation Technique (total respiratory impedence)

Based on a description by Du Bois *et al.* (1956), this tehcnique has found its greatest application in infants (Wohl *et al.*, 1969) and young children (Cogswell, 1973; Landau and Phelan, 1973), since little or no cooperation is required from the subject. The total respiratory impedence or resistance (Rt) is calculated from the relationship between pressure and flow at the mouth (or face mask) when flow is induced by a sinusoidal pressure wave.

The total impedence of the respiratory system comprises the vector sum of effective resistance (the pressure/flow relationship when pressure and flow are in phase) and effective reactance. The latter is the sum of two properties of the respiratory system: elastance and inertance. These are respectively 90° and 270° out of phase with flow (i.e. 180° out of phase with each other). At low\frequencies, elastance dominates, while at high frequencies inertance is an important contribution to respiratory impedence. As predicted, normal lungs behave like a simple linear (series) electrical model, exhibiting a frequency, the resonant frequency, at which elastance and inertance are equal in magnitude and therefore cancel each other out. At this frequency, 5–7 Hz in children, flow and pressure are in perfect phase and the total respiratory impedence represents the combined resistance to airflow of the lungs and chest wall.

The subject breathes through a pneumotachograph via a short low resistance tube which may be attached either to a mouthpiece or, for very young children, to a closely applied face mask (Fig. 1). The cheeks should be held, as for the panting manoeuvre, either by the patient, or an assistant standing behind. Mouth pressure, airflow and volume change may be recorded and analysed directly (Cogswell, 1973), with the signals superimposed upon those due to spontaneous breathing. A method of eliminating the effect of natural breathing (frequency less than 1 Hz) using a high pass electrical filter has been described (Milner, 1970). The method has an acceptable degree of reproducibility (within subject coefficient of variation 12%) in older children, although the scatter of normal values is wide in 4 and 5 year olds (Cogswell, 1973).

This method has several major defects. Firstly, the value of resistance is unrelated to lung volume, although this is also the case with many other indices of resistance to airflow. Indeed it is possible that the application of a 5–7 Hz pressure wave at the mouth might produce an increase in FRC in patients with lung disease. The second problem is that in the presence of lung disease, there may be no resonant frequency for the respiratory system as a whole. Under these circumstances, the total respiratory impedence will underestimate the flow resistance. A subtraction technique (Goldman *et al.*, 1970) has been applied to children in order to circumvent this effect (Landau and Phelan, 1973).

Forced Expiratory Manoeuvres

Peak flow rate. The low-range Wright peak flow meter (Airmed Ltd.), may be reliable in most children from the age of 2½ years and population standards are available for this age group (Milner and Ingram, 1970). The reproducibility of peak flow rate in this age group (a within-subject coefficient of variation of 8%) is not much more than in older subjects.

Partial expiratory flow volume curves. In an attempt to devise a relatively effort-independent test of airways function, Taussig (1977) has evaluated partial expiratory flow volume (PEFV) curves. Immediately after recording a period of quiet breathing, the subject is encouraged to blow out as hard as possible. From the flow-volume curve so produced, the maximum expiratory flow at FRC can be determined. In the pre-school age group, the within-patient coefficient of variation of 17%, and the variation for the group of 25% are similar to the poor values obtained for other indices of maximum expiratory flow. Moreover, many children are unable to perform the manoeuvre. It may be concluded that PEFV curves in pre-school children are very much dependent on cooperation and probably on effort too and are too imprecise either for population or individual studies.

SCHOOL CHILDREN

Most of the techniques available for adult lung function testing are directly applicable to children. In this section, emphasis will be placed on particular problems or particular applications in older children. A comprehensive set of normal values, for a range of commonly used lung function tests has been provided by Cogswell *et al.* (1975a,b,c).

Measurement of Airflow Obstruction

Peak Expiratory Flow Rate and Spirometry

Applications. These procedures are the primary means of measuring lung function in older children. They are rarely helpful alone as an aid to diagnosis. Spirometry and peak expiratory (PEF) flow manoeuvres are particularly useful in the assessment of the severity of airflow obstruction, as an objective means of recording the progress of a disease or as a measure of change in lung function during a provocation procedure. It should be noted that the FEV_1/FVC ratio of 75% does not distinguish between obstructive and "restrictive" lung disease in children. Because of the relatively great elastic recoil pressure in relation to their airways resistance the FEV_1/FVC ratio is normally over 90% in pre-pubertal children.

Equipment and techniques. Peak flow rate may be measured with one of the two Wright Peak Flow meters (Airmed), the standard adult model, or the low range, paediatric model suitable for children up to about 6–7 years. The flimsy, almost "disposable" Mini Wright peak flow meter (Airmed) is valuable for home monitoring. Calibration of peak flow meters should be performed dynamically because of the importance of inertial factors; there is a curvilinear relationship between the meter readings and flow rates during steady state flow.

There are three steps: (a) simultaneous pneumotachograph and PEF recordings are made with varying amounts of expiratory effort; (b) the pneumotachograph is calibrated with an accurate flow meter; (c) the calibration curve is used to check the accuracy of the PEF meter signals. An error of ± 10% may be acceptable for clinical purposes. The mini peak flow meter is usually used uncalibrated, for semi-quantitative clinical assessments of change in lung function.

Spirometry should be performed on equipment which, as previously mentioned (p. 298), gives a permanent record of the volume/time curve. The rather cumbersome wet spirometer has given way to the dry spirometer, allowing the simultaneous display of flow volume curves. Instruction of children before spirometry is extremely important (Brough *et al.*, 1972).

From the volume/time curve, the sensitive value of the mid expiratory flow rate ($\dot{V}$ 25–75), the mean flow rate over the second and third quarters of the forced vital capacity, can be calculated.

Reproducibility and sensitivity. Sensitive lung function tests permit the detection of the earliest changes in lung function in a child, and allow a distinction to be made between different pathological processes. For the purpose of following the progress of a disease, or of measuring change in response to treatment or provocation, the all important need is for a test of low variability. Errors due to the observer, the equipment and the subject may be summed in the within-subject coefficient of variation, which expresses the reproducibility of the test. The repro-

TABLE VII

Reproducibility and sensitivity of some tests of airways function in children

Lung function test	Reproducibility† Coefficient of variation (%)		Sensitivity* Abnormal results (%)	
	Normal population	Within-subject	Asthma	Cystic fibrosis
Peak flow rate	14	4	—	—
FEV₁	10	5	22	26
Airways resistance	27	11	39	26
FEF$_{25-75}$	20–30	8	50	32
FEF$_{50\%\ or\ 60\%\ TLC}$	30–80	15	62	60
CV (%VC)	45	24	25	21

† From various sources.
* From Cooper *et al.* (1974); a hospital-based but otherwise unselected group of children with asthma (120) and cystic fibrosis (85) were studied.

ducibility of some tests of airway function in children is shown in Table VII from which it is clear that PEF and indices derived from spirometry are amongst the most reproducible tests. Figures such as these should be considered before tests are embarked upon, and whenever change is being assessed. It is clear that even within the "normal range", changes in an individual patient's lung function may be significant. As previously mentioned (Table III) some tests are more reliable in adults than in children.

In choosing an appropriate test of airflow obstruction, not only should the reproducibility be considered, but also the purpose for which the test is being performed. The relative sensitivities of several tests, in two common conditions, asthma and cystic fibrosis, are given in Table VII. A compromise has to be made for any test of lung function, between reproducibility and sensitivity, based on this type of data. A useful discussion of the topic is provided by Nickerson *et al.* (1980).

Frequency of measurement; interpretation of results. Recurrent chest disorders in childhood tend to vary over short periods of time. Frequent observations with simple equipment are more helpful than the occasional measurement of batteries of subtle indices. By comparing the patient's own (and his parents') evaluation of his symptoms with the results of lung function tests, much can be learned about attitudes toward the disease in the family or about the patient's sensitivity (or adaptation) to disease (Rubinfeld and Pain, 1976). This can form the basis for education.

The measurement of peak flow rate at home, twice daily, is an established means of monitoring asthma. The results of such a period of monitoring can be interpreted in several ways: by trend analysis (e.g. Cusum analysis); by analysis of the degree of scatter (coefficient of variation in relation to the predicted within-subject variation); by calculation of the proportion of results below some arbitrary level of severity; or graphically. There is a need for standardization of these indices.

The Maximum Expiratory Flow Volume Curve: Tests of "Small Airways"

With the awareness that neonatal lung disease (Coates *et al.*, 1977), infantile bronchiolitis (Kattan *et al.*, 1977) and childhood asthma (Hill *et al.*, 1972) are all associated with long lasting changes in lung function, there has been renewed interest in the use of the most sensitive tests for detecting the earliest changes in the patency of small airways. Their value in paediatric practice has been questioned (Landau *et al.*, 1979).

Maximum expiratory flow volume curve. Information obtained by inspection of the shapes of curves must be interpreted in the light of the normal changes in shape during childhood (Fig. 3). In older children the curve has a characteristic shape being concave to the volume axis throughout the vital capacity. This may be because flow is limited towards RV by chest wall resistance, and not by frictional and convective forces within the airways. For this reason, even at low lung volumes, the maximum flow rate may never be truly independent of effort. This explains the poor reproducibility of the supposed effort-independent indices of small airways function $\dot{V}_{max\,50}$ and $\dot{V}_{max\,25}$.

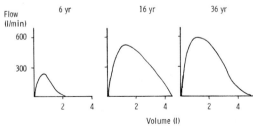

FIG. 3. Flow–volume curves: changes of shape with increasing age of the subject.

The variability may be reduced if MEFV procedures are carried out in a constant pressure plethysmograph, so that flow at the mouth can be related to the true change in lung volume (including gas compression), and to the absolute lung volume at which measurements are being made. Then, by expressing flow in the units "TLC/sec", indices of maximum flow at various proportions of VC or TLC are obtained which are independent of age or size (Zapletal *et al.*, 1969).

Because reproducibility is poor (Wiesemann *et al.*, 1981), the comparison of flow-volume curves performed in air and in He/O_2 mixture has been an unrewarding exercise in younger children. It has yet to be shown that indices derived from the MEFV curve in children are more useful than the $\dot{V}$ 25–75, derived from the flow–time curve. Little use has been made of the maximum inspiratory flow–volume curve (Zach *et al.*, 1980).

Closing volume; frequency dependence of dynamic compliance. Great demands are placed upon subjects during the measurement of these indices, hence the paucity of published standards for children, and the poor reproducibility (Table III).

Most studies of closing volume in childhood have employed modifications of the single breath nitrogen methods. Closing volume (as a proportion of VC) and closing capacity (as a proportion of TLC) reach a minimum in teenage and early adult life (Zapletal and Samenek, 1971; Mansell *et al.*, 1972). There is a progressive rise in closing volume with decreasing age in childhood. In the youngest children testable (7–8 years) the closing capacity may be less than FRC. When vital capacity is low, because of small size or reduction by disease, a sharp cut off marking phase IV may be undetectable. In disease, the increased slope of phase III also renders the distinction difficult. The few published standards for phase III slope in childhood suggest that the normal range (up to 2% N_2 per litre) is similar in older children (8–18 years) and young adults (Landau *et al.*, 1979; Hutchison *et al.*, 1981).

At breathing rates below 80 per minute, normal children do not exhibit frequency dependence of compliance. Little clinical use has been made of this test in childhood respiratory disease.

Bronchial Reactivity

Bronchial reactivity is the variability of the calibre of bronchi in response to stimuli which constrict and dilate their walls. Increased bronchial reactivity is the essence of asthma (Benson, 1979). A variety of stimuli, specific (e.g. antigens such as pollen) or non-specific (e.g. bronchoconstrictor drugs such as histamine) may be employed. Bronchial provocation with specific antigen is a technique normally performed by respiratory immunologists. This section deals only with non-specific bronchial reactivity testing.

Reactivity, and hence the outcome of tests, may be affected by drugs, environmental antigens and irritants, air temperature and humidity, recent exercise and recent respiratory tract infection or acute asthma. These should be avoided, or taken into account.

There is no generally accepted way of measuring the change in airways obstruction induced by a bronchial reactivity test. The choice of lung function test (e.g. airways resistance, FEV_1, peak flow rate) may influence results because some manoeuvres affect airway calibre. More importantly, differences in the baseline level of airways obstruction will affect outcome (see below). The construction of dose response curves to a particular stimulus is a way around this problem (c.f. Benson and Graf, 1977).

Provocation Tests

Exercise. Exercise induced asthma (EIA) is now known to be mediated by the airway cooling brought about by the hyperpnoea of exercise (McFadden and Ingram, 1979). To ensure reproducible results, exercise testing should be carried out under controlled conditions of air temperature and humidity. Suitable conditions are: temperature 18–20°C; relative humidity 50%. Under drier conditions, EIA may be excessively severe.

Six minutes of continuous running or walking on a treadmill at 6 Km h^{-1} and 8–10% slope is a standard method of provoking exercise induced asthma (Silverman and Anderson, 1972), but bicycle ergometry or free-range running may be quite as effective. In practice, the only safeguard required is the continued presence of the operator. Harnesses, emergency stop buttons and other safety devices are a hindrance and unnecessary in paediatric practice.

The parameter of lung function most often measured has been peak flow rate. Other parameters may be more sensitive (Haynes *et al.*, 1976) or give more information about the site of airways obstruction (McFadden *et al.*, 1977). The PFR should be measured every 2 min for the first 5 min after exercise, and thereafter every 5 min until recovery 15–30 min later. In children, the most severe bronchoconstriction occurs 3–5 min after stopping exercise, and a little later in adults. After exercise, there is normally a period of relative refractoriness to EIA of about 2 h

(Edmunds *et al.*, 1978), during which, however, histamine reactivity is unchanged.

Voluntary isocapnic hyperventilation. With the recent equating of exercise-induced and hyperventilation-induced asthma, it has been claimed that voluntary hyperventilation with or without cold air, may be a more simple and direct provoking agent, avoiding the extra stimuli and exercise. While this is appealing, some drawbacks should be taken into account:

(i) voluntary hyperventilation is neither natural nor, for children, easy to reproduce;
(ii) CO_2 must be added to the inspired air so that isocapnic conditions are maintained; this may have a direct effect on airway calibre;
(iii) the metabolic consequences of hyperventilation and exercise may be different;
(iv) while the effects on airway calibre of exercise and of hyperventilation may be similar, the mechanisms, which are ill-understood, may not be the same.

The equipment required for studying isocapnic voluntary hyperventilation may be simple (Kilham *et al.*, 1979), relying on the inhalation of room air of fixed temperature and relative humidity. CO_2 is added to maintain constancy of end tidal P_{CO_2}. Sophisticated equipment which provides air at less than $0°C$ and which is therefore free of water vapour, a more powerful stimulus to the airways, has been described by Deal *et al.* (1980). Dry compressed air is almost as effective in practice.

Children find it more difficult to maintain voluntary hyperventilation than adults do; moreover, their uneven respiratory rate and depth makes the smooth control of end-tidal P_{CO_2} rather difficult to achieve.

The simple measurements PEF or FEV_1 after hyperventilation are sufficient to detect bronchoconstriction. There are no paediatric population standards for hyperventilation-induced airways obstruction. However, with future study this technique may come to replace exercise testing.

Histamine and Methacholine challenge; bronchodilator inhalation. Histamine inhalation may be performed with a metered dosimeter or by continuous inhalation from a nebuliser (e.g. Wright nebuliser). There seems little to choose between the techniques, since both are equally reproducible (Beaupré and Malo, 1979), the importance being rigid standardization of technique. Younger children find it easier to breathe quietly from the mouthpiece of a nebuliser, rather than to be restricted to 5-breath aliquots of histamine aerosol.

A simple procedure is as follows (Cockroft *et al.*, 1977): serial dilutions of histamine acid phosphate in phosphate buffered saline are made up in the following concentrations: 0.03, 0.06, 0.125, 0.25, 0.5, 1, 2, 4, 8 mg ml^{-1}, (+16 and 32 mg ml^{-1} for normal subjects), together with a control solution. They may be stored, prepared, in a cool place in universal glass containers. The latter form the reservoir of the Wright nebuliser. Each in turn is attached to a Wright nebuliser, starting with the control solution, the starting dose depending on the patient's clinical state and response to control solution. Suggested starting doses are as follows:

(1) basal $FEV_1 > 70\%$, $< 10\%$ fall FEV_1 after control; (a) no regular treatment: 1 mg ml^{-1}; (b) intermittent treatment: 0.125 mg ml^{-1}; (c) continuous treatment: 0.03 mg ml^{-1}.

(2) basal $FEV_1 < 70\%$ or $> 10\%$ fall FEV_1 after control; all subjects: 0.03 mg ml^{-1}.

If in doubt, start with the weakest solution and work up slowly. The child breathes quietly through a short mouthpiece for 2 min. Peak flow rate or FEV_1 are measured 30 and 90 s later and the next dose administered 5 min after the previous dose. Increasing concentrations are administered until the PEF or FEV_1 has fallen by over 20% from the baseline value.

From a plot of PEF (or FEV_1) against concentration, the PC_{20} (provoking concentration producing a 20% fall in PEF or FEV_1) can be obtained by interpolation. Whether the dose of histamine should be expressed as an individual or a cumulative value has not been agreed. With the above technique, there is no cumulative effect. Values for PC_{20} have been obtained for some standardized procedures for normal children and for children with various respiratory disorders (Mellis and Levison, 1978; Noble-Jamieson *et al.*, 1982) and its reproducibility has been measured (Hariparsad *et al.*, 1983).

Methacholine challenge has been littled used in paediatrics. Standardized procedures (Juniper *et al.*, 1978) may easily be adapted.

Bronchodilator aerosol inhalation is certainly the commonest form of inhalation procedure. A rise in FEV_1 or PEF of more than 10% ten minutes after inhalation of salbutamol (ideally, nebuliser solution 0.5 mg in 2 ml water from a Wright's nebuliser) is said to indicate significant reversible airways disease. No chapter and verse can be quoted for this widely held belief.

Indices of Bronchial Reactivity

Ideally, an index of bronchial reactivity should be independent of the basal level of lung function. This is impossible in practice, except fortuitously, since changes in reactivity are themselves often associated with alterations in basal lung function (Empey *et al.*, 1976).

Change in reactivity ⟷ Altered lung function

It is probable that altered lung function in turn affects reactivity (Benson and Graf, 1977). Under normal circumstances, it would be impossible to sort out these factors without a measure of reactivity known to be independent of lung function.

When basal lung function is normal, or when tests are being compared in which basal lung function is identical prior to testing, then these simple indices are likely to reflect true changes in reactivity:

$$\text{Change in function} = \frac{\text{Basal value} - \text{Minimum value after challenge}}{\text{Basal value}} \quad \text{(Index 1)}$$

or

$$\text{Change in function} = \frac{\text{Minimum value after challenge}}{\text{Basal value}} \quad \text{(Index 2)}$$

An excellent discussion on the relative merits of these two indices and their statistical treatment, is given by Miller *et al.* (1975). In practice, for individual asthmatic children, bronchial reactivity by Index 1 is independent of basal lung function for exercise challenge (Silverman and Anderson, 1972) and for histamine challenge (Mellis *et al.*, 1978). Interestingly, in cystic fibrosis, a disease in which airways obstruction is not generally thought to be associated with significant hyperreactivity, histamine challenge produced the greatest change in FEV_1 (Index 1) in those children whose basal lung function was initially worst (Mellis and Levison, 1978).

Respiratory Muscle Function

Maximum Mouth Pressure

Equipment to measure the maximum and minimum pressures which can be developed during maximum expiratory effort from TLC and maximum inspiratory effort from RV, may simply be based on an anaeroid manometer (Black and Hyatt, 1969) or designed around strain gauge transducers and a chart recorder. It is possible to cheat by closing the glottis and blowing the manometer by pumping the cheeks. This can be prevented by allowing a controlled leak from the mouthpiece, so that a volume equal to a significant proportion of the mouth volume is lost during the manoeuvre. A mouth pressure sustained for 1 s should be reliable. Unfortunately, cheating during maximum inspiratory efforts can only be excluded by the simultaneous measurement of lung-volume. There are some paediatric standards (Reynolds and Heinz, 1983) with which the muscle power of children with neuromuscular disease may be compared.

Supine Vital Capacity

In normal children, the vital capacity is up to 10% smaller in the supine compared with the erect posture. This is due to an increase in the pulmonary capillary blood volume. In the presence of significant diaphragmatic weakness, the fall in vital capacity will exceed 10%. The interpretation is not straightforward in patients whose erect vital capacity is less than normal.

References

Beardsmore, C. S., Helms, P., Stocks, J., Hatch, D. and Silverman, M. (1980). *J. appl. Physiol.* **49**, 735–742.

Beardsmore, C. S., Wong, Y. C., Stocks, J. and Silverman, M. (1981). *Prog. Resp. Res.* **17**, 43–51.

Beardsmore, C. S. , Stocks, J. and Silverman, M. (1982). *J. appl. Physiol.* **52**, 995–999.

Beardsmore, C. S., Wong, Y. C., Stocks, J. and Silverman, M. (1982). *Med. Biol. Eng. Comput.* **20**, 657–660.

Beaupré, A. and Malo, J. L. (1979). *Clin. Allergy* **9**, 575–583.

Benson, M. K. (1979). *Br. J. Clin. Pharm.* **8**, 417–424.

Benson, M. K. and Graf, P. (1977). *J. appl. Physiol.* **43**, 643–647.

Black, L. F. and Hyatt, R. E. (1969). *Am. rev. resp. Dis.* **99**, 696–702.

Boon, A. W., Milner, A. D. and Hopkin, E. I. (1979). *Arch. Dis. Childhood* **54**, 492–498.

Brough, F. K., Schmidt, C. D. W., Dickman, M. and Jackson, B. (1972). *Am. rev. Resp. Dis.* **106**, 604–606.

Bryan, A. C., Mansell, A. L. and Levison, H. (1977). *In* "Development of the Lung" (Ed. W. A. Hodson), pp. 445–468. Dekker, New York.

Buckler, J. H. M. (1979). "A Reference Manual of Growth and Development". Blackwell, Oxford.

Coates, A. L., Bergsteinsson, H., Desmond, K., Buterbridge, E. W. and Beaudy, P. H. (1977). *J. Pediat.* **90**, 611–616.

Cockroft, D. W., Killian, D. N., Mellon, J. J. A. and Hargreave, F. E. (1977). *Clin. Allergy* **7**, 235–243.

Cogswell, J. J. (1973). *Arch. Dis. Childhood* **48**, 259–266.

Cogswell, J. J., Hull, D., Milner, A. D., Norman, A. P. and Taylor, B. (1975a). *Br. J. Dis. Chest* **69**, 40–50.

Cogswell, J. J., Hull, D., Milner, A. D., Norman, A. P. and Taylor, B. (1975b). *Br. J. Dis. Chest* **69**, 117–118.

Cogswell, J. J., Hull, D., Milner, A. D., Norman, A. P. and Taylor, B. (1975c). *Br. J. Dis. Chest* **69**, 118–124.

Cooper, D. M., Doron, I., Mansell, A. L., Bryan, A. L. and Levison, H. (1974). *Am. rev. Resp. Dis.* **109**, 519–524.

Cross, K. W. (1949). *J. Physiol.* **109**, 459–474.

Curzi-Dascalova, L. (1978). *Early Human Dev.* **2**, 25–38.

Deal, E. C., McFadden, E. R., Ingram, R. H., Breslin, F. J. and Jager, J. J. (1980). *Am. rev. Resp. Dis.* **121**, 621–628.

Doershuk, C. F., Downs, T. D., Matthews, L. W. and Lough, M. D. (1970). *Pediat. Res.* **4**, 164–174.

Dolfin, T., Duffy, P., Wilkes, D. L. and Bryan, M. H. (1982). *Am. rev. resp. Dis.* **126**, 577–579.

DuBois, A. B., Brody, A. W., Lewis, D. H. and Burgess, B. F. (1956). *J. appl. Physiol.* **8**, 587–594.

Dunnill, M. S. (1962). *Thorax* **17**, 329–333.

Edmunds, A. T., Tooley, M. and Godfrey, S. (1978). *Am. rev. Resp. Dis.* **117**, 247–254.

Empey, D. W., Laitinen, W. A., Jacobs, L., Gold, W. M. and Nadel, J. A. (1976). *Am. rev. Resp. Dis.* **113**, 131–136.

Fleming, P. J., Muller, N. L., Bryan, M. H. and Bryan, A. C. (1979). *Pediatrics* **64**, 425–428.

Fox, W. W., Schwartz, J. G. and Schaffer, T. H. (1979). *Pediat. Res.* **13**, 60–64.

Godfrey, S. (1981). *In* "Scientific Foundations of Paediatrics" (Eds, J. A. Davis and J. Dobbin). Heinemann, London.

Goldman, M., Kandson, R. J., Mead, J., Peterson, N., Schwaber, J. R. and Wohl, M. E. (1970). *J. appl. Physiol.* **28**, 113–116.

• Goldman, S. L., Brady, J. P. and Dumpit, F. M. (1979). *Pediatrics* **64**, 160–164.

Haddad, G. G., Epstein, R. A., Epstein, M. A. F., Leistner, H. L., Marino, P. A. and Mellins, R. B. (1979). *J. appl. Physiol.* **46**, 998–1002.

Van der Hardt, H. (1981). *Prog. Resp. Res.* **17**, 68–77.

Hariparsad, D., Wilson, N., Dixon, C. and Silverman, M. (1983). *Thorax* **38**, 258.

Haynes, R. L., Ingram, R. H. and McFadden, E. R. (1976). *Am. rev. Resp. Dis.* **114**, 739–752.

Helms, P. (1982). *J. appl. Physiol.* **53**, 698–702.

Helms, P., Hatch, D. J. and Cunningham, K. (1981). *Prog. Resp. Res.* **17**, 22–34.

Henderson-Smart, D. J. and Read, D. J. C. (1979). *J. appl. Physiol.* **46**, 1081–1085.

Hill, D. J., Landau, L. and Phelan, P. D. (1972). *Am. rev. Resp. Dis.* **106**, 873–880.

Hodson, W. A., Alden, E. R. and Woodson, D. E. (1977). *In* "Development of the Lung", (Ed. W. A. Hodson), pp. 469–496.

Hoffman, E., Havens, B., Geidel, S., Hopenbrouwers, T. and Hodgman, J. E. (1977). *Acta Paediat. Stockh. Suppl.* **266**.

Hutchison, A. A., Erben, A., McLennan, L. A., Landau, L. and Phelan, P. (1981). *Thorax* **36**, 370–377.

Juniper, E. F., Frith, P. A., Dunnett, C., Cockroft, D. W. and Hargreave, F. E. (1978). *Thorax* **33**, 705–710.

Kattan, M., Keens, T. G., Lapierre, J. G., Levison, H., Bryan, A. C. and Reilly, B. J. (1977). *Pediatrics* **59**, 683–688.

Kilham, H., Tooley, M., Silverman, M. (1979). *Thorax* **34**, 582–586.

Konno, K. and Mead, J. (1967). *J. appl. Physiol.* **22**, 407–422.
Krauss, A. N. and Auld, P. A. M. (1971). *Pediat. Res.* **5**, 10–16.
Landau, L. I. and Phelan, P. D. (1973). *Thorax* **28**, 136–141.
Landau, L. I., Mellis, C. M., Phelan, P. D., Bristowe, B. and McLennon, L. (1979). *Thorax* 217–223.
Mansell, A., Bryan, C. and Levison, H. (1972). *J. appl. Physiol.* **33**, 711–714.
Maxted, K. J., Shaw, J. and McDonald, T. H. (1977). *Med. Biol. Eng. Comp.* **15**, 398–401.
McFadden, E. R., Ingram, R. H., Haynes, R. L. and Wellman, J. J. (1977). *J. appl. Physiol.* **42**, 746–752.
McFadden, E. R. and Ingram, R. H. (1979). *New Engl. J. Med.* **301**, 763–769.
Mellis, C. M. and Levison, H. (1978). *Pediatrics* **61**, 446–450.
Mellis, C. M., Kattan, M., Keens, T. G. and Levison, H. (1978). *Am. rev. Resp. Dis.* **117**, 911–915.
Miller, G. J., Davies, B. H., Cole, T. J. and Seaton, A. (1975). *Thorax* **30**, 306–311.
Milner, A. D. (1970). *Lancet* **2**, 80–81.
Muller, N., Bulson, G., Cade, D., Whitton, J., Froese, A. B., Bryan, M. H. and Bryan, A. C. (1979). *J. appl. Physiol.* **46**, 688–695.
Nickerson, B. G., Lemen, R. J., Gerdes, C. B., Wegman, M. J. and Robertson, G. (1980). *Am. rev. Resp. Dis.* **122**, 859–866.
Noble-Jamieson, C. M., Lukeman, D., Silverman, M. and Davies, P. A. (1982). *Seminars in Perinatology* **6**, 266–273.
Olinsky, A., Bryan, A. C. and Bryan, M. H. (1976). *S. Afr. med. J.* **50**, 128–130.
Polgar, G. and Promadhat, V. (1970). "Techniques and Standards for Pulmonary Function Tests in Children". W. B. Saunders & Co., Philadelphia.
Radford, M. (1974). *Arch. Dis. Childhood* **49**, 611–615.
Reynolds, L. G. and Beardsmore, C. S. (1980). *Am. Rev. resp. Dis.* **121**, 395.
Reynolds, L. G. and Heinz, G. (1983). *Thorax*, in press.
Rigatto, H., Brady, J. and de la Torre Verduzco, R. (1975a). *Pediatrics* **55**, 604–614.
Rigatto, H., Brady, J. and de la Torre Verduzco, R. (1975b). *Pediatrics* **55**, 614–621.
Rubinfeld, A. R. and Pain, M. C. F. (1976). *Lancet* **1**, 882–884.
Ruttimann, U. E., Galioto, F. M., Franke, J. R. and Rivera, O. (1981). *Crit. Care Med.* **9**, 801–804.
Silverman, M. and Anderson, S. D. (1972). *Arch. Dis. Childhood* **47**, 882–889.
Stark, A. R., Goldman, M. D. and Franz, E. D. (1979). *Pediat. Res.* **13**, 250–256.
Stocks, J. (1977a). *Early Human Development* **1**, 285–309.
Stocks, J. (1977b). PhD Thesis, University of London.
Stocks, J. (1980). *Arch. Dis. Childhood* **55**, 17–21.
Stocks, J., Levy, N. M. and Godfrey, S. (1977). *J. appl. Physiol.* **43**, 155–159.
Stokes, G. M., Milner, A. D., Johnson, F., Hodges, I. G. C. and Groggins, R. C. (1981). *Pediat. Res.* **15**, 22–27.
Taussig, L. M. (1977). *Am. rev. Resp. Dis.* **116**, 1031–1038.
Taussig, L. M., Harris, T. R. and Leibowitz, M. D. (1977). *Am. rev. Resp. Dis.* **116**, 233–239.
Vanderghem, A., Beardsmore, C., Wong, Y. C. and Silverman, M. (1983). *Crit. Care Med.* (in press).
Wiesemann, H. and von der Hardt, H. (1981). *Respiration* **41**, 181–187.
Wong, Y. C. and Silverman, M. (1982). *Modern Problems in Paediatrics* **21**. (Karger, Basel).

Zapletal, A., Motoyama, E. K., van de Woestijne, K. P., Hunt, V. R. and Bouhuys, A. (1969). *J. appl. Physiol.* **26**, 308–316.

Zapletal, A. and Samenek, M. (1971). *Bull. European Physiopathologique Respiratoire* **7**, 139–147.

Zach, M. S., Schnall, R. P. and Landau, L. J. (1980). *Am. Rev. Resp. Dis.* **121**, 979–983.

SUBJECT INDEX

Page numbers in *italics* indicate references to figures or tables; *passim* means here and there throughout.

A

Acetylene in mass spectroscopy, 158, 159–160, 161
Acid-base balance
 arterial, 59
 and response to carbon dioxide, 251–252
Age, lung function and, 192, *193*, 209, 223
 in children, 295, 319, 320
Airways
 closure, 221–224
  and compliance, 191
 compression of, 204–206
 conductance, 200–202, 206–207
 obstruction
  in children, 318, 321–324
  and distribution of ventilation, 226
  mechanical properties of lung and, 192, 196–197, 200–210 *passim*
  test protocols and, 198, 234–245
 resistance, 185–188, 189, 199–203, 206–207
  in children, 299, 308–309, 311–313
Anaemia, 245
Anticoagulation of blood samples, 72
Apnoea
 in infants, test-induced, 305
 sleep, 265–267, 303
Argon
 in closing volume measurements, 222–223
 in mass spectroscopy, 161
 in nitrogen washout tests, 225

Arm cranking in exercise testing, 176, 288
Arterialization of ear
 for blood sampling in exercise, 284
 in oximetry, 97
Asthma
 and control of breathing, 251
 and exercise, 272, 321
 lung function testing in, 318–319
 mechanical properties of lung and, 192, *193*, 208

B

Back-pressure of carbon monoxide, 230, 235, 242–243, 246–247
Bag-in-box circuits, 13
 flow measurement in, 48–50
Balloons
 as gas reservoirs, 11
 gastric, 213–214
 oesophageal, 31, 36–37, 194, 213–214
  in children, 308–309
Bicarbonate, carbon dioxide transport as, 58–59
Blood gas analysis, 57, 59, 75
 automated, 68–69
 continuous, 85–103
 electrodes for, 59–62
  carbon dioxide, 82–84, 88, 93–96
  oxygen, 67, 78–80, 86–88, 92–93, 95–96
 in exercise, 282–283, 284–285
 gas chromotography and, 103–108
 infra-red absorption, 68

Blood gas analysis (*Cont.*)
  invasive, 85–90, 98–100, 107
  mass spectrometry and, 98–103
  non-invasive, 90–97, 102–103,
    107–108
  oximeter, 71–72, 81–82, 97
  oxygen content analyser, 67–68
  polarography, 67, 76–78
  samples for, handling of, 72–73
  tonometry and, 65
  Van Slyke and Neill method, 65–66
Blood pressure
  in exercise, 167, 281–282, 287
  in sleep, 264–265
Blood sampling
  in exercise, 167, 282–283, 284–285
  in sleep, 264
Blood volume, capillary, 241–243, 244,
    245
  in exercise, 247
  and posture, 298, 325
Body box, 31, 186–189
  airways resistance measurements,
    201–202, 311–313
  calibration, 40
  children and, 301, 304–306, 311–313
  flow measurements, 49–50, 188, 202
  lung volume measurements, 186–188,
    194–195, 196–197, 198–199,
    208–209
  in infants, 304–306
Breathlessness in exercise testing, 287,
    291
Bronchial reactivity, in children,
    320–324
Bronchial disease, mechanical
    properties of lung and, *200*
Bronchitis, chronic
  and control of breathing, 251, 252,
    264–265
  and distribution of ventilation,
    219–220, 226
Bronchodilator drugs, testing response
    to, 210
Bronchoscopy, mass spectrometry in,
    161, *162*

C

Calibration
  blood gas electrode, 60–62, 92

cycle ergometers, 177
  flow meters, 47, 50–53, 317
  infra-red gas analysers, 124, 125
  magnetometers, 20–21
  mass spectrometers, 149
  plethysmographs, 40, 301–302, 306
  pneumotachographs, 44, 274
  pressure transducers, 37–40
  spirometers, 16–17
  strain gauges, 19
  treadmills, 180–181
Carbon dioxide, *see also* Blood gas
    analysis *and* Gas analysis
  absorption, inclosed circuits, 12–13,
    116
  in blood, 57–59
  in control of breathing, 251–259, 264
  in exercise testing, 273–274, 276,
    283, 288–289
  monitoring in children, 314
Carbon monoxide
  analysis
    infra-red method, 120–123
    Van Slyke and Neill method, 66
  haemoglobin affinity for, 59
  in mass spectrometry, 158–160
  and oxygen-haemoglobin affinity, 58,
    71–72
  saturation, 59, 69–71
Carbon monoxide transfer factor, 227,
    229–230, 243–249
  and pulmonary capillary blood volume
    241–243, 244, 245
  in exercise, 247
  measurement of
    katharometers in, 118
    mass spectrometry in, 161
    rebreathing method, 238–240
    single breath method, 230–235
    steady state method, 235–237
  and membrane diffusing capacity,
    241–243, 244, 245
Carbonic acid and blood pH, 59
Cardiac output
  in exercise testing, 273, 276–277,
    282–284
  non-invasive measurement of, 158
Cardiovascular
  limits in exercise, 286–287, 290–291
  measurements in exercise, *280*,
    281–285

Catheterization
    for blood gas analysis, 85, 87,
        282–283
    in exercise, 167, 281, 282–283
    in sleep studies, 264
Chemoreceptors in control of breathing,
    251–252, 255, 259–261
Children, lung function testing in
    in infancy, 299–313
    pre-school age, 313–316
    principles of, 293–294
    problems of, 294–299, 305
    school age, 316–325
Circuits, respiratory
    for children, 296, 299–300, 304
    for control of breathing
        measurements, 253–254
    design of, 9–13
    for exercise testing, 274–276, 277,
        278, 279
    for helium dilution lung volumes,
        198, 224
    for single breath nitrogen test, 218
Closing volume, 221–224, 320
Compliance
    of lungs and chest wall, 185–186,
        190–194, 195–196, 201
        in children, 308, 310–311, 320
    of respiratory circuits, 10
Compression
    of airways in forced expiration,
        204–207, 208
    of gas, and measurement of flow,
        49–50
Computers in lung function testing, 8,
    255, 276, 299
    for calibration, 21
Control of ventilation, 5–6, 251–261
    in children, 303–304
    in sleep, 263–267
Cycle ergometers, 167–168, 174–178,
    288–289
    electromagnetically braked, 172–174
    friction braked, 168–172

D

Damping of pressure transducers,
    27–30
Dead-space
    anatomical, 220–221, 296

of flow meters, 43
    in respiratory circuits, 10, 274–275,
        296
    for children, 299, 304, 312
Deformity
    and chest wall compliance, 194
    and normal values, 295
Density of gas, and flow, 40–41, 44,
    48–49
Diagnosis
    exercise testing in, 272
    lung function tests in, 2, 294
Diaphragm, pressure measurements
    across, 213–214
Diffusing capacity
    of lung for carbon monoxide, 227,
        229–230, 243–248
    measurement, 118, 161, 230–240
    of lung for oxygen, 158–159, 228
    membrane, 241–243, 244, 245
Diffusion
    gas exchange by, 227
    in lung, 217, 221, 224, 226
    in transcutaneous monitoring, 91, 93
Distribution of gases in lung, 217–226
Drift
    in infra-red analysers, 123
    in plethysmography, 304
    with pressure transducers, 33, 38
    in mass spectrometers, 145, 149, 153

E

Elastic properties of lungs and chest
    wall, 189–203 passim
Electrocardiogram in exercise, 167,
    272–273, 280, 281, 290
Emphysema
    and control of breathing, 251, 252,
        265–266
    and distribution of ventilation,
        219–220, 226
    mechanical properties of lung and,
        192, 193, 200, 204, 208
Ergometers
    cycle, 167–178, 288–289
    treadmill, 167–168, 178–182, 321
Exercise testing, 271–272
    and carbon monoxide transfer factor,
        235, 237, 247

Exercise testing (*Cont.*)
  in children, 321–322
  conduct of, 288–291
  cycle ergometer, 167–178
  measurements made during, 272–285
  protocol, 285–288
  treadmills, 167–168, 178–182

                    F

Faintness in exercise testing, 287, 290
FEV_1, 209–210
  in children, 317–318
  in exercise testing, 272
  in provocation testing, 322, 323
Fibrosis
  cystic, lung function testing in, 318,
    324
  pulmonary, mechanical properties of
    lung and, 192, *193*, 196
Flow measurement
  calibration, 50–53, 317
  in children, 296, 299–301, 314,
    319–320
  compliance of circuits and, 10
  differential pressure systems, 40–44
  dynamic factors in, 26
  electronically sensed methods, 45,
    264–265
  in exercise testing, 274, 275
  expiratory, 47, 207–208, 317
  gas composition and, 48–49
  gas compression and, 49–50
  from spirometers, 44–45
  in whole body plethysmography,
    49–50, 188, 202, 208–209
Flow rates
  in airway resistance measurements,
    312
  in children, 296, 299, 316, 319–320
  in closing volume measurement, 223
  in forced expiration and pressure,
    204–208
  in forced inspiration, 206, 208
  peak expiratory, 47, 207, 317
Flow sensitivity
  of infra-red analysers, 124
  of katharometers, 114–115
  of oxygen analysers, 127, 129

Flow-volume curves, 207–209, 319–320
  partial, 316
Forced expiration, 185–186, 203–211
  in children, 316, 316–320
Forced oscillation method of measuring
    resistance, 203
  in children, 315–316
Fragmentation in mass spectrometry,
    133, 141, 154–155
Functional residual capacity
  compliance and, 190–193, 195–196
  measurement of, 196–197, 198, 306

                    G

Gas analysis, *see also* Blood gas analysis
  emission spectral, 130
  infra-red, 119–125, 314
  Lloyd-Haldane method, 62–64
  mass spectrometry, 131
    applications, 155–164
    electronic improvements, 150–155
    principles, 131–139
    specifications, 139–150
  paramagnetic, 126–128
  polarographic, 128–129
  thermal conductivity, 113–119
  zirconia, 129
Gas chromotography in blood gas
    analysis, 103–108
Gas composition, and flow, 46, 48–49,
    52
Gas compression, and flow, 49–50
Gas exchange, 3–5, 227
  and age in children, 295–296
  carbon monoxide transfer factor, 227,
    229–230, 241–248
  measurement, 230–240
  in exercise, 273
Gas meters, 17–18
Gas mixing, *see* Mixing

                    H

Haemoglobin
  and blood gases, 58, 69–72, 76, 80,
    81–82
  and carbon monoxide transfer factor,
    229, 241, 243, 244–246

Haemorrhage, intrapulmonary, 240, 246
Halothane, in mass spectrometry, 102, 103
Heart disease
  and control of breathing, 252
  exercise testing in, 271, 272, 281, 287
Heart rate in exercise testing, 272–273, 281, 286–287, 289, 290
  workload related to, 174–175, 179
Height, lung function related to, 294–295
Helium
  analysers
    katharometer, 113–119, 198
    mass spectrometer, 159–160
  in closing volume measurement, 222–223
  dilution techniques, 113, 115–118, 196–198, 224, 232–233
  in children, 306
Histamine challenge in children, 322–323
Humidity, see also Water vapour of gas
  and blood gas analysers, 65, 68
  and flow, 46, 48, 202
  and gas analysis, 130
  of inspired gas
    and exercise induced asthma, 321
    in open circuits, 12
Hyperventilation
  in exercise, 287, 289
  provocation testing by, 322
Hysteresis in pressure measurement, 25, 39, 302, 313

I

Infra-red gas analysers, 119–125, 314
Isotopes, in mass spectrometry, 142, 158–159, 164

K

Katharometers, 113–119, 198
  in gas chromotography, 105, 116

L

Leaks
  in plethysmography, 304
  in respiratory circuits, 9–10, 117, 198, 253–254
Linearity
  in flow meters, 43–44
  of gas meters, 18
  in jerkin plethysmography, 22
  of mass spectrometers, 144
  of nitrogen meters, 130
  in pressure measurement, 25, 28, 33, 38
  in thoracic displacement measurement, 18–19
Lloyd-Haldane method of gas analysis, 62–64
Lung volumes, 185, 196
  and airways resistance, 200
  and carbon monoxide transfer factor, 232–233, 234–235, 240, 244
  in children, 296, 299–303, 304–306, 325
  closing volume, 221–224, 320
  and compliance, 190–193, 195–196
  in forced expiration, 204–211, 320
  in forced inspiration, 206, 208
  helium dilution measurement, 113, 115–118, 196–198, 232–233
    in children, 306
  and pressure recording, 211–212
  by thoracic displacement, 18, 20–21
  in exercise, 277–280
  by whole body plethysmography, 186–188, 194–195, 196–197, 198–199, 208–209
    in children, 304–306
Lungs, mechanical properties of, 185–186, 189–211 passim, 315
  in children, 295–296

M

Magnetometers, 19, 20–21
  for children, 303
Mass spectrometry
  in blood gas analysis, 98–103
  in gas levels in tissue, 99
  in respiratory gas analysis, 131

Mass spectrometry (*Cont.*)
  applications, 155–164
  in bronchoscopy, 161
  electronic improvements, 150–155
  principles of operation, 131–139
  specifications, 139–150
Maximum mid-expiratory flow, 210
Mechanical properties of thorax, lung
    and airways, 185–214 *passim*,
    315
  and age in children, 295–296
Mixing, gas
  in lung, 217, 219–226
  in respiratory circuits, 10, 198,
    275–276, 301
Muscles, respiratory
  in children, 303–304, 324–325
  and pressures in thorax, 190, 197,
    211–214
  weakness of, 196, 208, 211

N

Neonates
  blood gas monitoring, 85–88, 90–96,
    104
  lung compliance in, 311
  thoracic gas volume in, 297–298, 303,
    303–304, 304–306, 312
Nitrogen
  analysis, 63–64
  meters, 130
  single breath test, 217–223, 320
  washout test, 224–225
Normal values
  for carbon monoxide transfer factor,
    248
  for children, 294, 310, 316, 323, 325

O

Obstruction, airways
  in children, 318, 321–324
  and distribution of ventilation, 226
  mechanical properties of lung and,
    192, 196–197, 200–210 *passim*
  and test protocols, 198, 234–235

Occlusion pressure, 261–263, 308
Oesophagus, pressure measurements in,
    30–31, 36–37, 194–195, 213–214
  in children, 306–309, 313
Oximeters, 71–72, 81–82, 89–90, 97,
    285
Oxygen *see also* Blood gas analysis *and*
    Gas analysis
  in blood, 57–58, 59
  and carboxyhaemoglobin formation,
    241–242
  consumption, in exercise testing,
    273–274, 282–283, 288–289
    and type of ergometer, 167, 168,
    175, 179
  content, 75–76, 90
  control of breathing, 252–255,
    257–263
    in sleep, 264–265
  diffusing capacity for, 228–229
  and exercise, 271–273, 282–283, 287
  and katharometers, 115–118
  saturation, 58, 69–72, 76, 80–82,
    89–90, 97
  and ventilation, 259

P

Pain, chest, 7, 287, 290–291
Paramagnetic oxygen analysis, 126–128
Patient co-operation
  in carbon monoxide transfer factor
    measurement, 234
  in children, 297
Peak expiratory flow rate measurement,
    47, 207
  in children, 316, 316–319
  in exercise testing, 272, 290, 322
  in provocation testing, 322, 323
Perfusion
  tissue, and transcutaneous oxygen, 96
  ventilation
    and carbon monoxide transfer
      factor, 234, 244, 247–248
    imbalance, 7
pH, blood, 57–59
  and control of breathing, 251–252
  electrodes, 59–62, 88–89
  and oxygen saturation, 69

Plethysmography
  barometric, 302, 303
  impedance, 21, 303
  inductive, 20, 21, 302
    in exercise, 280
  jerkin, 22, 301–302
  whole body, 31, 186–189
    airways resistance measurements,
      201–202, 311–313
    calibration, 40
    in children, 301, 304–306, 311–313
    flow measurements in, 49–50, 188,
      202
    volume measurements, 186–188,
      194–195, 196–197, 198–199,
      208–209
    in infants, 304–306
Pneumotachographs, 25, 30, 40–44,
    254–255
  for children, *300*
  in exercise testing, 274
  heating of, 48, 202
Polarographic oxygen analysis
  in blood, 67, 76–78, 87, 92
  gaseous, 128–129
Posture in child testing, 297–298,
    307–308, 313, 325
Predicted values, *see* Normal values
Pressure, barometric and blood gas
    analysis, 68
Pressure, static
  and muscle strength, 190, 197,
    211–214, 324–325
  occlusion, 262–264, 308
  and respiratory disease, *200*, 201
  in thorax, 189–192, 199
    in forced expiration, 204–207,
      208–209
Pressure flow curves, 205–207
Pressure measurements
  alveolar, 199, 201–202
  in children, 296, 306–309, 313, 315,
    324–325
  compliance of circuit and, 10
  dynamic factors in, 26–30
  at mouth, 30, 199, 201–202, 203,
    213, 324–325
  oesophageal, 30–31, 36–37, 194–195,
    213–214
    in children, 306–309, 313

static factors in, 25–26
  transdiaphragmatic, 213–214
  transducers, 32–36; 37–40, 296
    in whole body plethysmography, 31,
      186–189, 197, 198–202
    in children, 304–305
Pressure-volume curve
  of chest wall, 196
  of lungs, 190, 191–193, 194–195
  of respiratory muscles, 211–212
Provocation testing in children,
    321–323

Q

Quality control with blood gas
    electrodes, 60–62, 65

R

Rebreathing manoeuvres
  for airway resistance in children, 311
  for carbon monoxide transfer factor,
    238–240
  in exercise testing, 277, 283
  for pulmonary capillary blood flow,
    158
  in ventilatory control measurements,
    256, 259, 261
Reproducibility in lung function tests,
    1, 297, *298*, 315–320 *passim*,
    323
Reservoirs for open circuits, 11, 275
Residual volume
  airway patency at, 223
  calculation of, 196
Resistance
  airways, 185–188, 189, 193, 199–203,
    206–207
    in children, 299, 308–309, 311–313
  of flow meters, 43
  pulmonary, in children, 313
  respiratory, in children, 314–316
  of respiratory circuits, 11, 29,
    274–275
    for children, 396, 299–300
Respiratory disease
  blood gas monitoring in, in neonates,
    85

Respiratory disease (*Cont.*)
and control of breathing, 251, 252
in sleep, 263, 264–267
and distribution of ventilation,
219–220, 223–224, 226
exercise testing in, 272, 287, 290
mechanical properties of lung and,
192, *193*, 196, 200–210 *passim*
in children, 310–311, 315–316
symptoms of, 6–7
and test protocols, 198, 234–235,
240, 255
tests of, in children, 317–319,
321–324
Response times
infra-red analyser, 124
katharometer, 114–115, 119
mass spectrometer, 132, 134,
142–144, 163
for blood gas analysis, 98, 99–100,
103
nitrogen meter, 130
paediatric equipment, 296
Rotameters, in flow calibration, 51–52

S

Safety in exercise testing, 176–177, 180,
290–291, 321
Saturation
carbon monoxide, 59, 69–71
oxygen, 58, 69–72, 76, 80–82, 89–90,
97
and ventilation, 259
Signal-to-noise ratio
of mass spectrometers, 144–148,
156–158, 160–163 *passim*
in paediatric work, 296
Sleep studies
in children, 297–298, 314
control of breathing in, 251, 263–267
Smokers, carboxyhaemoglobin levels in,
59, 230, 246–247
Solid state detectors in gas analysis,
125
Solubility, gas, in blood, 57, 59, 163
Spirometers, 13–17
in flow measurement, 44–45, 208
Stethographs, 18–19

Strain gauges
mercury in silastic, 19
unbonded coil, 32–33

T

Temperature
and blood gas analysis, 61, 65, 68, 73
transcutaneously, 91–92, 93–96, 97
body
and exercise blood gases, 285
and oxygen-haemoglobin affinity,
58, 91
gas, and flow, 46, 48–49, 202
and gas analysis, 129, 156
of inspired gas
in exercise induced asthma, 321
in open circuits, 12
and whole body plethysmography,
189, 202, 304
Thermal conductivity analysers,
113–119, 198
in gas chromotography, 105, 116
Thoracic displacement, measurement
of, 18–20
in exercise, 277–280
in sleep, 264, *265, 266*, 303
Thoracic gas volume
and flow, 209
in neonates, 297–298, 303–304,
304–306, 312
from whole body plethysmography,
186–188, 189, 197, 198–199, 202
Thorax, mechanical properties of,
185–186, 189–194, 196, 211–214
Tidal volume measurement
in infants, 299–302
by thoracic displacement, 18
Time constants
of pressure transducers, 34–35, 37
and response time, in mass
spectrometers, 143
Tonometry, blood, 62, 65
Total lung capacity
calculation of, 196
from plethysmography, 199
and carbon monoxide transfer factor,
244
elastic properties of lungs and, 192,
193, 196

Transducers, pressure, 32–36
  calibration, 37–40
  in flow measurements, 40–44
  for children, 296
Treadmills, 167–168, 178–182, 321

V

Valve boxes, 12, 274–275
  for children, 304–305
Vasoconstriction on exercise, 282
Vasodilation and transcutaneous blood
  gases, 91
Van Slyke and Neill method of gas
  analysis, 65–66
Ventilation, 2–3
  in children, 299–304, 314
  control of, 5–6, 251–261;
    in sleep, 263–267
  distribution of, 217–226
  and exercise testing, 167, 271–280,
    282–283, 289
  -perfusion imbalance, 7
    and carbon monoxide transfer
    factor, 234, 248
  rate, and measurement of carbon
    monoxide transfer factor,
    236–237
Vibration
  and infra-red carbon dioxide analysis,
    125
  and whole body plethysmography,
    31–32
Viscosity of gas, and flow, 40–41, 48–49

Vital capacity
  and carbon monoxide transfer factor
    measurement, 235
  elastic properties of lung and, 196
  in forced expiration, 207–209, 209,
    317
  and posture, 298, 325
Volume measurements, *see also* Lung
    volumes *and* Thoracic gas
    volume
  gas meters, 17, 254
  in open circuits, 11–12
  by pneumotachograph, 254, 274, 296
  spirometers, 13–17, 254
Volume-time curves, 209–211, 317

W

Weight, body, and energy output, 167
Workload, 285–286
  on cycle ergometer, 167, 168–174
  on treadmills, 179
Wright peak flow meter, 47, 317
Water vapour, *see also* Humidity
  absorption of, for gas analysis, 116,
    124, 127, 129
  in infra-red carbon monoxide
    analysis, 120, 123, 124
  in mass spectrometry, 132, 150–152

Z

Zirconia oxygen analyser, 129